Holland Larson
3/79

THE FIRST ENCOUNTER:

The Beginnings in Psychotherapy

To Bill—and all his students, past and future

THE FIRST ENCOUNTER:
The Beginnings in Psychotherapy

William A. Console, M.D.
Formerly Clinical Professor of Psychiatry
State University of New York,
Downstate Medical Center,
Brooklyn, New York

Richard C. Simons, M.D.
Professor of Psychiatry
University of Colorado Medical Center,
Denver, Colorado

Mark Rubinstein, M.D.
Clinical Assistant Professor of Psychiatry,
State University of New York,
Downstate Medical Center,
Brooklyn, New York

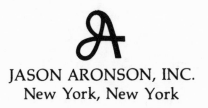

JASON ARONSON, INC.
New York, New York

ACKNOWLEDGMENTS

This book would not have been possible without the support and encouragement of Dr. Herbert Pardes, then chairman of the Department of Psychiatry of the Downstate Medical Center, State University of New York, Brooklyn, N.Y. and his successor, Dr. Robert Dickes. Their generosity in making available to us the resources of the department was invaluable.

We would like to express our deepest gratitude to Mrs. Dorothy Console and Dr. David Console for their support of the book at a time of great personal loss and sorrow for them, to Mrs. Helene Ellinger for her devotion and dedication throughout every phase of the preparation of the manuscript, and to the 1974 class of first-year psychiatric residents at the Kings County-Downstate Medical Center for their courage, honesty and commitment in the tape-recorded sessions. We also owe a special debt of gratitude to the patients who agreed to participate in the videotaped interviews with Dr. Console.

Many other individuals helped to make this book a reality. Mr. Martin Nathanson, Mr. Barney Thau and Mr. Herbert Jacobs provided valuable technical assistance with audio and visual equipment. Dr. Milton Berger and Mr. Pat Corbitt graciously provided us with a tape recording of a presentation that Dr. Console made at the South Beach Psychiatric Center on November 2, 1973 that formed the basis for Chapter Two of this book. Ms. Gerri Bavaro, Mrs. Rita Morales, Mrs. Marilyn Zwerin and Mrs. Edith Rubinstein typed many pages of manuscript, and Mrs. Libby Cohen, Mrs. Dorothy Braunstein, Ms. Vera Krassin, Mrs. Doris Main, Mrs. Helen Weissman, Mr. Jake Fass and Mrs. Bertha Spector helped with many other details.

We would like to express particular appreciation to Dr. Robert Langs, for his responsiveness to this undertaking, and to our publisher, Dr. Jason Aronson, for his enthusiasm, his encouragement, and his many helpful criticisms and suggestions.

Finally, we thank our wives—Barbara and Bette—for their support, patience and love.

Richard C. Simons, M.D.
Mark Rubinstein, M.D.

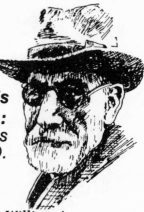

Classical Psychoanalysis
and Its Applications:
A Series of Books
Edited by Robert Langs, M.D.

Langs, Robert
THE TECHNIQUE OF
   PSYCHOANALYTIC
   PSYCHOTHERAPY, VOLS. I
   AND II

THE THERAPEUTIC
   INTERACTION, TWO-
   VOLUME SET

THE BIPERSONAL FIELD

Kestenberg, Judith
CHILDREN AND PARENTS:
   PSYCHOANALYTIC
   STUDIES IN DEVELOPMENT

Sperling, Melitta
THE MAJOR NEUROSES AND
   BEHAVIOR DISORDERS IN
   CHILDREN

Giovacchini, Peter L.
PSYCHOANALYSIS OF
   CHARACTER DISORDERS

Kernberg, Otto
BORDERLINE CONDITIONS
   AND PATHOLOGICAL
   NARCISSISM

OBJECT-RELATIONS THEORY
   AND CLINICAL
   PSYCHOANALYSIS

Console, William A.
Simons, Richard C.
Rubinstein, Mark
THE FIRST ENCOUNTER

Nagera, Humberto
FEMALE SEXUALITY AND THE
   OEDIPUS COMPLEX

OBSESSIONAL NEUROSES:
   DEVELOPMENTAL
   PSYCHOPATHOLOGY

Hoffer, Willi
THE EARLY DEVELOPMENT
   AND EDUCATION OF THE
   CHILD

Meissner, William
THE PARANOID PROCESS

Horowitz, Mardi
STRESS RESPONSE
   SYNDROMES

Rosen, Victor
STYLE, CHARACTER AND
   LANGUAGE

Sarnoff, Charles
LATENCY

Series Introduction

William Console was an example, par excellence, of a special type of psychoanalyst. Such men earn their reputations as superlative psychoanalytic teachers and clinicians, largely on a local level and almost entirely through their direct interactions with psychiatric residents and psychoanalytic candidates. As these pages attest, Dr. Console was remarkably sensitive both to the needs of his students and to the concerns and processes within the patients they studied together. Many considered him a "clinician's clinician" and all who worked with him—I, personally, was most fortunate to be among them—benefited greatly in many important ways from his analytic wisdom. It is more than evident, then, that we are all deeply indebted to Drs. Richard C. Simons and Mark Rubinstein for having conceptualized this book with Dr. Console and for having completed the writing of it following his death. There is much to be gained in observing this fine psychoanalyst at work and in following the development of a group of psychiatric residents over the course of a year. It is therefore with great satisfaction that I welcome this work to the Series. It stands as an illustration of the sagacity of the quiet and unsung psychoanalytic clinicians who tend to prefer direct communication to the written word, and who have substantially enhanced the standing of classical psychoanalysis and its broad clinical applications.

Robert Langs, M.D.

Contents

THE FIRST ENCOUNTER:

The Beginnings in Psychotherapy

CHAPTER ONE

The Use of the Initial Interview in the Teaching of Psychotherapy

Richard C. Simons, M.D.
Mark Rubinstein, M.D.

Beginning many years ago, Dr. William Console brought the force of his personality and his unique style to the teaching of psychiatric residents and psychoanalytic candidates at the Kings County-Downstate Medical Center in Brooklyn and at the Downstate Psychoanalytic Institute. Avoiding abstract theoretical discussions, he placed great emphasis on the very first contact with a patient. Over the years he became more and more impressed with the wealth of diagnostic and prognostic data that could be obtained from a carefully conducted initial interview. At the same time he considered it absolutely essential that an empathic alliance between patient and therapist be established by the end of the initial interview.

Thus he had little difficulty in reconciling the controversy (1-3) that has existed over the years in regard to the most effective approach to the initial psychiatric interview. The opinion of one group of authors (4-10) is that the primary goal of the initial interview should be the diagnostic and prognostic evaluation of the patient. The assessment of the interviewer-patient interaction and the establishment of a therapeutic alliance should remain secondary to this primary goal. Another group of authors (11-18) would reverse these goals, placing primary importance on the therapeutic relationship through the encouragement of a spontaneous unfolding of the patient's associations, with as little interference by the interviewer as possible.

Dr. Console saw no conflict here. He felt that both goals were of equal importance, and that to place one ahead of the other was to ignore the fundamental principles of dynamic psychiatry and psychoanalysis (19, 20). One must always evaluate everything that transpires in the interaction with a patient, and in the initial interview this can be accomplished only by active and searching questioning. Otherwise one can come to the end of the first interview and know a great deal about the presenting symptoms, but next to nothing about who the patient really is—his background, his family, his developmental history, his education, his work and sexual relationships, his strengths and assets and creative potential, his accessibility to psychotherapeutic work—in other words, his past and his possible future. However, such active and searching questioning can only be meaningful and helpful if it takes place in the context of a relationship of trust and confidence, one that always respects the patient's anxieties and the various defenses that are called upon to deal with those anxieties.

Thus, inappropriate activity and questioning on the part of the interviewer can only heighten the patient's anxiety and prevent the communication of important data. At the same time, inappropriate silence or passivity on the part of the interviewer will also frighten the patient. Gill, Newman and Redlich, in their important book, *The Initial Interview in Psychiatric Practice*, generally side with the proponents of the less directive interview approach. Yet they comment as follows on the failure of some interviewers to pursue actively certain material:

"The technique of quickly leaving painful subjects often is interpreted by the patient as a reluctance to attack major difficulties. A patient's anxiety may even be heightened by the feeling that if the therapist is fearful, the problem must be serious indeed. A bold attack which shows that the therapist knows what he is about, that he can lay his finger on the trouble and is not afraid, may not only be very reassuring but may go far toward helping the patient overcome the ever-present tendencies to evasion, whether these are conscious or not."

Dr. Console would have vigorously agreed with this observation. He taught his students to heed a patient's every word, to listen to every syllable or pause, to observe every movement, gesture and facial expression—and at the same time to obtain as broad a landscape of information as possible in the first interview. Otherwise, how else can one proceed intelligently with the patient? How can one make a rational recommendation—even if the recommendation is to return for a second interview—without some sense of both the intrapsychic and the external reality of the patient? And if this knowledge is not obtained in a manner that inspires the patient's trust, hope and confidence, if an alliance has not been established by the end of that first meeting, then it will not really matter how much one knows about the patient. Because he may never return.

At some point over the years Dr. Console's method of teaching and supervision began to be referred to as "microanalysis." He became known as a legendary teacher who, when supervising a resident psychotherapist or an analytic candidate, would listen to the first few words of the session, and then stop the presentor and spend many minutes fruitfully discussing the implications of those first few words by the patient. This approach was especially dramatic in seminars and continuous case conferences, where he would demonstrate over and over again that the unconscious is comprehensible, and that the subsequent course of an entire session and sometimes even of an entire treatment can often be predicted on the basis of a patient's first communciations.

His emphasis on detail and his extraordinary ability to extract from the smallest shred of evidence a larger and more coherent picture of a person, earned him something of a reputation as a "Sherlock Holmes of the mind." Perhaps a vignette will make this point. Several years ago, in a small Hispanic neighborhood on the upper West Side of Manhattan, a series of five horrible crimes occurred. Four young boys were sexually mutilated and murdered. The fifth boy escaped alive. The killer inflicted multiple stab wounds, not haphazardly but symmetrically, and then cut off the penises of these young boys, including the penis of the boy who escaped. The nine-year-old boy who escaped told the police that he had been forced to suck on the man's penis prior to his own being cut off. The assumption was that the same thing happened with the other four boys, who were unable to escape and were stabbed to death. The community had become frantic and the news media had dubbed the murderer *The West Side Killer*. These events took place suddenly over the course of a few months, and enormous pressure was placed on the police to apprehend the murderer.

The police were mystified. The suddenness of the onset of events, the lack of substantive clues as to the killer's identity, and most of all, the bizarre and seemingly incomprehensible precision and sameness of each murder left them bewildered and frustrated. The fear in the neighborhood mounted as each passing day left the killer still at large. It was partly in desperation that the police sought Dr. Console's advice, as they were experiencing a growing awareness that ordinary logic and deduction would not suffice in such a uniquely horrible pattern of crimes. They sought to understand intellectually what they intuitively recognized as meaningfully repeated behavior.

Dr. Console listened as the three detectives from the New York City police department presented their case. They described to him the specific details of the sexual mutilation, facts that were never published in the newspapers for fear of causing complete panic among the people. After he had listened carefully to all the facts in the case, he then asked to see the on-site photographs of the dead bodies. They were not pretty pictures, but Dr. Console studied them carefully, and in doing so, he noticed something that had puzzled the police. In each photograph the boy's body was nude or partially disrobed, and *each body was lying face down. In each and every case the boy had been wearing sneakers. The boy's sneakers had been removed, and had been neatly placed alongside the body, upright, paired, and pointing in the same direction.*

At that point Dr. Console and the police made the following deductions. Since the murders all occurred after five o'clock in the evening, say between 5 P.M. and 10 P.M., the murderer was probably a man employed in some marginal kind of work. In any event, his work was of such a nature as to permit him to roam freely in the neighborhood at that time of day. Dr. Console further deduced from the location of the bodies on rooftops and in cellars, that each victim had been lured there by the man and had not suspected his true motives, especially since after the first murder all the children had been warned to avoid strangers. Thus, it was reasonable to speculate that the man was probably known by sight to many in the neighborhood and was perhaps a janitor or porter or some other person of inconspicuous appearance, whose presence in the neighborhood would be unquestioned at that hour of the day.

But what of the many stab wounds and the sexual mutilation, and what of the sneakers placed in such a precise fashion beside the bodies? Dr. Console speculated that the murderer had himself once been sexually abused, possibly penetrated anally, and very likely many times; hence the multiple stab wounds. This abuse may have occurred at the hands of a sadistic older man or brother, at which time, Dr. Console conjectured, the then young boy was forced to lie, face down on a bed, *alongside which he saw his own two sneakers on the floor.* And this same boy, now a man engaged in an orgy of mutilation and death, was inflicting upon these youngsters a distorted and lethal version of his own earlier experiences.

He further speculated that the sudden onset of this behavior was the result of the man's having recently sustained a loss or some other threat to his tenuous psychic equilibrium. Perhaps he had lost his mother or sister or wife, someone who had been a stabilizing or organizing force in his life, and who had sustained his precarious sense of masculinity. With the loss of such a woman, he was in the throes of a homosexual panic and a murderous rage. If these speculations were true, then Dr. Console reasoned that this man was, in his own horribly maladaptive way, attempting to make sense of and reorganize what for him was a growing feeling of fragmentation and disintegration, and that he was probably following the case closely in the daily press. Hence, a well-publicized statement by the police that they had discovered a recognizable pattern in all the murders and that they were close to cracking the case, might be just the impetus necessary for this man to regain his equilibrium. Upon reading this news, he might murder no more. The police followed this recommendation and the murders abruptly came to a halt. The killer was never apprehended and, as far as is known, has never killed again. We shall, of course, never be able to determine the accuracy of Dr. Console's speculations unless the murderer is someday found. But they do have the ring of truth. At least three hardened detectives, experienced in the ways of homicide, immediately thought so.

Thus Dr. Console was able to convey to his students an appreciation for the fact that within a single word there may be a world of meaning, and that with a simple gesture a patient may tell us volumes about himself and his world. But even with this focus on detail, Dr. Console never lost sight of the totality and individuality of the human being.

With the advent of videotape techniques, Dr. Console's methods of teaching became even more vital and alive. Here was an opportunity for him to record sessions with patients visually, and to subject his recordings to the scrutiny and microscopic dissection of his students, as his students' accounts of their sessions had been scrutinized by him all the previous years. It was a teaching technique to which he passionately devoted the last four years of his life.

In November of 1973 Dr. Console gave a talk on these techniques, specifically involving the use of videotaped initial interviews in the teaching of psychotherapy. The response on the part of the audience was overwhelming. He was basically a very shy man who published very little during his lifetime. It seems that he never fully appreciated the fact that what for him was an ordinary and everyday approach to understanding a patient, became for others a masterful and richly dynamic model for the understanding of human behavior. As a result of the interest generated by this talk, he asked us to collaborate in the writing of a paper detailing the advantages of this method of teaching. In very short order it became clear to all three of us that a book would be a far more appropriate format in which to present the richness of this data.

At first we were unsure of how best to proceed. It was our wish to demonstrate the advantages of these teaching techniques and to detail, if possible, the evolving psychological sophistication of a group of first-year psychiatric residents. We then conceived the basic idea of this volume. If we were to demonstrate the quality and the interactional processes of this kind of teaching and learning, why not simply record the events exactly as they occurred and then transcribe them? This then is what we did.

Beginning in September 1974 one of us (Dr. Rubinstein) sat in on Dr. Console's weekly meetings with the first-year residents in psychiatry at the Kings County-Downstate Medical Center in Brooklyn. Dr. Rubinstein recorded each meeting, and then transcribed the session immediately afterwards. Over the course of the year, five videotaped initial interviews by Dr. Console were studied in detail. The transcription of the previous week's session was read separately by each of us and then discussed by the three of us in a regular weekly meeting that preceded the next session with the residents. Issues that we felt warranted more attention were discussed, but there was no attempt to structure ahead of time any of the meetings with the residents.

It had been our original intention when it came time to edit the transcribed sessions and to write the book, that we would include "interpolated remarks" throughout the discussions of the various cases. It became obvious at virtually every point at which the videotape machine was stopped and a discussion ensued, that there was ample opportunity for extensive commentary on the dynamic and genetic material that had emerged about the patient. We could also have made many comments about the learning processes that were unfolding during the sessions, but we quickly abandoned the idea of commenting about the residents, either individually or as a group, even though this detailed account of the proceedings yields fascinating data for the reader concerning problems in education in general and the teaching of psychotherapy in particular. Later on we also abandoned our original intention of inserting annotated comments about the patients into the text. We did this because we felt that such comments would interrupt, visually and ideationally, the conversational flow of the case discussions as they appeared on the printed page, and also because they would dampen the vividness and the spontaneity of the discussions.

Let us now proceed to Dr. Console's thoughts about the use of videotape in the teaching of psychotherapy, and then hear from the patients themselves.

References

1. Dickes, R., Simons, R. C., and Weisfogel, J. Difficulties in diagnosis introduced by unconscious factors present in the interviewer. *Psychiatric Quarterly* 44: 55-90, 1970.
2. GAP Report No. 49. Reports in Psychotherapy: Initial Interview. *Group for the Advancement of Psychiatry*. New York. 1961.
3. Rosen, V. H. The initial psychiatric interview and the principles of psychotherapy: some recent contributions. *Journal of the American Psychoanalytic Association* 6: 154-167, 1958.
4. Finesinger, J. E. Psychiatric interviewing: some principles and procedures in insight therapy. *American Journal of Psychiatry* 105: 187-195, 1948.
5. Hendrickson, W. J., Coffer, R. H., and Cross, T. N. The initial interview. *Archives of Neurology and Psychiatry* 71:24-30, 1954.
6. Menninger, K. A. *A Manual for Psychiatric Case Study*. New York: Grune and Stratton, 1952.
7. Saul, L. J. The psychoanalytic diagnostic interview. *Psychoanalytic Quarterly* 26: 76-90, 1957.
8. Stone, L. The widening scope of psychoanalysis. *Journal of the American Psychoanalytic Association* 2: 567-594, 1954.
9. Tarachow, S. *An Introduction to Psychotherapy*. New York: International Universities Press, 1963.
10. Whitehorn, J. C. Guide to interviewing and clinical personality study. *Archives of Neurology and Psychiatry* 52: 197-216, 1944.
11. Coleman, J. V. The initial phase of psychotherapy. *Bulletin of the Menninger Clinic* 13: 189-197, 1949.
12. Deutsch, F. The associative anamnesis. *Psychoanalytic Quarterly* 8: 354-381, 1939.
13. Deutsch, F., and Murphy, W. F. *The Clinical Interview. Volume I.* New York: International Universities Press, 1955.
14. Fromm-Reichmann, F. *Principles of Intensive Psychotherapy*. Chicago: University of Chicago Press, 1950.
15. Gill, M. M., Newman, R., and Redlich, F. C. (in collaboration with Sommers, M.). *The Initial Interview in Pychiatric Practice*. New York: International Universities Press, 1954.
16. Knight, R. P. Evaluation of psychotherapeutic techniques. In

Psychoanalytic Psychiatry and Psychology, Volume I, ed. R. P. Knight and C. R. Friedman, pp. 65-76. New York: International Universities Press, 1954.

17. Powdermaker, F. The techniques of the initial interview and methods of teaching them. *American Journal of Psychiatry* 104:642-646, 1948.
18. Sullivan, H. S. *The Psychiatric Interview.* New York: Norton, 1954.
19. Stevenson, I. The psychiatric interview. In *American Handbook of Psychiatry, Volume I,* ed. S. Arieti, pp. 197-214. New York: Basic Books, 1959.
20. MacKinnon, R. A., and Michels, R. *The Psychiatric Interview in Clinical Practice.* Philadelphia: W. B. Saunders, 1971.

CHAPTER TWO

The Use of Videotape in the
Teachinging of Psychotherapy

William A. Console, M.D.

Of all residents in medical training, the psychiatric resident occupies a unique and somewhat unenviable position. At the end of his training he is probably the least equipped and the least confident of any of his colleagues in other specialties, in regard to his ability to treat patients and to meet the realities of psychiatric practice.

The internist, the surgeon, the dermatologist, the radiologist, the obstetrician and the pathologist all finish their training with two things—a reasonable sense of completion, and a fairly secure conviction that they can take care of most of the conditions that will come their way. It is rare for the psychiatrist finishing his residency training to feel either of these things; to feel both is virtually nonexistent. The vastness of the subject matter, the nature of resistance, the complexities of transference and countertransference, the use of the self as an essential tool in the treatment, and the slowness of change are all in sharp contrast to the day-to-day experience of residents in any other medical discipline.

There is considerable contrast as well in the method of teaching. Interestingly, residents in other specialties frequently express their envy of the intensity of the didactic instruction which the psychiatric resident receives. They seem to feel that excellence of training depends on the frequency of meetings with the faculty. And indeed, in most teaching hospitals, psychiatric residents follow a schedule that is not vastly different in either form or substance from that of college and medical school. A glance at such a schedule is revealing. It usually presents the work week divided into various hours—some devoted to history-taking, psychodynamics, psychopathology, and principles of psychotherapeutic technique; and others showing assignments to various wards or outpatient clinics. It is all very reminiscent of the medical school schedule. So training in psychiatry is in the nature of a continuing experience of being schooled and thus, in many ways, is a continuing infantilization.

In this connection, I find the recent elimination of the internship as a prerequisite for psychiatric residency training particularly unfortunate for the psychiatrist, because it seriously delays his beginning to feel like a doctor. The move directly from medical school to psychiatry residency deprives the resident of the growth opportunities inherent in primary patient care and the responsibility for making life-and-death decisions.

This state of affairs unwittingly nurtures the narcissism of the instructor, and reinforces and perpetuates the teacher-pupil relationship rather than encouraging a new colleagual one. Too frequently this becomes an exercise in versatility—an opportunity for the teacher to display his own brilliance with fast, penetrating insights. And all too often, it leaves the resident with a feeling of despair. How can he ever hope to match that kind of performance?

This touches on a critical difference between psychiatric training and all other medical training, and suggests the role that videotape techniques can play to reduce the magnitude of that difference. In all of residency training except psychiatry, the resident observes firsthand how his older and more experienced colleague functions with his patients. He observes and participates in the surgeon's, the obstetrician's, the internist's history-taking, examination and treatment. The manner in which these experienced physicians function in the outpatient clinic or on the ward is not essentially different from the way they function in their offices. There is no need for them to reconstruct from memory the manner in which they developed the history, how they sorted out the important and unimportant findings, the steps by which they arrived at a diagnosis, and their reasons for having prescribed the treatment that they did. The resident can be at their side every step of the way. This is not so in psychiatry.

The fundamental nature of psychotherapy tends to preclude the presence of a third person. What we do in our offices is covert and shrouded in mystery. When we try to reproduce and describe our history-taking and our therapeutic techniques, we encounter many difficulties. Our memories are faulty and are made more so by our amnesia concerning the mistakes we made and by our desire to smooth the rough edges and give our listener a coherent account—an account which almost invariably has an element of self-serving deletions and alterations. Some of this is unavoidable because it is inherent in any secondhand account.

The resident listening to such a rendition marvels at its smoothness. He envies the coherence with which the dynamics seem to unfold and he marvels too at the precision of the therapeutic interventions. He is overwhelmed by the appalling contrast between this and his own painful and stumbling performance with his patients. He believes that his teacher's therapy sessions move on well-oiled wheels, unerringly, to that brilliant, succinct interpretation which brings with it insight and cure. His teacher does very little to disabuse him of this notion. So the psychiatric resident has very little opportunity to observe his teacher at work. The model presented to him is not a working model but is rather a verbal description of how the model is supposed to work.

It is clear that television and the television camera could give us an opportunity to make up for some of these shortcomings of psychiatric training. It can give us an account of what actually takes place between patient and doctor, without concern for the fallibility of memory. We are given an account, not only of every word, but of every inflection and every gesture. And it is given us in a form that can be observed and studied in its original state, over and over again.

However, it was not these considerations I have just sketched that led me to the use of videotapes in teaching. My original use of the technique was in a course designed to help the residents formulate treatment goals early in their contact with patients. Too frequently, the resident found himself inextricably tangled in what had deteriorated into an interminable and unproductive relationship with a patient. It was my feeling that by using videotaped initial interviews, I could help the resident establish some beginning goals, deal realistically with how much might be done in treatment, and recognize what might be foolish to pursue.

In this process I became aware that the initial interview lends itself to teaching at all levels. With residents I have used it in the first year of their training, to help them deal with some of the fundamental aspects of the patient-doctor relationship. I have tried to do this with techniques calculated to elicit the important aspects of the history. I have also tried to focus on and help the residents observe the dynamic interchange that occurs, to show them what a resistance really is, to indicate the living quality of transference and countertransference, and to understand the implications of these phenomena.

Let me make a few comments concerning some of the technical matters involved. First, I want to say that I have always insisted on using a single camera for both the doctor and the patient. This is in contrast to some videotape techniques where a split screen is used. I have deliberately avoided this. My desire has been to give the resident an awareness of the living quality of the interview and of the dynamics of the interchange. It is my feeling that to have a split screen, or to have the camera focus simply on the patient and not on the doctor, leads to a fragmentation of this process. It lends, in my opinion, a quality of disembodiment when the doctor speaks— disembodiment in the sense that his voice seems to come from nowhere. So that, while we might use close-up views of the patient at times, I encourage the technicians to keep these views to a minimum and to focus in the main on both people involved in the interview.

Sometimes, by the way, it is difficult to keep the technicians in check. I think that technicians are often tempted to try to emulate their colleagues at the football and baseball games—with multiple views, close-ups, instant replays and superimposed images. So again, I have often had to insist on a relatively simple view of the two people so as to demonstrate best the ongoing dynamics of the interchange.

Let me also mention that the interview as taped usually runs for about fifty minutes. In the course that I give, the sessions are one-hour long and once a week. It usually takes six to eight one-hour sessions with the first-year residents to analyze microscopically and appreciate fully the implications of almost every word and indeed virtually of every sentence of the interview.

I would now like to present a short segment of a tape. This is an interview with a young woman. Later I will clarify some of the vagueries of the situation.

(The videotape machine is turned on. The patient and Dr. Console are seen sitting in their respective chairs. The patient is a young, somewhat obese woman who appears to be in her late teens. She is dressed in a casual shirt and dungarees. There are two streaks of paint on her dungarees. She appears tense and distraught.)

Dr. Console: What happened today that you fell?

Patient: I took the train here and then I was going to take the number ten bus and I was running across the street. They were painting the curb yellow and I stepped on it and I went flying. My back hurts. And . . . the police came and they took me to the hospital and when we got here—they just left. First they said "go here—go there," and I was just wandering around in the hallway. So I went to the nurse and asked to see a doctor because my back was hurting and she said that all the doctors were in a conference. And I said, "What am I supposed to do?" She looks at me like I'm crazy that I'm asking a question like that and she says, "What's the matter?" I said, "I hurt my back." And she's looking at me like you wouldn't believe and she said, "Well, all the doctors are in conference now." I said, "All of them?" She said, "All of them are in conference. They have to learn. They learn in the conference room." So then she sent me someplace else and that's when I saw Dr. Rubinstein . . . and then I came here.

Dr. Console: That's too bad. Why did you go to Dr. Rubinstein in the first place?

Patient: Well, I was seeing a counselor at the university and I wanted to continue seeing somebody, you know. She left a message at Kings County Hospital, which she also gave me. She wanted me to continue seeing somebody. You're not

supposed to see the same person for more than a term and I
was seeing her for more than two terms already and she said
that I should come here and she gave me your number and I
called up.

Dr. Console: Why had you sought counseling originally?

patient: Because I'm not happy. It's just that I'm generally
depressed and it just seems that my life doesn't work out.
(*pause*) I know I'm going to be more emotional now than
before because my back just started to hurt. (*voice cracks and
tears appear in her eyes*)

Dr. Console: (*softly*) I'm sorry . . .

Patient: There are things like this—everything builds up and
I really feel like crying. It's just that things don't work out and
I don't know why. I don't know what I'm doing and it just
seems like I don't get what I wan . . . I don't get anything—and
I don't know why.

Dr. Console: You said "not get what I want." What do you
want? What thoughts do you have about the "things that I
want"?

Patient: I've never had a real relationship with a man.

This young woman had an appointment for a videotape
interview and she came twenty minutes late. She came late, with
her dungarees smeared with yellow paint. And as she described to
me in this segment of the interview, she was running for the bus
and had not noticed that the curb had been or was being painted,
and she stepped on it and went flying through the air. There was a
commotion and the police came and brought her to the hospital.
While at the emergency room of the hospital, really only across the
street from where we were supposed to have our interview, there
was an unfortunate circumstance of no doctor being available.
They were all in conference and apparently the urse did not feel
that the patient's physical state warranted her interrupting them.
The patient was ambulatory and in no apparent pain. In any event,
she finally found her way to the interview room and we began the
session in the manner just presented.

So this tape was made. I have now shown it to two successive
groups of residents—two consecutive years. The residents are

instructed to ask me to stop the tape at any time so that we can discuss anything that was said. At the point in this tape where the patient said, "I know I'm going to be more emotional now than before because my back just started to hurt"—if you recall, my comment was, "I'm sorry." The residents yelled for me to stop the tape. I had made the statement in a very soft voice, one that was barely audible on the tape. We rewound the tape a few feet and replayed it. Lo and behold . . . I had said to the patient, "I'm sorry." The residents were *appalled*. "You said, 'I'm sorry' to a patient?" They could not believe what they had heard. They were absolutely flabbergasted. I asked them what they would have preferred me to say. This, to them, was the veritable destruction of all technique . . . to say "I'm sorry" in the face of the patient's complaining about something that was too painful too bear.

Yes, I was aware, as were the residents, that this was not the real reason that she was going to cry. I was aware that she was about to describe some of her real feelings—feelings that were painful for her—and that she had to defend herself and say that if she wept it would not be because of what she was telling me . . . it would not be because of the content of her thoughts and feelings as they would relate to her whole life; but that if she cried it would be because of the pain in her back. The residents had been perceptive enough to see this and understand that the patient's tears would follow because of the psychic and not the physical pain. But to confront her with this in the initial interview would have been foolhardy and stupid. Rather, I chose an empathic statement which was also a true statement. . . . I *was* sorry that she had fallen and was experiencing this pain, and that we had gotten off to a late start in our talk.

I mention this episode in some detail because if it were not for the videotape technique, it would be extremely unlikely, in my trying to reproduce the session verbally and present it to the residents, that I would have included this interchange in my account, because it was so simple and natural a thing for me to have said. I would never have made a point of remembering and relating it to the residents. I would never have been able to demonstrate this small interchange and its implications. And I would therefore have missed the opportunity of making clear to the residents in the most vivid fashion, that the psychotherapeutic stance which we encourage—that of relative anonymity, of avoiding a social relationship and so on—does not preclude being human.

Allow me to make one other point that relates to what I have been discussing. This involves the idealized view that the resident gets of his teacher's psychotherapeutic work, as I mentioned before. The videotape technique can effectively counter this misconception. Let me illustrate this to you from this same segment of taped interview with the young woman.

I know very little about these patients when they come for the interview. I instruct the resident just to bring the patient, a patient whom he feels will be somewhat verbal and who will consent to being filmed. Thus, I did not know this young woman's age at the time of the interview. She looked quite young, maybe sixteen or seventeen, was dressed casually, and spoke in an almost childish manner.

When I first showed this tape to the residents, I stopped it at precisely the point at which the patient said, "I've never had a real relationship with a man." I then said to the residents, "Now watch carefully because I'm going to make a mistake here." Again, they were appalled. *"You . . . make a mistake?"* It was almost beyond belief for them that I could make a mistake and here they were about to view it on television. Well, it turned out that I did not make the mistake but I honestly thought that I had.

The mistake that I thought I had made was one that would have been a colossal blunder had I made it. After she said, "I've never had a real relationship with a man"—my recollection of the interchange had been that my next question to her was something in the nature of, "Well, how old are you?" That would have been a terrible mistake because it would have revealed considerable hostility and prejudicial feelings toward her. Remember, I was under the impression that she was sixteen or seventeen . . . she was twenty-two by the way . . . and in asking her that question at that moment, I would really have been saying to her . . . "What do you mean you've never had a real relationship with a man? You're only a kid. What the hell right do you have to expect such a thing at your age?" Fortunately I did not do this. A few minutes later she mentioned something about "When I was nineteen," and then I asked her age.

Thus, the fidelity of the recording speaks for itself and this is a great advantage for the residents in their attempt to grapple with this mysterious and shrouded process called psychotherapy. With videotaped initial interviews we can say to the residents, "Here it is . . . at least in its beginnings," and we can show the process of psychotherapy to them as it actually unfolds in the very first encounter with a patient.

CHAPTER THREE

The Roach Woman

Dr. Console: The story is probably apocryphal, but nonetheless it is told again and again, that when someone wants to become a reporter, his editor explains that in writing a story he will have to include *who, what, where, when, why* and *how.* So the reporter goes out on his first story with these questions in mind and writes his story.

Now, in an initial interview, *you* will have the task of the cub reporter going out on his first story, with some modification, particularly in the order of these questions. The "who," however, is always first. Who is this person? And what does this person come for? So the first need is to identify the patient and to identify the complaint . . . the chief complaint.

We will go on from that point to answering, as best we can, all of the other questions, but assigning to them a slightly different importance. The reporter is writing a story; we are taking a history. We have an advantage over the reporter, in that the chances are very great that he has only a one-shot opportunity. Having gotten his story, there is very little else to be done in the way of follow-up. In our situation, however, we are going to enter into a treatment relationship with the patient and will have many other opportunities to fill in the history, because we are taking history throughout the course of treatment.

But I want to concentrate on that very first interview that you have with your patient and try to demonstrate how very far indeed you can go in just one interview toward answering those six questions—*who, what, where, when, why* and *how.*

(The videotape machine is turned on. The patient, a young white woman in her mid-twenties, and Dr. Console are seen entering the room and taking their seats. While entering, the patient has been talking. Her initial words are inaudible.)

Patient: . . . a few questions. What are you going to ask me?
Dr. Console: I'm going to ask you why you've come to the clinic so as to find out what your difficulties are and try to help you with them.

Dr. Console: All right. So, this is one of those situations in which, as the patient enters the door, she makes some comments. She begins to talk. In a general sense, beyond the circumstances of this specific room with its camera lens and microphones, when you see a patient for the first time, and he or she starts to talk to you while walking into the room, you have to make one conjecture. You have to come to a tentative conclusion. What might that be?
Dr. Marcus: That the patient is very nervous—anxious.
Dr. Console: That the patient is anxious! The chances are very great that this is the first *direct* evidence of the patient's anxiety. Now in the artificial situation of a video studio with all the equipment, there's a little additional anxiety. But even in a consultation room such as you will have a few years from now, with all its high-class furniture, there will still be some people who will immediately start to talk. They're revealing their anxiety. I don't recall the specifics of this young woman's question as we walked in, but it was in the general nature of asking me what was going to happen; what was I going to do? And I told her what I was going to do.

Dr. Console: I'm going to ask you why you've come to the clinic so as to find out what your difficulties are and try to help you with them.
Patient: Well, I came because I had a terrible fear of roaches.

Dr. Console: "I came because I had a terrible fear of roaches."
Dr. Clarke: I don't think that anyone would come to the clinic

because of a fear of roaches. I think it's implicit that there's much more, but that's the ways she visualizes it. She presents it as a fear of roaches.

Dr. Console: Yes, I think that is a very apt and accurate comment. The chances are not very great that a person would seek psychiatric help in the face of a single fear. What about the word "terrible"? She didn't say, "I have a fear of roaches." She said, "I had a *terrible* fear of roaches."

Dr. Clarke: It certainly gives it a pressured, driven quality.

Dr. Console: Yes. She confers upon it a particular intensity. A *terrible* fear of roaches. And you suggest, as I understand you, that we have some confirmation of our original conjecture, that she started talking because she was anxious. She is expressing her anxiety in the word "terrible."

> *Dr. Console*: You *had* a terrible fear of roaches?
> *Patient*: Well, I haven't seen any for quite some time. . . .

Dr. Console: She said, "I *had* a terrible fear of roaches." I asked her about this and she said "Well, I haven't seen any for quite some time." What do you think about that?

Dr. Alper: The first question that comes to my mind is, why did she come to the clinic now?

Dr. Console: Yes. Why did she come to the clinic if she hadn't seen one in some time? What assumptions can we make? Does she anticipate seeing them again and she now wants some prophylaxis? Or, are we going to get a further story regarding other things that are distressing to her? Now at this point, in light of her chief complaint, what are we thinking of diagnostically? What diagnosis have we tentatively made? That the patient suffers from what?

Dr. Kent: Anxiety.

Dr. Zimmer: A phobia.

Dr. Console: A phobia! Anxiety you can say about everybody. Whenever someone comes to see you, you can assume that he's anxious. But when you say "phobia," the anxiety becomes more specific—the chief complaint is a phobic one.

Patient: I haven't seen any for quite some time but I imagine it will happen again.

Dr. Console: When did you first become aware of this?

Patient: Oh—a couple of years ago.

Dr. Console: How old are you?

Patient: Twenty-five.

Dr. Console: So, I've established two things: that she's twenty-five and that she's been aware of this fear for a couple of years. Now, what does "a couple of years" mean? Suppose instead, she had said, "Let's see, today is the twenty-seventh of September . . . it's almost two years now." Do you note any difference between the diffuseness, the vagueness, if you will, of "a couple of years" as opposed to the specificity of "two years ago"?

Dr. Redley: Well, when someone says, "I'd say it was just about a few years ago," the next thing I would like them to be able to do is to pinpoint an event or situation that they feel was connected with it. I would like the patient to describe more.

Dr. Console: And in wanting her to do that, what would you do?

Dr. Zimmer: Ask her . . . just say something like, "Two years ago?"

Dr. Bond: I would be hoping that she would say, "I first became afraid of roaches while I was at so-and-so's house, on July fourth and so on."

Dr. Console: Well, let's stay with the hypothesis that I've offered you. That instead of saying "a couple of years" . . . and a couple is really very vague . . . I'm asking, if the patient *had* responded to my question with "two years ago," what would you do? Why not ask her, "What happened two years ago?" In other words, please erase from your conception of technique the device of repeating the patient's last two words with a rising inflection in your voice and an expectant expression on your face. If the patient says, "two years ago," ask what happened two years ago.

Dr. Console: And a couple of years ago, what happened?

Patient: I just saw a few roaches (*laughs nervously*) and I became terrified.

Dr. Console: Terrified . . .as though what? What might happen?

Patient: I really don't know—they just leave me terrified.

Dr. Console: She used the word "terrible" before and now the word "terrified." These are highly charged words. Now if we're talking about tigers and the patient says, "I was terrified" . . . your natural response is "me too." If a tiger was running after me, I would be terrified. But a roach? "I was terrified"? There's an intensity here that we're going to have to elucidate. We're going to have to get some idea of what she's talking about. So it was a couple of years ago that she saw roaches. Well, how does that ring to you in terms of the facts of life? She's twenty-five years old.

Dr. Alper: She's never seen them before?

Dr. Console: She is suggesting that she's never seen them before. Now I wonder, under what aseptic conditions was this girl brought up that she went through twenty-three years of life and never saw a roach? And a couple of years ago, she saw one, was terrified and continued to be terrified thereafter . . . about a roach? So, at some point, I'll have to inquire . . . "Tell me, where in the world do you come from?"

Patient: I really don't know. They just leave me terrified. I just shake all over. My knees get weak . . . the last time, I broke out in hives.

Dr. Console: Actually?

Patient: Yeah (*laughs*).

Dr. Console: "I just shake all over. My knees get weak . . . the last time, I broke out in hives." What about that? What is this patient demonstrating in terms of the physiological responses to anxiety?

Dr. Chassen: Conversion?

Dr. Console: All right . . . I would prefer to say here . . . a tendency to somatize. A tendency to respond to anxiety somatically. Now, if you see a patient who, during the course of the first two minutes of an interview, indicates a tendency toward somatization, what questions might come to mind as you think of her as a therapy patient?

Dr. Marcus: If she tends to somatize her anxiety, less of it would be available as a tool to work through conflict.

Dr. Console: Precisely. After all, your treatment is not going to be to prescribe an antihistamine or Nupercaine for itching . . . or anything of that sort. The only thing we prescribe is language . . . talking back and forth. And Dr. Marcus' point is quite correct. The suggestion here is that this woman has a tendency to make a response with a bodily reaction, rather than to communicate her anxieties verbally.

> *Patient*: Yeah (*laughs*). I don't understand it. I know logically they can't hurt me.

Dr. Console: Now what about her next comment? She said she broke out in hives, but then said, "I don't understand it. I know logically they can't hurt me." If we had moved in the direction that Dr. Marcus suggested, namely to concern ourselves about the alacrity with which she indicated a tendency to somatization, what has she done now, by saying, "I don't understand it. I know logically that they can't hurt me"?

Dr. Redley: She could be thinking in terms of the cockroaches having bitten her to produce the hives. . . . She may have had that connection somewhere in her mind.

Dr. Console: But she says they *haven't* bitten her. She says in effect, "They haven't touched me, so why would I break out in hives?" I'm suggesting that she's moving in the opposite direction . . . in the direction of reflecting. If we want to get real high class about this, we can say she's moving in the direction of indicating the capacity for ego-splitting. That means that someone is able to stand aside and look at himself in a given situation. This is what she's doing. This is a plus. It doesn't sound as bad as it did originally. At first, there was a somewhat more primitive quality to it, and by virtue of its primitivity, much more difficult to reach in psychotherapy.

> *Patient*: I don't understand it. I know logically they can't hurt me.
>
> *Dr. Console*: But you say that it's been some time since you've seen the roaches.
>
> *Patient*: Yes. I don't see them very often.

Dr. Console: When was the last time that you saw them?

Patient: A couple of months ago. When I first came to the clinic

Dr. Console: Oh I see. You first came to the clinic a couple of months ago?

Patient: Right.

Dr. Console: And what happened?

Patient: I had seen some roaches and I had gotten all upset again, and a friend of mine who comes here suggested that I come also.

Dr. Console: So you came, and . . .

Patient: I was interviewed. . . . Since then I haven't seen any, so I don't know (*laughs*).

Dr. Console: You were interviewed and what were you told about treatment?

Patient: I was told that I would be interviewed three times and evaluated, and that I would come twice a week for treatment. I didn't hear anything about that until Dr. Roberts called me last week.

Dr. Console: All right, so here we have to deal with the machinery of the clinic. A patient comes and there is an artificial distinction between the diagnostic and the treatment portions, as though they're two different things. And in the clinic, they are different things for most people because one person is assigned to do the diagnostic interview and the case is often assigned to someone else for treatment. This artificial demarcation will not exist in your practice. You'll see the person; you'll do the diagnostic; and you'll treat the patient. You won't say to the patient, "Well look, the first sessions are diagnostic, then we start treatment." Because the moment you see a person, treatment has started. A relationship has begun. Now, I think she's answered Dr. Alper's question about why she's come at this point. She's come now because she was called now, after she had first called on her own. So her motivation sounds pretty good. She wanted help but the wheels turn slowly at the clinic and she had been waiting for treatment. So, it's not that there's some strange reason for her having waited these months. She comes now because nobody notified her before this.

Dr. Clarke: There's one question that came to my mind.

Dr. Console: Yes?

Dr. Clarke: It seems that this patient is quite suggestible. She came to the clinic only because a friend suggested this to her.

Dr. Console: Well, I think you may be making the mistake of taking the patient's early words at face value. You will find that most people are aware of inner stress, but going to a psychiatrist is only for "crazy" people. Then someone comes along and says, "Hey, I went . . . or my cousin went . . . and was helped." This may be just the little extra support that the patient needs to make the decision which he or she may have been struggling with for some time. So, it can be unfair to patients to decide that there's some capricious reason for their seeking help. You will hear very commonly of a friend influencing the patient, but you will learn later on in the treatment that the patient had been worrying about his problems for a very long time and that he just needed a little extra push to help him take the step toward treatment.

Dr. Console: I see. So you were really waiting to hear from the clinic all these months?

Patient: Yes.

Dr. Console: Nothing happened until just recently?

Patient: Right.

Dr. Console: Now tell me about yourself. Tell me about how this roach business goes.

Patient: It doesn't seem to make much sense. A couple of years ago I saw one for the first time. I think it was the first time I'd ever seen a roach. Because I don't remember ever seeing one before.

Dr. Console: Where have you lived? (*The residents begin laughing*).

Dr. Console: You see, this is a startling statement in a way. She talks like a Brooklyn girl. At least, she's from the general metropolitan area and she does not look to me like Nelson Rockefeller's daughter. So . . . how does it come about that she never saw a roach until she reached her twenties?

>*Dr. Console*: Where have you lived?
>*Patient*: A private house.

Dr. Console: Do you find that an interesting response? I asked her where she'd lived and she answered "a private house."

Dr. Clarke: Well, you know, roaches are not found in private houses. They're usually in projects.

Dr. Console: All right. Her view seems to be that roaches are in apartments, tenements, projects, whatever, but that "a private house" confers a certain immunity. What is she establishing beyond that for us?

Dr. Clarke: I would say she's separating herself from other sorts of people.

Dr. Console: Yes . . . she is separating herself from a lot of people. Now, what is this? Is she being snooty? Does she have some fantastic, narcissistic idea about herself so that she's separating herself from the common people? How can we explain this? What I see her doing is establishing a kind of socioeconomic hierarchy. I see her establishing the fact that she came from a private house, which means that her parents could afford one, and that her mother was a good housekeeper. In this sense, she is not riffraff but rather comes from a clean, honorable, middle-class, good housewife, good mothering situation.

It sounds like an awful lot of assuming, doesn't it? You may be struck by the manner in which we are trying to put together threads and strands of information and weave it into this woman's story. And yet this is exactly the process that must go on in your mind from the very first moment of the initial interview. It would appear at first glance that our situation is vastly different from that of the reporter in that people come to us; we don't go after them. They come to us because they have a story to tell. That is, they have a complaint. . . . They are bothered by something and they are seeking some kind of help. But as time goes by, we will see that there is a great similarity between our task and that of the reporter. Because even though the patient comes to us with some willingness, there is also an enormous amount of what we might characterize as unwillingness and inability to tell the story.

Now when we refer to that inability, we're really talking about
resistance. We're talking about the patient's need to defend
himself . . . the inherent need to present himself in the best
possible fashion, and to avoid presenting himself in the worst
fashion. This leads to his distorting the story. In the beginning, we
listen. We try to remember what the patient has told us, but we
leave the door open so that, as time goes by, these original facts, as
given, will undergo very real changes. As his resistance decreases,
as we make an effort to help reduce this resistance, the patient
becomes more and more able to tell us everything and his capacity
to remember becomes greater. His willingness to confront himself
with the events of his life increases.

> *Patient*: A private house. In Brooklyn, in Flatbush. You
> know, I've always been a little afraid of bugs of any kind.

Dr. Console: So we have the additional information now that
indeed she has lived in Brooklyn. In a private house to be sure. And
. . . she has never seen a roach. In terms of what we know of the
facts of life, this represents a rather curious circumstance. However, she then adds, "I've always been a little afraid of bugs." What
are your thoughts about that statement? I'm asking you to use
what you know about people in general. The statement, "I've
always been a little afraid of bugs" is what? A remarkable
statement or a common one? Which would it be?

Dr. Kent: A common one.

Dr. Console: Yes. I mean this is a very ordinary thing. Would you
say anything about the matter of gender here . . . comparing men
to women in regard to a fear of bugs.

Dr. Marcus: Well, I think it would be more common in women.

Dr. Console: Yes, I think this is a statistical fact. If it is, how are we
going to account for the fact that generally women tend to have
greater feelings about bugs than men? Men may appreciate
equally the fact that bugs are dirty vermin, but the chances are
very great that men will not develop the same intensity of
response, the same kind of anxiety, when confronted with bugs as
women do.

Dr. Clarke: Isn't it a fact that in this society, a man is supposed to be very forceful and strong in these matters and is expected to be protective?

Dr. Console: All right, so you are suggesting that it really is a cultural phenomenon having to do with the commonplace concept that men are supposed to be tough and not be bothered by these things. I would say that probably plays a part, but I don't think it's the reason for the really striking difference that Dr. Marcus has suggested. I think there are other reasons for it. Reasons that pertain, very simply, to being a man as opposed to being a woman. . . to the differences between the sexes.

Dr. Meyer: Well, I don't know. . . . Are you suggesting that . . .

Dr. Console: I'm not suggesting anything (*The residents begin laughing*). I don't want to suggest a blessed thing. I just want to suggest that you give this some thought, that's all.

Dr. Meyer: I'll give you my fantasy.

Dr. Console: That's more honest.

Dr. Meyer: That bugs are some kind of symbol for something else . . . some sort of universal symbol, one that women would be more frightened of than men would be. Maybe they're symbolic of penises or something.

Dr. Console: Well, I would say that if we're going to limit ourselves this way and say that, to women, bugs are symbolic of penises . . . women don't think a helluva lot of men (*group laughter*). I'm not suggesting that Dr. Meyer is way off base. I think he's on the right track, but not with the precision that I would prefer.

Dr. McDermott: Bugs typically come in and out of crevices and are also dirty, horrible things, unlike . . .

Dr. Console: Unlike penises? (*more group laughter*). Well, let me interrupt you to say that your first statement that bugs come in and out of places is very true, so that if we are to think in terms of the woman and her concern about this . . . what is her concern? That they're coming out of places or they're going into places?

Dr. McDermott: Into places.

Dr. Console: That they're going into which places?

Dr. McDermott: Her places.

Dr. Console: That's right. Her places. Really, her *place*. Now you are all familiar with the difference between the sexes in the matter of the mouse in the room. And what difference is there? It's characterized in cartoons everywhere. The man's reaction is "get rid of this thing" or something like that, but the woman's reaction is what?

Residents: To jump up.

Dr. Console: To jump up on the chair and do what?

Residents: Hold her knees together.

Residents: Stay off the ground

Dr. Bond: To hold her dress down.

Dr. Console: (*standing with knees together and hands over groin*). To protect herself (*group laughter*). So her statement that "I've always been a little afraid of bugs" may very well represent a derivative of what we have developed in these past few minutes. Now let's see if this speculation is confirmed by the data.

> *Patient*: I've always been a little afraid of bugs of any kind . . . somewhat afraid, but not to that point. And then I saw the roach and I went crazy.
>
> *Dr. Console*: And this was when, you say?
>
> *Patient*: A couple of years ago. It's not clear in my mind exactly when.
>
> *Dr. Console*: And you were living where? With your family?
>
> *Patient*: Yeah. I was living with my husband in our apartment.
>
> *Dr. Console*: In an apartment . . . just the two of you?
>
> *Patient*: Right.
>
> *Dr. Console*: And this was daytime, nighttime . . . when was it?
>
> *Patient*: I think it was evening . . . I went into a panic.
>
> *Dr. Console*: Was your husband there at the time?
>
> *Patient*: No, he wasn't.

Dr. Console: So, it was toward evening and her husband was not there when she first saw the roach and went into a panic. Why did I take the pains to establish that her husband was not there? What could you anticipate had her husband been present? Would she have had the same reaction or would it have been a lesser one?

Dr. Farber: Lesser.

Dr. Console: Why?

Dr. Farber: With her husband not present, sexual desires could not be satisfied.

Dr. Console: Sexual desires could not be satisfied. . . . Are you suggesting that she was in such a state that she couldn't wait a little while longer, until her husband came home?

Dr. Farber: She could have felt guilty about having had sexual feelings . . . on an unconscious level.

Dr. Console: Well, if we want to talk about an unconscious level, might it not be really a matter of vulnerability? Whatever her unconscious desires were, her vulnerability to this invasion, to this attack, however she feels it, would be much greater without her husband there. With him present, she would feel protected.

> *Dr. Console*: He was not.
> *Patient*: It's much better if he is, it's not so bad.
> *Dr. Console*: Why is that?
> *Patient*: I guess he pampers me . . . he comforts me. He'll always kill it. When he's not there it's much worse.

Dr. Console: So you see, if he's there he kills it. He comforts her and she feels much better. In other words, "He protects me from this invasion . . . from this danger. Without him there, I feel more vulnerable."

> *Patient*: I went to a hypnotist. I got cured.
> *Dr. Console*: And?
> *Patient*: It seemed to work, because I didn't see any after that.
> *Dr. Console*: What did the hypnotist do?
> *Patient*: Well, he put me under hypnosis. It didn't seem very—it wasn't very deep but it was enough to help my fear of it.
> *Dr. Console*: How many times did you see the hypnotist?
> *Patient*: Four times.
> *Dr. Console*: Four times. And on each occasion he hypnotized you and then what?
> *Patient*: I was all right then, but (*laughing*) then I didn't see a roach for a long time after that. So I can't be sure, you know. And then the last time . . .

Dr. Console: That's a perfectly good cure. She saw the hypnotist four times. He hypnotized her and she was then all right, because she never saw a roach afterwards. This is very much like the patient whom I treated who had a tax-free income of about two hundred thousand dollars a year, and who had a subway phobia. But she never took subways, because she had a chauffered car. So, she had a subway phobia. It was of no consequence.

> *Patient*: And then the last time I saw one . . . that's when I came to the clinic.
> *Dr. Console*: How long have you been married?
> *Patient*: Six years in February.
> *Dr. Console*: Six years in February (*pause*). Can you tell me about yourself. Where you come from and where you've grown up?

Dr. Console: Now, five minutes of the interview have gone by. We have learned about her chief presenting complaint. With it, we've picked up some other pieces of information. That she is twenty-five years old. That she is married, and has been married for about six years. That she lives with her husband in an apartment and so on.

It is time now to move away from the chief complaint. We have the beginning of the "who." Who is this person? We have the "what" she came to the clinic for. Now in my desire to answer all the other questions, but to answer them in the context of the *person*, I have switched from specific questions about the chief complaint to the question which I will put in various forms with different people. It adds up simply to this:

Look, *I want to know who you are*. I want to know where you come from. I want to know what your development has been. I want to know as much as possible about the experiences you have had since childbirth. In the course of that, I will want to know about your family. I will want to know about your mother and father and your brothers and sisters, and indeed your grandparents as well. Where you fit in the line. What your relations with your parents are and have been. What your experiences were in the matter of growing up. What your experiences have been in grade school, in high school, college . . . whatever. I want to know, in getting this developmental story, what your sexual development has been like. I want to know about masturbation. I want to know about your early sexual contacts and experiences. I want to know about the process of your falling in love and marrying, and about what went into your making this particular choice, because this decision, this object choice in marrying someone, is not something that is made lightly. It is not a function of circumstance. It is in response to very specific needs. And when I begin to get the answers to all of these questions, I'm going to know why this woman has the chief complaint that she does, and what it probably represents.

In other words, I'm saying to you, that when you are interviewing a patient, do not get caught up in the chief complaint. Listen to it. Satisfy yourself that you have some understanding of it and then move on to the broad picture. In what context does this particular complaint appear in this person? Hence, the question that I have asked. With another person I might say, "Give me a brief chronology of your life. Tell me about yourself as best you can remember from the very beginning." And you will notice that if the person starts off by saying, "I was born in so-and-so, and I went to such-and-such high school," I will gently stop him and indicate that there's an enormous period of time between being born and going to high school. What took place in between? I will bring him back in an effort to get a chronological, developmental account of what his life experiences have been. This is the only way I can understand the patient. This is the only way, I believe, that anyone can really understand the patient.

> *Dr. Console*: Can you tell me about yourself? Where you come from and where you've grown up?
> *Patient*: I grew up in Brooklyn.
> *Dr. Console*: You were born in Brooklyn.
> *Patient*: Right . . . and when I was three years old the family moved to a private house. And I lived there.
> *Dr. Console*: Until when?
> *Patient*: Until I was nineteen.

Dr. Console: Until your marriage. And then . . .

Patient: Then I moved to New Jersey for a couple of years . . . to an apartment. Then I came back to Brooklyn. I went to school in Brooklyn. Catholic schools. I always went to Catholic schools.

Dr. Console: Can you tell me something about your family?

Dr. Console: All right. She responded to my question with these somewhat disparate, isolated facts. But they are revealing. She told us something about moving from here to there. She was married at nineteen. That she is or was Catholic. That she had gone to parochial school, which has many implications for us. But, she has not satisfied me in the matter of providing me with a chronology of development vis-a-vis having a father, mother, brothers and sisters. So I asked her to tell me about her family.

Dr. Console: Can you tell me something about your family?

Patient: My father had a small business. . . .

Dr. Console: Now, is there anything significant here? My question and her answer.

Dr. Alper: For what it's worth she chose to mention her father first.

Dr. Console: OK. My question was about her family. This is characteristically what I will do unless I have good reason to ask specifically about a particular parent. She mentioned her father first. What do you think about that?

Dr. Marcus: I really don't know for certain, but I would think that most people will begin by mentioning the mother.

Dr. Console: Why would that be?

Dr. Marcus: Because the mother is the primary caretaker and the first love object for us all.

Dr. Vis: I'm not sure I agree. I think that in certain societies, almost everyone would mention the father first. It would depend upon the role that men and women play and how dominant a man is supposed to be in a particular culture.

Dr. Dulay: I think that most women would mention the mother first and describe her. She's the person with whom a woman patient will have to identify.

Dr. Console: I think that all of you have made very perceptive points. The only observation that I want to add is that it's important to note whom the patient chooses to mention first, the mother or the father. It has a great deal of meaning. I don't know if I would state that there's a general rule . . . that men will mention one parent first as opposed to women. It depends mostly on the individual situation of the patient and what his or her relationship to the parents have been. But make a mental note of whether a patient mentions the mother first or the father.

> *Patient*: My father had 'a small business . . . a candy store. When I was younger, in my younger years, he didn't do so well, and then he got his own business. And . . . my mother is a housewife.

Dr. Console: In terms of what we've been discussing, notice that she gives a moderately elaborate description of her father, followed by a terse statement, "My mother is a housewife." This is what you will see characteristically, that a particular parent is mentioned first and described in more detail. In this case, it's the father.

Dr. Vis: In certain societies, I think virtually everyone will mention the father first. He is the more dominant and powerful figure. I think that there are great societal determinants.

Dr. Console: I appreciate the fact that there are these cultural differences, but be aware that we will ultimately come down to the fact that no matter what the culture is, so long as there is a mother, a father, and a child, certain things are inevitable. What I am going to try to help you understand is that our major concern has to do with the primary and original culture. By this I mean the family. A father, mother, brother and sister. This is the first culture to which we are all exposed and it is its influence that is of the greatest consequence to us in understanding people's problems.

> *Patient*: And my mother is a housewife. And I have three sisters and a little brother.
> *Dr. Console*: Three sisters. And you're the oldest?
> *Patient*: Right.
> *Dr. Console*: How was it, being the oldest child?

Patient: Well, at first I found it was fun . . . and then, as the others got older, it wasn't that much fun anymore.

Dr. Console: We've established that she is the oldest of five siblings . . . three sisters and a brother, all younger than she. And we know that the firstborn occupies a special position in the family and my questions at this point have to do with learning something of what her experiences and her attitudes were in relation to this. She says that at first it was fun, but as they grew older, it wasn't so much fun. Do you have any thoughts as to what she might be telling us?

Dr. Vis: Initially she would have been the sole recipient of the attention of her parents. But as more siblings came along, that attention would have diminished.

Dr. McDermott: The older child usually has power over the younger ones and tells them what to do . . . tends to do unto the younger as has been done unto him. This is apparently quite pleasurable for the older child. But when the younger ones reach a certain age, it's much harder to push them around . . . to tell them what to do. Perhaps that's why it was not as much fun for her.

Dr. Console: You have suggested then that it falls to the oldest child to act in what capacity, vis-a-vis the younger children?

Dr. Meyer: Kind of like a surrogate mother.

Dr. Console: Kind of like a mother, particularly if the first child is a girl. So in those terms, what might she be denoting in the change from its having been pleasurable when they were small to its becoming less so when they became bigger?

Dr. Meyer: She moved. Her position changed from being a mothering figure and having a special relationship with her parents, to just being one of the girls in the family . . . having to compete for the same attention. My fantasy had more to do with her position relative to her father. We already speculated about her feelings about penises. . . . Well, we talked a bit about the symbolic value . . . the symbolism of the roaches. Thinking along that line and perhaps extending it, could it be the primary position with the father that she's really talking about?

Dr. Console: I would suggest that her fear of roaches has very little to do with what we're talking about. Any patient in this position could easily say the same things she has said regarding her younger siblings. That it was fun when they were smaller and she was acting in the capacity of a mother. As they grew older and became more self-sufficient, her functioning as a mother to them would have been attenuated. As you suggested, they became more equal as siblings compared to the situation where she was the big girl and they the little kids. She's describing a change that took place over the course of many years.

> *Dr. Console*: So you went to grade school and to high school ... Catholic schools. And when you finished high school what did you do?
> *Patient*: Well, I went to work for the telephone company ... a clerical job. I went to school at night.
> *Dr. Console*: School at night?
> *Patient*: College ...
> *Dr. Console*: With what in mind?
> *Patient*: A degree.
> *Dr. Console*: A degree.

Dr. Marcus: I was hoping she'd be more specific.

Dr. Console: How do you mean "more specific"? What could be more specific than this piece of paper ... a degree? (*group laughter*).

Dr. Kent: Most people who go to school do so to study or learn a particular field or area rather than just to get a piece of paper ... particularly if they go to night school. It reminds me of the jokes we used to tell each other in undergraduate school about women getting their MRS degree. That sort of thing (*group laughter*).

Dr. Console: What's the implication of this joke?

Dr. Kent: The implication was, sexist though it may have been, that women go to school to get married. To find husbands.

Dr. Console: All right, this is one of the implications. That the aim is to get married. We have to concern ourselves with what *this* woman has told us. When I said, "With what in mind?" she answered ... "degree."

Dr. Iglesias: It seems to be very important for her self-esteem. She has to prove in some way that she's worth something. In her childhood she occupied an important position in the family hierarchy. She was third in command and when the other kids grew up, she lost that command and became just another one of them. Now she says that she wants a degree. This is something tangible to prove that she's worthwhile.

Dr. Console: Yes. And what about the emphasis we placed upon the idea that she lived in a *private house*? I'm asking you to put all this together. This is something of an unusual response to the question I asked her. I expected an answer such as, "I wanted to teach," or "I wanted to become an executive assistant or a supervisor at the telephone company," or "I wanted to learn business," something like that. I think that this is what Dr. Marcus alluded to when he mentioned her lack of specificity. But I insist that she was quite specific . . . "degree." And I think that Dr. Iglesias' analysis of the situation has considerable merit. That this has to do with her image of herself—of her feeling of esteem about herself, and that a degree becomes a badge. It denotes accomplishment.

Dr. Farber: To tie it in with a fear of bugs and the question of phallic symbols . . . the degree could represent the acquisition of the lost penis. The penis that she wasn't born with.

Dr. Console: Well, I have to remind you that these are all ideas that *you* have brought up . . . phallic symbols and such. Now that's a theoretical conjecture which may or may not have validity, but on the basis of the information that we have thus far, I would prefer that we try to stay within the limits of the actual material that has been presented. I feel that at this point, she has presented us with the idea that she really doesn't think a helluva lot of herself, and that the degree would bolster her self-esteem.

Dr. Rubinstein: It's important for us to be able to speculate, but equally important not to burden a patient with our conjectures until we can support them. It's essential that we be able to use our imagination—as long as we keep our associations to ourselves.

Dr. Console: Indeed you must learn to speculate, to begin to feel comfortable with all of your fantasies about a patient. I want you to feel free to bring out any idea that occurs to you. Don't dismiss it. Let's try it on for size and see how it fits.

Patient: I didn't do very well in college. I had (*inaudible*) . . . (*nervous laugh*).

Dr. Console: Had you done well in high school?

Patient: Oh . . . all right—C's. I was an average student, you know (*pause*). My sisters all did better than I did.

Dr. Console: And when did you meet your husband?

Patient: Working at the telephone company. I had gotten a promotion. I was sent to an office in Manhattan and I met him there.

Dr. Console: What was he doing?

Patient: He was working in the boiler room. . . .

Dr. Console: In response to the question, "How did you meet your husband?" she says, "I got a promotion. I was working in Manhattan." Obviously this is a real promotion! Transferred from Brooklyn to Manhattan! What heights beyond that can you reach? (*group laughter*). And she met him there. What was he doing? "He was working in the boiler room."

Dr. Chassen: Well, I was struck by the fact that we were talking about her self-esteem. She takes this opportunity for advancement and goes to Manhattan, and then she marries the man in the basement . . . goes down, in a sense, to the boiler room.

Dr. Console: So you're suggesting that there might be some significance in the manner in which she has given us the information . . . namely, going from the idea of a promotion to meeting her husband who was working in the boiler room. You say that you're struck by it and whenever you're struck by anything, give it thought. If ever a patient says something that causes a reaction inside of you, the question you have to ask yourself is, "What is going on? What can this possibly mean?" If the patient says something that sounds strange, you must say to yourself, "I have to get an explanation for this . . . so that it is no longer strange and it fits in with what I know."

Dr. Bond: It seems to me that it's a strange way to introduce one's husband. I mean that most women, I think, would try to glorify their husbands' work.

Dr. Console: You mean you would have felt better if she had said, "I met him. He was a subterranean engineer" . . . or something like that (*group laughter*).

Dr. Bond: I would think maybe a plumber or an electrical engineer.

Dr. Console: All right, there's a certain quality here which raises questions in your mind. She just mentions that he was working in the boiler room . . . nothing else.

Dr. Bond: Yes . . . after she builds up everything else.

Dr. Console: Yes. This is what I referred to as the juxtaposition of, "I got a promotion, went to Manhattan . . . and he was in the boiler room."

Dr. Clarke: Dr. Bond's question is pretty valid. We don't really know yet, but this man could be an engineer in the boiler room. That's information we didn't get yet . . . exactly what his position was.

Dr. Console: Absolutely . . . it could be but it hasn't come out yet.

Dr. McDermott: She had what seemed to be an embarrassed smile on her face after she said that he was working in the boiler room.

Dr. Console: That's a good observation. Let's look again and see (*the tape is replayed*).

> *Patient:* He was working in the boiler room (*long pause during which she looks uncomfortable and smiles*) . . . I guess I should say that that appealed to me.
>
> *Dr. Console:* Why did that appeal to you?
>
> *Patient:* I don't know why . . . (*laughs*). It just did. It seems strange.

Dr. Console: Notice, I'm silent. She had indicated some discomfort after stating that he was working in the boiler room. I'm not going to let her sweat, but I'm not going to jump right in either. I gave her a moment to follow up on this and she did. By herself. She said, "I guess that appealed to me." "Why did that appeal to you?" "I don't know. . . . It seems strange." We can put this in the category of some kind of reflective capacity. She could just as readily, having made these statements, have gone on to something else. At the very least, it suggests that she wonders, that she has some questions about all of this. This is of consequence. It is meaningful, in an initial interview, to find someone who is willing to volunteer the idea, "You know . . . this is strange . . . this is not an ordinary, straightforward, everyday sort of thing." She has thought about this.

> *Patient*: I don't know why (*laughs*). It just did. It seems strange. Like the engineers around. They were there. People like that, you know. I really didn't care for them.

Dr. Console: "There were engineers around, and people like that. I didn't really care for them."

Dr. Farber: I think a boiler man is filling a void. Filling a void . . . a furnace, sort of womblike. And the boiler man feeds it.

Dr. Console: Why can't an engineer fill a void? An engineer *erects* things (*group laughter*). An engineer *makes* things.

Dr. Farber: I wonder if he fills things constantly. Constantly satisfying the furnace (*more laughter*).

Dr. Chassen: My associations are to boiler rooms. What crawls around in basements and boiler rooms? Cockroaches and mice . . . lowly, dirty things, crawling in and out of furnaces and crevices.

Dr. Bond: Maybe she's the kind of woman who would be much more impressed by the so-called masculine type, than by the educated engineer.

Dr. Console: It's possible, but is every engineer aesthetic?

Dr. Vis: I think that by disregarding the highly qualified person, she has boosted her self-esteem. She can disregard the person in the higher position and feel better about herself.

Dr. Cohen: Yes, one way of boosting her self-esteem is to date someone who's recognizably lower than she. She can reject the engineers, and date the boiler-room man.

Dr. Dulay: Maybe the boiler-room man resembles father.

Dr. Console: This is a woman who said that she was going to college for a degree. I tried to infer from this that she needs some kind of a badge. If you need a badge, then you don't think very much of yourself. This woman really has a low sense of self-esteem. She is not worthy of, and could not deal with, could not measure up to the educated man . . . the engineer. She was picking someone whom she felt was more her size. So this object choice is in keeping with her low estimation of herself.

> *Patient*: But there was something about Don that I cared for.
> *Dr. Console*: Well, let's see if we can find out what it was. You said that you went out with the engineers and you didn't care for them.
> *Patient*: I think I felt more confident in going out with my husband. I suppose he didn't think he was so wonderful as the engineers, that he wasn't so great. They seemed to feel that they were bestowing a gift on me by taking me out.

Dr. Console: Now what are we going to do with that. "I think I felt more confident"—with someone at a lower level. "My husband didn't think he was so great as the engineers, who thought that they were great." What mechanism is she using?

Dr. Farber: Rationalizing.

Dr. Console: A little more specifically.

Dr. Chassen: She's saying that her husband is going to have the same view of himself as we think that she has of herself . . . that he is not going to feel that he is as great as the engineers.

Dr. Console: She says specifically that he didn't think he was so great. It was the engineers who thought that they were great.

Dr. Zimmer: I think there's also the expectation that her husband was going to put her on a pedestal, which the engineers wouldn't do. Her husband would increase her self-esteem.

Dr. Console: My question is, if the boilerman would put her on a pedestal, why make the assumption that the engineer would not do the same? Here's a girl, well . . . she's slightly plumpish, but, as we used to say in Brooklyn . . . she's got a nice *built* and everything. Why wouldn't somebody fall in love with her, idealize her and put her on a pedestal? Isn't that what falling in love is all about?

Dr. Alper: I think that she's using projection here and putting her feelings about herself onto the engineers. In other words, "I don't feel that I'm so wonderful, therefore, they're doing me a favor by taking me out."

Dr. Console: Absolutely. The mechanism involved is a projection. The engineers would think they were so great? No . . . this is *her* idea. *She* thinks that they're so great . . . too great for *her*. Her statement that she didn't care for them is the rationalization that Dr. Farber mentioned, but this follows the projection. The projection is the more important aspect of what is taking place here. She's imputing to *them* the feelings that *she* has about them . . . the feelings of being high and mighty. We have no evidence whatsoever that they think so well of themselves.

In fact, if we think about engineers . . . or at least when I went to school, the engineers were the guys who walked around with slide rules and who wouldn't know what to do with a girl if they tripped over one (*group laughter*). They were socially inept. Now those of us in the College of Arts and Sciences . . . we knew the score (*group laughter*). Those engineer guys didn't study English and history. They just knew how to use a slide rule, and how to build a bridge or lay a road . . . a *road* (*group laughter*). They were the least capable in the area of easy, heterosexual relationships. So that if she really knew the score, she would have known that her chances with an engineer were very, very good, because engineers don't think much of themselves in this sphere.

> *Patient*: . . . bestowing a gift on me by taking me out (*laughs*).
> *Dr. Console*: And your husband, was he Catholic too?
> *Patient*: Yes, but he wasn't religious. He's divorced.
> *Dr. Console*: How old is he?
> *Patient*: He's thirty-four.

Dr. Console: All right, so we now have some additional information. What about these facts? Do they strike you in any way?

Dr. Marcus: He's more experienced, more fatherly maybe. Being nine years older and divorced he's significantly older than she is. She could possibly be looking for a father figure.

Dr. Console: All right. If we want to think in these broad and popular terms, because people on television always talk about "father-figures," we are impelled by this information to wonder about the fact that she is married to an older man who has previously been married. Dr. Marcus suggests the quality of the older man's "experience." This may suggest her looking for someone who is more versed in the matters of the world, rather than a contemporary. In a way, this probably reflects something about the father, who at least in her childhood, seemed omniscient. She could go to him with any question and he had an answer. Most fathers answer the questions . . . right, wrong, it makes little difference.

Dr. McDermott: As a divorced man he may also be someone else's marital reject and this would be appropriate for a woman who wants someone who is not all that high up.

Dr. Console: Well, of course, we don't know that he was a marital reject, but it's an interesting speculation to make. You keep it in mind and let's wait and see what she's going to tell us about that.

Dr. Meyer: At this point I would also wonder how her parents felt about her having married an older, divorced man.

Dr. Console: Suppose I asked her at this point, "How did your parents feel about this?"

Dr. Meyer: I don't think you should ask that at this point. I would be wondering about it but it would not be wise to comment.

Dr. Console: Why wouldn't you comment on it at this point if you were wondering?

Dr. Meyer: Because I think that would be making a statement as to your feelings about her marriage . . . a value judgment.

Dr. Console: What would you very likely convey to her with this question?

Dr. Meyer: I think you would convey your disapproval of the relationship.

Dr. Console: Absolutely. You would be unwittingly, in *her* eyes, aligning yourself with the establishment, with the adult world. She already imputes this to you. It has no relation whatsoever to your age. Your position puts you there. What we are trying to do is get her story, uninfluenced and unimpeded by any suggestion that we are making a judgment. A judgment that she would undoubtedly hear as critical, because the chances are that her Catholic parents were not overjoyed at the prospect of their daughter marrying a divorced, older man. This is a perfectly valid assumption. Therefore, you don't have to ask about that. Asking would be doing the opposite of what you're trying to do . . . namely to establish a therapeutic or working alliance with her. Asking this question would be moving in the direction of an adversary relationship.

> *Dr. Console*: He was divorced at the time you met him?
> *Patient*: Right.
> *Dr. Console*: Do you know anything about his first marriage?
> *Patient*: Yes—some things. He does make some comparisons and I learned a little bit about it.
> *Dr. Console*: What did you learn about it?
> *Patient*: Well, he tried very hard. . . .

Dr. Console: What is she going to tell us?

Dr. Clarke: That it was the first wife's fault that the marriage ended in divorce.

Dr. Console: In other words, he did what he could to keep the marriage going but the first wife mucked it up in some way. So he wasn't quite a reject.

> *Patient*: Well, he tried very hard. She was a strange person. She cared a lot about money and clothes, you know, not interested in her child.

Dr. Console: The first wife was a strange person. She cared a lot about things like money and clothes. What about that?

Dr. Redley: That's certainly not defining what's strange about her.

Dr. Console: Yes . . . what's strange about this? How does this make a woman a strange person? How does this make a man a strange person? How does this make anyone a strange person, other than perhaps a monk who has taken a vow of poverty and chastity? As far as the rest of the world is concerned, are these not perfectly unstrange interests to have? So, what might she be doing here?

Dr. Farber: By saying these things, she implies that she herself is noble and self-sacrificing . . . that she is doing without much of what she wants.

Dr. Console: Remember that her statements are in the context of describing the relationship between the husband and his first wife, and that it ultimately ended in divorce.

Dr. Alper: Well, she's protecting her husband, saying that his first wife was strange and that it was all her fault.

Dr. Console: That is what she's doing. She is saying to us, "My husband is not a bad man. He did not heave this woman out capriciously. The marriage was not dissolved without good reason." She's trying to establish that her husband is a good and honorable person but he made the mistake of marrying this mercenary creature.

> *Patient*: . . . money and clothes, you know, not interested in her child. Things like that. And then—in fact, she was going to a psychiatrist.

Dr. Console: "In fact, she was going to a psychiatrist." So what are we going to hear?

Dr. Rubin: That the former wife was crazy. The husband was OK and that whatever happened was her fault . . . that she was not all there.

Dr. Clarke: It may also denote what this woman thinks about going to a psychiatrist. If to go to one means that you're crazy, what is she doing here then?

Dr. Console: Absolutely. And at some point you're going to have to ask that question. How soon I asked it, I don't remember. Let's watch and see.

> *Patient*: And then, in fact—she was going to a psychiatrist. And he told them that it was hopeless, that she couldn't be cured very fast. That's about all I really know about it.
> *Dr. Console*: Were you wary about coming to see a psychiatrist?
> *Patient*: No. I'm comfortable with the idea. I have friends who do it.
> *Dr. Console*: What other fears or concerns do you have?

Dr. Console: Now what am I doing here? I asked her about other fears or concerns. I am looked for further phobic manifestations because it is rare to find a patient with a single phobia. The story of the phobic patient resembles the throwing of a pebble into a lake, where a series of rings expands outward and outward.

In our language what that means is that in the face of a phobic anxiety, the patient erects a defense. The defense characteristically takes the form of avoidance and for a while the patient is able to overcome the phobia by this avoidance mechanism. But the underlying pathology and the need to defend are still there. So the phobia spreads.

You may have a woman come to see you. She may describe to you how, one day, a number of months ago, she was in the butcher shop and she was suddenly overcome by a feeling of dread and then panic, and had to get out of there. She thereafter discovers that she is unable to go to the butcher shop. So she stops going and, for a while, avoids the anxiety. Then the anxiety occurs in the grocery store... then the vegetable store... then the supermarket and it gets wider and wider until she becomes more and more restricted.

> *Dr. Console*: What other fears or concerns do you have?
> *Patient*: I'm afraid—uh—girls my own age. I mean, not fear like with the roaches, where I shake or anything like that, but I'm not comfortable with them. ....

Dr. Console: So, again, I had asked her about any other possible phobias and she stated, "I'm not comfortable with girls my own age."

Dr. Clarke: She doesn't seem to feel that she's worth anything. Competing is just not her style. She must feel that she can't win.

Dr. Console: Anybody want to venture beyond that?

Dr. Parker: This reminds me of the situation with her sisters, where as they became older and got closer to adulthood, she didn't like it. She backed off.

Dr. Console: You certainly have to wonder why she said this. This is a rather striking response to my general question about other fears or concerns. Now she says, "It's not like the fear of roaches .... but I'm uncomfortable with girls my own age. With *girls* my own age." Now, when a patient makes two consecutive statements or sentences, there is a connection between them and there is a suggestion of equivalency between them, despite the patient's categorical denial. "It is not like the fear of roaches but I'm uncomfortable with girls my own age." You must start to think that it *is like* the fear of roaches, and not that it is different. She had to put them together with that negative ... but in your thinking, you have to contemplate that the negative is put there specifically as a defensive maneuver and that she is establishing an equivalency.

> *Patient*: I'm not comfortable with them. You know, I fear going into a group with them. Job interviews, things like that.
> *Dr. Console*: What about that?
> *Patient*: Well, I fear I'll be judged.
> *Dr. Console*: You say "girls my own age." ... Does this mean that young men your own age you don't fear?
> *Patient*: No ... I get along fine there.

Dr. Alper: It leads me to speculate that there might be some sort of sexual material here. . . .

Dr. Console: What sort?

Dr. Alper: Very deeply repressed homosexual fears or wishes, that might surface into consciousness when she's with a group of girls.

Dr. Farber: It might seem that with girls her own age, there's more competition for what roaches represent. This could be another aspect of it. We're back to the idea of women feeling dissatisfied with not having a penis. They might be competitive with each other to try to get it back. So this might have something to do with competition.

Dr. Console: Note the specificity here. "I am uncomfortable with girls my own age." Now Dr. Alper suggests that there is something sexual behind this. Then he gets up his courage a little more and he says that there may be something "homosexual" about this. And Dr. Farber now moves away from the idea of a potential attraction to girls, against which she must defend, and thinks in terms of competition. That she tries to avoid competing with girls her own age. Now, on the basis of what we know so far, is there any feeling that one is a more likely circumstance than the other? Is it more likely that we're in Dr. Alper's camp or in Dr. Farber's camp?

Dr. Vis: I think it's more likely that we're dealing with what Dr. Farber said. She specifies girls her own age. I think that if she had homosexual wishes or fears, she would be uncomfortable with women of any age. We also know that she has a low sense of self-esteem and that she would probably find it difficult to compete.

> *Dr. Console:* You think you may not have this feeling with men?
>
> *Patient:* Yes.
>
> *Dr. Console:* In the job interview, however, it doesn't make any difference whether it's a man or a woman.
>
> *Patient:* I feel at ease usually when I see someone who can put me at ease.
>
> *Dr. Console:* How does someone put you at ease?
>
> *Patient:* You know, by smiling . . . and I end up doing OK. There is something else lately . . . for a while I was afraid that my husband was being unfaithful, which is a little bit silly. . . .

Dr. Console: "One other little thing . . . recently, not all the time, I was afraid my husband was being unfaithful." In the context of what has gone before, what might we begin to feel now?

Dr. McDermott: That has two possible explanations. One is that she still feels so inferior that even her husband, who was the boiler-room man, would prefer someone else, or, she's having fantasies of him with other women, which has homosexual implications. She's imagining the same man with her and with some other woman.

Dr. Console: Well, you're saying that she's *imagining* the man, the same man with another woman. What information do we have that enables us to leave out the word "imagine"?

Dr. Parker: He's divorced, we already know that.

Dr. Console: The man was already married and *had* another woman. So that if she is imagining this . . . if this is her fantasy, we also have the knowledge that it was, at one time, a fact as well. Now, what about that?

Dr. Marcus: I think we're still dealing with the previous question concerning her fear and discomfort around women—whether it's an unconscious homosexual fear or a fear of sexual rivalry. Her fear that her husband might be unfaithful would tend to substantiate her discomfort around women as arising out of a fear of sexual rivalry.

Dr. Console: That she would then be competing with other girls?

Dr. Marcus: Right.

Dr. Console: Now, let me bring up a fundamental principle of psychotherapy. Your approach to this specific material indicates good common sense. We have the picture, thus far, of a young woman who doesn't seem to think an awful lot of herself and who married the man in the boiler room. Then came the material that she's uncomfortable with girls her own age and that this does not obtain with men or boys her own age. Then came the occasional fantasy that her husband may be unfaithful to her. In attempting to put this together you are using good common sense in speculating that her discomfort may be due to the danger of losing him to another woman, a danger reinforced by the fact that she already knows that there was a prior marriage that didn't work out and that this could be her fate as well. That an attractive woman might come along and win him away.

And I say that this is good common sense. But the point that I want to make is that "good common sense" is going to lead us down the garden path. It is going to lead us into trouble because common sense is fine if we are dealing with purely conscious matters. But in dealing with our patients we are dealing with the unconscious. And you are going to have to make an enormous shift, a very significant shift in your way of thinking. That means, you're going to have to abandon good common sense and put in its place good *uncommon* understanding of human psychological functioning.

The analogy that I have made on many occasions is the change from driving an automobile to flying an airplane. Now all of you know how to drive an automobile. You have acquired a great deal of common sense about how to deal with this machine. If you were to fly an airplane and apply the same common sense that you derived from operating an automobile, which also moves you from one place to another, you would wind up very dead.

In an automobile, you are safer if you go slowly. As you go faster, the danger of an accident or loss of control increases. In an airplane, the opposite is true. So long as you go fast, you're safe. When you begin to slow down, you're in trouble. In an automobile, the closer you are to the ground, the better off you are. In an airplane, the farther away you are from the ground, within limits, the safer you are. When you approach the ground, you're in trouble.

If you were to take flying lessons, you would learn the mechanics of an airplane. You have a stick and if you push the stick forward, the nose of the plane goes down. If you pull it back, the nose goes up. You have a rudder-bar or its equivalent, and if you want to turn one way, you push with one foot and if you want to turn the other way, you push with the other foot. These are the rudiments of flying. Now, if you are flying and you go a little too slow and the plane starts to stall, the nose drops and you will find yourself moving toward the earth. In that situation, the common sense that you carry over from your previous experience would tell you, "I have to get the nose up, and I do that by pulling back on the stick." And if you do that, you'll go into a spin; you'll crash and you'll be killed.

Curiously, in the face of this danger, you push the stick *farther forward*. You do the opposite of what common sense tells you to do. Because by pushing the stick forward you increase flying speed. As you increase flying speed you increase lift, you increase control and then, at the appropriate speed, at what seems to be the dangerous crashing speed, you ease back on the stick and the plane straightens out and goes on. So what I am saying to you is that in learning psychotherapy, you are going to move from a terrestial set of common-sense rules to an atmospheric one in which these rules are no longer valid. And we will see shortly how this obtains in the matter of the conclusion that this woman is afraid that someone will take her husband away. That's good common sense. But that's not what she's telling us.

Patient: I was afraid that my husband was being unfaithful, which is a little bit silly because he really wasn't (*laughs*).

Dr. Console: So now she's added "which is a little bit silly because he really wasn't." Having said that, she has established clearly that this is a fantasy. She says that there are no facts to substantiate it and thus it is very clearly in the area of fantasy. If it is fantasy, we have to wonder what function it serves in her psychic economy. What role does it play? People don't say or feel things for nothing. There are reasons. There's a reason for her to entertain the fantasy that her husband is fooling around elsewhere.

Patient: It's just that I ran into all these little things that were happening. He's really not like that . . . it's kind of strange.
Dr. Console: When was this? You say for a while . . . how long back?
Patient: It was right after I had the baby, and I was very unhappy for a while. Well, he was going to school at night. During the day I can't get in touch with him because he works all over the city. . . . So I guess it was a kind of loss of contact. And . . . a lot of my friends were breaking up—it all gets me sad.
Dr. Console: And you say you had this fear. Does it make you sad. Do you think about it? Get down about it?
Patient: Oh sure.
Dr. Console: Why do you think that is?
Patient: I don't know. I think I always told him that if he's ever unfaithful, that's it—it's over. Maybe I'm afraid of that. I don't want to lose him.
Dr. Console: Any idea that it makes you angry?
Patient: Uhm . . . to a certain extent

Dr. Console: Now, what am I pushing here? Do you sense anything?
Dr. Alper: I'm wondering. When she talks about the fear that he might be unfaithful and tells him that if he's ever unfaithful "that's it." . . . How much is a fear and how much is a wish? She doesn't seem to get very angry about all this and I think the lack of anger goes along with its being a wish.

Dr. *Console*: Well, there are two aspects here. I asked her if this made her sad and she said that it did. But did you feel there was any great conviction in her response? Remember, I had to *ask* her if this made her sad.

Dr. *Alper*: Not at all . . . very little conviction.

Dr. *Console*: Then I turned to the feeling of anger and she's not even really angry about it. So where does this fit into what we've developed so far?

Dr. *McDermott*: It sounds as if she's having a somewhat satisfying fantasy, with minimal feelings of sadness or anger.

Dr. *Console*: A reasonable' speculation. I was asking these questions because I felt that these feelings were lacking in her. Dr. McDermott goes even further and suggests that perhaps the thought gives her some kind of gratification. And this may be so.

> *Patient*: Uhm—to a certain extent. It does make me angry. It makes me, uh, I don't know. It hurts my pride. Yeah, it makes me angry.
> Dr. *Console*: Do you see very much of your family?
> *Patient*: Yes.
> Dr. *Console*: You live near them?
> *Patient*: Yes, I do.

Dr. *Console*: As you can see, I switched the topic. She's told us about her thought of her husband's possible infidelity and I got her to elaborate on that a little. But it was my feeling that she was not ready to continue to elaborate on this point, and so I'm turning back to fundamentals. What is, was, and has been the situation in your life? How did you relate to the rest of your family and how did they relate to you? I want further information. Let's see what we get.

> Dr. *Console*: And you have a child, one year old?
> *Patient*: Yes.
> Dr. *Console*: Boy or girl?
> *Patient*: Girl. (*There is a pause here*).
> Dr. *Console*: Why do you think you waited such a long time? It's been six years now and you had a child after five years.

Patient: Well, I think at first we weren't really in a position to do so. We were enjoying life. I didn't feel any need for a child until—you know, we had a very good relationship and we were just enjoying our lives.

Dr. Console: Notice that I waited a fairly long time to see if she would spontaneously elaborate. She didn't. There's no point in just sitting there and glaring at each other, permitting the situation to deteriorate into a contest of who's going to talk first. So I asked her this rather pointed question about why she and her husband waited so long to have a child. Her response was that they were enjoying themselves and they didn't feel they had any need of a child. Any thoughts about that?

Dr. Kent: Well, we have to wonder how much of a good time she and her husband were having. We know that for at least the last two years she has had the phobia. She may have wanted the baby to cement the bond ... to keep what may have been a deteriorating relationship from getting worse.

Dr. Console: Yes. Regrettably this is a very common finding. When a marriage starts to get rocky and uncomfortable, when there is more than the usual amount of strife, the woman may make the decision to have a baby. This may be, as Dr. Kent suggests, an attempt to cement the marriage. But what are some of the dangers that a person making such a decision may be overlooking? Specifically here, where the child is a girl?

Dr. Iglesias: There's the danger that the child may be viewed by the mother as a competitor for the husband's affection.

Dr. Console: This is a very common consequence. That now the woman, who had been troubled and who wanted to create this "cement" in the marriage, may find herself having created more trouble in that she may now feel unloved and envious. The husband comes home and the first thing that he does is rush to the child, pick her up, play with her and bestow his love and attention upon her. To make it even more striking, he may neglect to do the simple things he had done prior to the arrival of the child. He can forget to say hello. He may go right to the child and not even greet his wife in the customary way, with a kiss and so on. So, as Dr. Iglesias suggested, this unwitting sort of competition, brought about by the husband's reinforcing the uneasy situation that obtained prior to the child's arrival, may really have a terrible effect upon an already troubled marriage.

> *Patient*: And that's why we waited. We were just enjoying ourselves and felt that for a lot of practical reasons we couldn't afford it and all that.
>
> *Dr. Console*: And when you had the child, this good relationship . . . having good times, seemed to have changed?
>
> *Patient*: Right. When I got pregnant.
>
> *Dr. Console*: When you got pregnant, you felt that it started to change?
>
> *Patient*: Yes.
>
> *Dr. Console*: What did you notice?
>
> *Patient*: I got depressed. I was trying to get pregnant, but I ended up crying when I found out that I was.
>
> *Dr. Console*: What were your feelings at that time?
>
> *Patient*: I don't know.
>
> *Dr. Console*: That you wanted to get pregnant and yet when you learned that you were pregnant, you cried.

Dr. Console: Any thoughts about that?

Dr. Bond: It certainly would have to do with whatever her expectations were concerning having a baby.

Dr. Console: Yes, what about that?

Dr. McDermott: Well, there are often people who have unrealistic expectations of something that they want to attain. Once the goal has been achieved the fun no longer exists. This could have been the case with this patient, that once the goal of becoming pregnant had been reached, there was little left in the way of sexual enjoyment. These things vary from couple to couple but many couples, when trying to have a baby, increase the frequency of intercourse, and when the baby is conceived, the sexual activity may drop back to its previous level.

Dr. Console: So you're suggesting that once the procreational function has been served, the recreational function tends to drop out?

Dr. McDermott: Right.

Dr. Console: Well, what might a pregnant woman begin to fear about motherhood?

Dr. McDermott: It might restrict her.

Dr. Console: Yes. It's going to impair her mobility. It's going to mean, among other things, that she cannot go freely here and there. She cannot just leave the house. There's a child there. The child brings with it joy and happiness, but responsibilities as well. So, we would have to consider this woman's reluctance to have a child as a reflection of her feeling that she and her husband were having a good time and that this could all change with the responsibility of a child.

> *Dr. Console*: That you wanted to get pregnant and yet when you learned that you were pregnant, you cried.
>
> *Patient*: All those responsibilities coming out. I guess there is a strange relationship between my husband and me.
>
> *Dr. Console*: What were his attitudes at the time? Do you recall?
>
> *Patient*: Oh—he was happy about it.
>
> *Dr. Console*: Were your parents?
>
> *Patient*: They were overjoyed. It was their first grandchild.
>
> *Dr. Console*: Tell me more about your mother and your father.
>
> *Patient*: Well my mother is a good mother. She keeps a good home. She loves all her children. She's a good wife, keeps the house decent. She's sarcastic at times . . . and a little bit cutting. She can insinuate. But you know, it's really that she's just trying so hard. I don't think she realizes sometimes how she can hurt. And my father . . . he's great. He's very crabby and does a lot of yelling but it doesn't matter.

Dr. Console: Now we have a very brief description of some of the characteristics of the mother and the father.

Dr. Farber: She describes her parents in mostly good terms.

Dr. Console: What's the part that's not in such good terms?

Dr. Farber: I don't recall.

Dr. Console: The father does a lot of yelling. The mother is described as being a good housekeeper and so forth, but she's also described as sarcastic and cutting. That's pretty bitter medicine . . . sarcastic and cutting. Father on the other hand . . . well, he's crabby and yells, "but it doesn't matter." Let's go back to the original introduction where she mentioned her father first and gave more of an elaborate description of him than of the mother. She had described them in that order. With what we've just heard, what can we now say regarding her feelings about her father and her mother? At the very least we would have to say that she has the capacity to let her father's crabbiness and yelling slide off her back, but this is not so with the mother. "She's cutting and sarcastic."

Dr. Meyer: She seems to expend a great deal of effort in minimizing her feelings about her parents.

Dr. Console: Wouldn't we expect that? We're not dealing with a woman who floridly despises her parents. She still loves them and so she describes some of their good qualities. She's being a little protective. However, despite her protectiveness, a glimmer of resentment toward the mother comes through.

> *Patient*: He's very crabby and does a lot of yelling but it doesn't matter. He would never hurt you with sarcastic remarks.

Dr. Console: There's some more confirmation. She defends the one dislikable quality that she describes in her father, but doesn't defend her mother's sarcastic and cutting tendencies. You will often find that the parent of the same sex as the patient is the parent with whom the patient has had the greatest difficulty in getting along . . . at least on a superficial level. If the patient is a woman, you're going to hear a similar story to the one that this patient presents. And, if your patient is a man, the most likely description of the situation that you'll hear is: "My mother is all right. She understands me . . . but my father just doesn't understand me and we have great difficulties." What I am saying is that in many, many patients, you will hear derivatives of what we refer to in "high class" language as the Oedipus complex.

Dr. McDermott: What about the situation where a patient clearly expresses more positive feelings about the parent of the same sex and negative ones about the parent of the opposite sex? It does happen.

Dr. Console: It would be significant. And we would want to find out why this is so for a particular person and why his or her story doesn't follow the general run of things.

Dr. Console: You mean he could make sarcastic remarks but he wouldn't do it?

Patient: Sure he could, but he wouldn't make them. His crabbiness isn't hard to take. He means well . . . "do this, do that . . . don't let such and such happen." You know, nothing insulting or that isn't well meant.

Dr. Console: How old are your sisters? Who's next and so on?

Patient: Uh . . . twenty-one . . . nineteen . . . sixteen. And my little brother is seventeen.

Dr. Console: Twenty-one. So there are four or five years between you and the next one.

Patient: Right.

(During this segment of the tape, there have been long pauses, with the patient rarely picking up a question and elaborating.)

Dr. Console: Now I want you to observe these pauses. My intention, or really my hope, is that she'll pick up and continue her narrative. But this is the first time I've ever seen this woman, and there are going to be some very measured pauses. I'm not going to sit for any length of time and let this girl sweat and become anxious. You will hear, during your training, the term "stress interview." Please, do not let that be your goal.

Dr. Console: What was your social life like when you were younger? Did you have much fun?

Patient: Oh—I went out a fair amount. It was fun. Mostly Friday and Saturday nights. Nobody that was steady for a long period of time. I had two different boyfriends. When I was fourteen and when I was sixteen.

Dr. Console: Did your parents object to this?

Patient: Well, they weren't crazy about it, but they really didn't try to get in the way.

Dr. Console: They didn't try to stop you . . . they didn't say, "You can't do it"?

Patient: Yeah.

Dr. Console: What national origin are your parents?

Patient: Italian.

Dr. Console: Italian. Was Italian spoken at home?

Patient: No.

Dr. Console: No. They were born here?

Patient: Yes. My father speaks Italian but my mother doesn't. He likes to speak Italian when he sees someone that he knows speaks it well.

Dr. Console: Your grandparents speak Italian then . . . they were born in Italy?

Patient: Yes, my father's parents were both born in Italy. My mother's parents . . . I'm not sure.

Dr. Console: What has all this got to do with the price of cheese? All these questions, national origin . . . Italian . . . where were the parents born? Were the grandparents born here? When and why did they come to this country?

Dr. Kent: When she had been talking about the boy that she had been seeing, you wanted to find out how her family felt about it.

Dr. Alper: She mentioned that she had few restrictions placed on her.

Dr. Console: Yes. I was trying to establish how old-fashioned or modern her parents were. If they had been foreign, then there's a good chance there would have been difficulties. They might have objected to a fourteen-year-old girl going out on a date. In a more general sense, the matter of ethnic origin or family background is of great importance. It helps form an understanding of the "who" . . . who is this person? There should be no doubt in your mind that family attitudes and customs are going to influence our patients and their attitudes. The flavor of the household is going to be markedly different for a second generation girl of Italian extraction than for a fourth generation girl of Irish or other descent. While these two people will have to negotiate the same milestones in a developmental sense, the hopes and the expectations of their respective families will enormously influence the ease or difficulty with which they will do so.

Dr. Console: So they weren't really old-fashioned Italians?
Patient: No.
Dr. Console: They didn't make a big fuss over a fourteen or fifteen-year-old daughter going out?
Patient: No . . . my father seemed to mind it more than my mother. Sometimes he would get a little upset over it, but not much. It was the fatherly kind of thing. He really didn't mind it much. My mother objected a bit more. She didn't mind me going out either, except she wanted me to go out with a lot of different people.
Dr. Console: Why did she want you to go out with a lot of different people?
Patient: Well, for the normal reasons, you know, you're supposed to play the field, get some knowledge before you choose anyone. But in those days, it seemed you had to have a boyfriend.
Dr. Console: So at least in the matter of going out they weren't terribly strict.
Patient: No . . . they weren't at all.
Dr. Console: And what were the arrangements in things like hours? When you would go out, when were you supposed to come back?
Patient: As long as it was reasonable it was OK. There were curfews and stuff like that . . . it was all OK.
Dr. Console: And what about your social life at that time? You went with relatively few boys?

Dr. Console: This is a general maneuver that I will ask you to observe with great care. Despite the fact that this is a twenty-five-year-old married woman with a child, I'm moving very gently and moving chronologically into an account of her psychosexual development. When the patient is talking about high school and about her dates, inquire about those dates. What was the nature and the degree of intimacy that occurred? What were her early responses? What was the masturbatory history? All this can be elicited very easily if you approach it in this gentle and chronological fashion. This is very important. I think it is the best method to use in order to make an inquiry into the patient's psychosexual development.

> *Dr. Console:* . . . You went with relatively few boys?
> *Patient:* Yes, because I went with them for a while.
> *Dr. Console:* For a while?
> *Patient:* For a long time.
> *Dr. Console:* And with each of these, what developed, that you went with them for a while?
> *Patient:* Not much when I was going out between thirteen and fourteen. It was pretty uneventful. I went out with one boy between thirteen and fourteen, and then another one between fifteen and sixteen. It was about two years each time . . . the two fellas. And . . . both of them were unfaithful. And both of them came back.
> *Dr. Console:* Unfaithful in what sense? That they went out with . . .
> *Patient:* That they went out with other girls, right. One of them was very ugly, very shy, very nervous. It's hard to imagine that anyone would have wanted to go out with him.

Dr. Console: Now, she has characterized one of them as being very ugly, very shy and very nervous, and as someone to whom you would never expect other girls to be attracted. Is this of any consequence to us in the light of what we know about this woman?

Dr. Zimmer: Well, it's very similar to the feelings she had in regard to her husband . . . working in the boiler room. She seems to be more comfortable with a lesser type of man.

Dr. Console: So now we know more about her choice of the man in the boiler room. She chose him in preference to the engineers because they constituted a threat to her. She fantasized them to be articulate and educated, and therefore not interested in her. So that her choice of the man in the boiler room is not happenstance, as nothing is happenstance in human functioning. Particularly, nothing is happenstance in the area of object choice, in the matter of picking a wife or a husband. As I like to put it, marriages *are* made in heaven, meaning that they are a consequence of the partners mutually concluding at some level in their minds that they will complement each other. Each is seeking something in the other person.

Now, in many circumstances, what they are seeking in the other person is a particular personality that meshes, or interdigitates with their own. That is, a seriously masochistic woman will look for and find a sadistic man. A sadistic, aggressive woman will look for and find a masochistic, passive man. And this way, it works out. They form what you might call a neurotic "pact." And here we would have to say that not all neurotic choices in marriage are doomed. There are people who spend their lives in a marriage where the *currency of love is fighting*.

It will not be unusual for you to hear from a patient how the couple was arguing about the spouse's behavior at a party ... looking at other men or women, this or that ... and there's a big, knock-down, drag-out fight. They are virtually brawling. They may be disrobing to go to bed and are calling each other names, and then they get into bed and everything is just great. It becomes almost the prerequisite to being able to have intercourse. A moment of love must be preceded by hours of sadomasochistic interaction.

Dr. Farber: If one of the members of this marriage goes into therapy, can't it ruin the marriage? If the husband, for instance, enters therapy and recognizes and understands his sadism and then alters his behavior, the marriage will be ruined.

Dr. Console: Well, I wonder about the choice of the word "ruined." That is to say, if one of the people goes into treatment and loses the need to be either masochistic or sadistic, then the marital relationship becomes untenable. In that sense, the marriage is changed by virtue of one of the partners becoming moderately healthier. This is not an uncommon fear for a spouse to have. A woman can have the fear that when her husband goes into treatment, he'll dump her. A man can have the same fear if his wife enters treatment. It is not uncommon to find that the spouse who is not in treatment does many things in the service of sabotaging the treatment . . . to abort it and to preserve the old relationship. But, getting back to our patient, I do feel that we now have whatever confirmation we needed in the matter of this woman's impaired self-esteem and its influence on her object choices.

> *Patient*: And the other one was very handsome. If I had opened my eyes I would have seen.

Dr. Zimmer: I think she means that she would have seen that she wasn't worthy of him.

Dr. Console: She would have seen that he was a handsome man and that he would therefore prefer another girl. So we have a second confirmation of the original idea that the more attractive engineers would have constituted a threat to her.

> *Dr. Console*: Well, after these two, who came next?
> *Patient*: My husband.
> *Dr. Console*: Your husband.
> *Patient*: Well, there were lots of guys in between, before my husband, but most of them were wise guys and nothing developed.
> *Dr. Console*: So that until the time that you met your husband you never really got seriously involved?
> *Patient*: No.
> *Dr. Console*: And you never got intimately involved?
> *Patient*: No.
> *Dr. Console*: No sexual intimacy?
> *Patient*: Not really. Nothing to speak of.
> *Dr. Console*: Not really.

Dr. Console: See the progression here. Seriously . . . intimately . . . sexually. You have to build gradually. Despite the fact that she's married, to zero right in may strike the patient as somewhat presumptuous on your part. For one thing, be aware that with the level of sophistication today, most people who come for treatment think that we're only interested in their sexual lives. Don't confirm that. Don't reinforce that idea by behaving in that fashion. Go gradually. Inquire about the social life and social involvements. Approach the concept of closeness and intimacy, then the sexual. And she says, "Nothing to speak of." That's a fairly common response. What is she really saying?

Dr. Alper: "Nothing that I feel comfortable talking about."

Dr. Console: Yes . . . that's exactly what she means. "I don't want to speak of this any further."

> *Patient*: I went out with some boys for a while but not for a long time. I considered them just friends. Some of them were serious about me, but I wasn't very serious.
>
> *Dr. Console*: Then you're suggesting that the first one with whom there were intimacies was your husband?
>
> *Patient*: My husband.
>
> *Dr. Console*: And how did that occur? How was it? . . .
>
> *Patient*: Well, I asked him (*laughs*), you know, because I felt that it was time that I learned what's going on.

Dr. Console: So, we establish at this point that her first really intimate experience, that is, actual intercourse, took place with her husband. Or her husband-to-be. Furthermore, she asked him. What do you think about that?

Dr. Marcus: It says something about the kind of man he is. He seems quite passive and lacking in initiative and didn't take the first step. She had to ask him.

Dr. Console: Yes. Remember, this is a man who has been married before and from her point of view, this must have had a multiplicity of meanings. It suggested, among other things, that she was picking someone who was experienced, someone who could introduce her to sex. And she states very clearly that their sexual relationship did not start as an expression of his ardor . . . but that she asked him.

Dr. McDermott: One possibility of her marrying someone who had been married before is that this is the opposite of her fear. She is taking away from some other woman, rather than having another woman take away from her.

Dr. Console: I think you have to modify that a bit. Recall that the first marriage broke up because the wife was psychotic, or at least that's what the patient believes. The quality of her taking him away from the first wife is greatly attenuated. I think that here you're using a fairly acceptable concept and trying to squeeze the patient into it. We shouldn't do that. We have to come to our conclusions on the basis of what our patients have told us . . . on the basis of what comes from them, rather than having preconceived notions into which we fit the patient.

Dr. Rubin: Her having to ask the husband to have sex with her again points to her low sense of self-esteem. She couldn't entice him.

Dr. Console: This may have been the case. Her charm was not working and she had to take the initiative.

> *Dr. Console*: You say that you asked him. Exactly what do you mean?
>
> *Patient*: I said, "Would you like to show me?" At first I kind of saw him like a friend. He was teaching me how to play the guitar. He seemed too old to marry. He was twenty-eight at the time. So I asked him. I said, "You know, I don't know how to do it . . . could you show me how?" (laughing). As a friend, you know. So he was gentle and nice. . . .

Dr. Console: Now that's an interesting bit of detail. "We were going out as friends and he was teaching me how to play the guitar and I told him I didn't know how to play this instrument either. Show me how." How do you feel about that?

Dr. Zimmer: There are two things that I think might be going on. One of them is that she's trying to tell him, "Listen, I don't value sex very highly. It's not important to me. It's the same as teaching me how to play the guitar." And the second thing I'm thinking of is that she's really saying to him, "I'm really desperate. Even though I have no intention of marrying you, I really want some sex."

Dr. Kent: She's treating it as an asexual thing. There's a denial of it.

Dr. Console: There's considerable denial of the meaning that this has for her. Her analogy to playing the guitar is revealing. "He was teaching me to play the guitar, so while you're teaching me that, teach me this other thing also." If there is denial here, then we have to disagree with Dr. Zimmer's last point that sex isn't terribly important to her. You don't have to deny something unless it's very important and makes you feel uneasy.

Dr. Meyer: It suggested to me also her saying to him, "Teach me how to be a woman. I just don't know anything about being a woman." I wonder how this relates to her self-esteem. She's really out of touch with her feelings. It's hard to imagine how she managed to stay so naive, knowing that adolescent girls usually have many discussions about these things. She must have had some ideas about sex. Another thing that struck me was the infantile quality of the experience. It reminds me of the games that children play . . . "Let's compare our genitals."

Dr. Console: Yes, it does suggest the "doctor game"—"Let's look at each other and examine each other." And Dr. Meyer also makes the point that at one level the patient is saying, "Teach me to be a woman," and that this represents her low level of self-esteem. Would you care to speculate as to what else it might mean . . . what other idea might be involved in such a request?

Dr. Iglesias: This reminds me of her need for the degree, as though it was a badge of accomplishment. She becomes worth something as a woman.

Dr. Console: Well, you're elaborating on Dr. Meyer's conjecture here, that it is still in the area of her self-esteem and that she needs another badge. But might there be something else?

Dr. Vis: It could be that she has doubts about her femininity. She has to have her sense of femininity reassured by having a sexual relationship with a man.

Dr. Console: Yes. I think it is valid at this point to expand upon the very analogy that she gave us. That if she doesn't know how to play the guitar and he's giving her guitar lessons . . . and then she asks him to teach her how to have sex, that she wants lessons in how to be a woman. So it may be that she has doubts as to whether she is one, or how much of a woman she might be. In other words, there are more profound reasons for her behavior than simply the issue of her self-esteem.

Dr. Meyer: I wondered also, earlier we were talking about a possible homosexual concern . . .

Dr. Console: Yes. This was brought up. . . .

Dr. Meyer: . . . and I was thinking that implicit in this situation is the idea, "Show me or tell me how your wife used to do it."

Dr. Console: Might be. We don't know how much of an interest she has or had in the events of his former marriage, but your speculation is a valid one. People commonly express this kind of interest in the experiences that the spouse has had.

Dr. Farber: In a way she was taking the masculine role by asking him.

Dr. Console: OK, she was taking an active posture here, although she was putting it in a passive way. And let us be alerted to the fact that very commonly, a seemingly passive attitude may have an enormously active and aggressive aim. For instance, imagine a kid of twelve or thirteen. He's had a hell of a difficult time with his father for many years, and the old man is always slapping him around. It gets to the point where the boy decides that if the father slaps him for anything, he'll just stand there and won't permit a tear to come to his eye and won't say a word. So, he becomes passive and receives this punishment without an active response, but is being subtly aggressive because he knows that the lack of response on his part is going to further infuriate the father. He is being terribly aggressive by just doing nothing.

Patient: . . . so he was gentle and nice (*long pause*).

Dr. Console: It was all right?

Patient: Oh, it was horrible (*laughing*). It took a long time.

Dr. Console: What was horrible?

Patient: Before he could penetrate. It took months.

Dr. Console: So he went to show her, and it took a long time before he could penetrate. Any thoughts?

Dr. Meyer: She said it was "horrible." If she had used the word "terrible," then it might have related back to her statement about the fear of roaches. Another thing . . . it's quite aggressive to make him wait such a long time to penetrate.

Dr. Console: That's a very aggressive piece of behavior indeed. She says, "Show me," but then it takes months before he can show her. She could be saying to him, "How inept you are that you're not able to penetrate."

Dr. Kent: It would be an aggressive act if she made him wait that long to penetrate. But we don't know that he was kept waiting. Maybe he was impotent. We've already commented on his apparent lack of initiative.

Dr. Console: That's a very good point. But I don't get the feeling that is what she's describing here. She would establish that she was all right and he was defective if that had been the case. I think that what she's saying suggests that he is trying and has an erection and is simply unable to get in . . . because she's not letting him.

> *Patient*: I don't know why it's like that. I even have trouble with examinations. . . .

Dr. Console: So she suggests that there's an antecedent history and that she has had some trouble with examinations, meaning of course, examinations by a doctor. We are going to get the story of the inability of a gynecologist or a general practitioner to insert a vaginal speculum into her.

> *Patient*: I even have trouble with examinations . . . problems like that. I don't know . . .
> *Dr. Console*: Do you feel yourself kind of tighten up?
> *Patient*: Yes, and I can't help it.

Dr. Meyer: You've commented about how you pause and wait for her to continue and how she won't. Since she said that she has trouble being examined by a doctor, I'm wondering if these pauses are a reflection of the same problem.

Dr. Console: You're probably right. At an unconscious level, virtually anything I say to her can be perceived as a penetration by me. We do talk about someone making a penetrating remark. This woman may very well perceive my questions as a penetration, as though the words are invading her.

Dr. Rubinstein: And she's exposing herself here.

Dr. Console: Indeed, to being examined and penetrated.

Patient: I talk to myself logically. I try very hard. And still I freeze up. I just can't help it.

Dr. Console: So now she has made a statement which in many ways will always be crucial to us in our work. She says, "I've talked to myself," meaning, "I've told myself, look . . . this is silly. It shouldn't be. I shouldn't behave this way. I shouldn't react this way." And yet, when it comes down to it, she tightens up. Her reaction is the same. She is saying that common sense and logic, ordinary, good, reasonable logic is not enough. It doesn't change anything. I say again, her hairdresser could easily say to her, "Come on. What's the matter? Relax, it'll be all right". And she can say, "All I have to do is relax." But the situation arises and she cannot relax. Because the conflict is in the *unconscious*. The conflict is not in consciousness. And wherever appropriate, it is our task to help make the unconscious conscious. So that then she might be able to deal with it. This is an extremely important point that she's making. She tells us that she tries to dissuade herself from this anxiety. She uses reason and logic. She knows it's silly and foolish and that it shouldn't happen this way. But every time, she tightens up. Because the reasons are beyond her.

Dr. Console: And it still happens sometimes, now?
Patient: Well, during examinations.
Dr. Console: During examinations.
Patient: Not really with my husband. I—uh—sometimes I'm still scared. I'm still frightened for some reason. But, you know, it's not any sort of problem, you know. There'll just be a momentary tightening, you know, and then I'm all right.

Dr. Console: So the manner in which she said this tells us that it's a current problem even though she tried to limit it to gynecologic examinations. Which means that should she go for an examination, she's going to scream bloody murder before the gynecologist can insert even the smallest speculum into her. She says, "I'm still frightened for some reason," which she changes to "But you know, it's not any sort of problem . . . just a momentary tightening." She's being evasive and trying to tell us that this is past history . . . "Let's forget about it." But it isn't past history. It's operative at this very moment and has been right along.

> Dr. Console: But you say, "I'm still scared. I'm still frightened." Now you've used these words . . .
> Patient: I just realized that . . . (pause).
> Dr. Console: What did you realize?

Dr. Console: What happened? I was about to make a comment and she interrupted me to say, "I just realized." I was going to point something out to her. I had said, "You've used these words," but I never finished the sentence. I was going to say, "You've used these words *before*."

> Patient: I just realized that . . . (pause).
> Dr. Console: What did you realize?
> Patient: That I used them about the roaches too. I said that I'm scared and frightened.

Dr. Console: "That I used the same words about the roaches." There was no need for me to finish my statement because she interrupted me. She made the connection herself. We are observing an example of a sudden insight. The connection she made is very clear. That all of the feelings about being penetrated by her husband, the tightening and being scared, are in some way connected with her original complaint, her original words, "I have a terrible fear of roaches." Does anybody want to expand on that?

Dr. Meyer: Well I just want to say that it was my impression that she wasn't really struck by the fact that she had used the words "scared" and "frightened" before. I think that she was struck by her realization that the feelings are the same. I think that's why she's really excited about the insight.

Dr. Console: Excited about it in what sense?

Dr. Meyer: Well, I think that she's enjoying finding that out.

Dr. Console: It's a discovery! She's excited in the sense that it's a discovery. It's likely that she had never entertained the thought that there might be a connection between her fear of roaches and her sexual behavior with her husband. Now for the first time, she is suggesting that there is a similarity. And when you hear of a similarity you must think in terms of an equivalency. So, we're putting an equal sign there.

> *Patient*: That I used them about the roaches too. I said that I'm scared and frightened. I don't know if it really could be.

Dr. Console: So, having had the insight, she backs off a little and says, "I don't know." With the insight there is a threat and the patient defends.

> *Dr. Console*: But there's something in both situations and you suggest that you don't know what it is. You say, "I'm scared" . . .
> *Patient*: I'm scared that they're going to hurt me, you know.

Dr. Console: So I said to her, "In both situations you don't know what it is" and she said, "I'm scared they're going to hurt me." She has made another equivalency and another equal sign can be put there.

> *Dr. Console*: The roaches?
> *Patient*: The roaches . . . I don't *know* what I'm scared of.

Dr. Console: Now she is again backing away and defending. She states that she's afraid that her husband is going to hurt her but that she doesn't know what it is she fears with the roaches. What are we going to think about that? Are we too going to have our doubts, or do we feel that we know what she fears about the roaches?
Dr. Alper: It's a very similar fear, but in symbolic terms.
Dr. Meyer: I would also say that there are probably more things attached to this than just the fear of being penetrated, and that the roaches actually symbolize a whole constellation of things.
Dr. Console: Yes, I think that it would be an enormous exaggeration at this point to impute to her an order of insight

which now puts this all together. If that happened you would be working a modern miracle. It's going to take weeks and months of working on this issue to help her see that these two things are very intimately related. She is still dealing with them as though they are two disparate fears which have some accidental quality of commonness. And you're perfectly right in anticipating that a whole constellation of ideas are condensed in the roach . . . and what the roach will do and how this relates to what her husband does, and its meaning for her. So, as you say, this is something that would have to develop gradually over a long period of time. But again I would make the point that the insightful thought that occurred to her in this interchange, is, in the long run, of considerable significance.

> *Patient*: The roaches—I don't *know* what I'm scared of. I'm just afraid that they're there. I wouldn't know if they were there. You know, they could be any place in the house and you don't *know* if they're there. You can't see them hiding.
>
> *Dr. Console*: If you can't see them hiding, how is it that it's so bad?
>
> *Patient*: Well, I'm uncomfortable. I know they must be there. I know that . . . that they'll come out. And now, I hate to walk into my kitchen to try to cook dinner. I can't open my cabinets. I just get that feeling. It's frightening. So that's why I moved out. We're in the process of moving.
>
> *Dr. Console*: You're actually in the process of moving?
>
> *Patient*: Yes.
>
> *Dr. Console*: With the idea that there won't be any roaches in the new place?
>
> *Patient*: Well, I'm going to a two-family house. It's easier to control if you happen to see a roach there. Our lease isn't up yet on the other place and in fact, we probably would have stayed another year if it hadn't been for the roaches.
>
> *Dr. Console*: Well, you say that in a two-family house it would be easier to control.
>
> *Patient*: Yes. There, if I see a roach, I'll get those bombs, you know. . . .

Dr. Console: What are you laughing about, Dr. Zimmer?

Dr. Zimmer: Well, I'm afraid of her bombs (*group laughter*).

Dr. Console: Television advertises insect killers with big explosions. Raid . . . BOOM! But in this circumstance, you don't have to be influenced by television because Dr. Zimmer's reaction is a valid one. For a one-inch-long insect . . . she's going to *bomb* it. What does this suggest as to how she feels about the magnitude of the threat?

Dr. Zimmer: It has to be met and countered with an enormous amount of power.

Dr. Console: The magnitude of the threat must be of an overwhelming nature, if she needs to control it with bombs. You know, it reminds me of the time shortly after the Japanese surrender when it became known that we had a small stockpile of atomic bombs left over. I remember reading a piece in the *New York Times* about a farmer who had written to the War Department asking for a couple of these bombs . . . as war surplus . . . because he had some tree stumps that he couldn't get out too easily. Could they sell him a few atomic bombs to dislodge those tree-stumps? (*group laughter*).

Dr. Marcus: I think that another indication of the magnitude of her fear is the fact that she had to move a year earlier than expected. That's quite an upheaval and indicates how frightened she must feel.

Dr. Console: Yes, you are denoting one of the fundamental characteristics of the phobia, and that is the environmental manipulation in order to avoid the phobic situation. So, if a person is afraid of an object, he moves away from it. But it won't hold water. It won't hold water because the difficulty is an intrapsychic one that the person takes with him, wherever he goes.

> *Patient*: . . . and bomb my house and my neighbor's apartment. That'll be the end of 'em. In the apartment there's no way . . .
>
> *Dr. Console*: You mean they can come from anywhere?
>
> *Patient*: Oh, any apartment. In a large building you just can't control them.

Dr. Console: So, to go back to what you observed . . . you used the word "scared" or "afraid" . . . afraid of what?

Patient: Well, with my husband I'm afraid that it's going to hurt when he penetrates.

Dr. Console: And this despite the fact that on many occasions you've had this experience and it has not hurt.

Patient: I know, it's really silly. I know.

Dr. Console: Well, silly is one way of describing it. But isn't it more than that? You *know* that it's not so terrible. Maybe the first time it did hurt, but with each subsequent occasion, you seem to have something of the same idea—that the penetration is going to hurt.

Patient: Yes.

Dr. Console: When in fact, you know that there were scores of times that you were penetrated and it didn't hurt.

Patient: Right.

Dr. Console: What am I doing?

Dr. Marcus: You're trying to show the incongruity between her persisting fear and what's really happening. She's had intercourse many times and things worked out all right, yet she still has the fear.

Dr. Console: All right.

Dr. Redley: In a sense, she feels that her fear of cockroaches is irrational but that her fear of penetration is not irrational. So you're pointing out that her fear of penetration is as irrational as is her fear of cockroaches.

Dr. Console: Yes. This is one of the things I'm doing. I want to focus on her own awareness that she knows from experience and yet her experience does not dispel the fear that it's going to hurt. She is quite specific about the persistence, the regularity and the consistency of this response.

Now I want to make another point. On two occasions Dr. Redley has addressed herself to the issues at hand, and have you noticed anything about her language?

Dr. Alper: I don't know if it's worth anything but the fact is that she referred to the bugs as "cockroaches."

Dr. Console: You don't know that it's worth anything? (*group laughter*).

Dr. Alper: Well, many people might tend to refer to them semantically that way.

Dr. Console: OK. Now, *this* woman has been quite specific. It's "roaches, roaches, roaches." Now I have a personal difficulty here because when I was a boy growing up, they were not "roaches." They were "*cock*roaches." Dr. Redley had used the word "cockroach" once before, even though the patient had not. Now, she does it a second time and I'm compelled to point this out to you. Maybe, as Dr. Alper says, it has no significance but we have to question it.

Dr. Rubinstein: But maybe it's worth something (*group laughter*).

Dr. Console: It's worth something, yes. And it becomes worth more in the context of her statement to the effect that, "With my husband, it's a fear of penetration, but with the roaches, I don't know what it is." Now, my feeling is that as a child, the word she would have heard around the house was "cockroach." That is what her parents probably called it.

Dr. Meyer: She was talking about the roaches and you brought her back to the sexual problem. It occurred to me that you were trying to make a connection, to reinforce the parallel that was there.

Dr. Console: I don't think I was doing that. I think she's talking about both areas and I'm staying there with her. I don't think I'm introducing anything to her . . . coming out of left field. True, she says that she knows that the fear with her husband is a fear concerning the pain of penetration, and I asked about the roaches. By the way, notice that I didn't say, "What about the *cock*roaches?" I might have given the whole story away if I had said that. She might have been shocked into an insight for which she was not ready and did not want at the time.

Dr. Cohen: Do you feel the need, to use Dr. Meyer's word, to "reinforce" insight on her part?

Dr. Console: No. I am not concerned with reinforcing insight in an initial interview. My concern is more for the capacity of the person to pick up on or recognize whatever insightful connections emerge. Can she pick up on it and carry it further? This then

becomes a very good sign in terms of the suitability of the patient
for long-term, insight-oriented psychotherapy. This is referred to
as "psychological-mindedness," or the capacity for insight on the
part of the patient. This is not a patient who would come in and
say, "Look, I have headaches and they occur when I eat spinach.
They have nothing to do with how I think or feel." With such a
patient you would feel that the capacity for insight is minimal. In
this woman there is a good deal of evidence that such a capacity is
present and can be developed and enhanced. So I'm not reinforcing
anything. I'm only testing her capacity to take the next step.

Dr. Iglesias: Although I learned that the correct word for this
insect is "cockroach," when I came to this country I found that
many Americans shorten it to "roach."

Dr. Console: In other words, they cut part of it off! (*group laughter*).

Dr. Iglesias: I've noticed that men and women of all ages tend to
shorten it. I rarely hear the word spoken as "cockroach."

Dr. Console: What about in Spanish . . . "*cucaracha*"? In Italian . . .
"*cockarochali*"? In many languages it's a double word. My fantasy is
that as a child the word she would have heard was the longer
version. This is, of course, my conjecture. I make it in light of the
material that has emerged thus far in the interview.

> *Dr. Console:* When in fact, you know that there were scores
> of times that you were penetrated and it didn't hurt.
> *Patient:* Right. It's not total. But when I go for an internal
> examination, it *does* hurt. They use some instruments . . . I'm
> terrified of the instruments.
> *Dr. Console:* Terrified of the instruments . . .
> *Patient:* I am, yes, you know . . .

Dr. Cohen: I wonder if she's referring, indirectly, to the
examination that she's undergoing in the interview. I get the
feeling that she felt a little pushed. A little examined.

Dr. Console: A little penetrated. She might very well.

Dr. Rubinstein: Well, no matter which examination she's referring
to, she said, "I'm *terrified* of it."

Dr. Console: Yes. This is the point that I wanted to make. She said,

"I'm terrified of the instruments." I felt it would be gilding the lily if I said to her, *"Terrified* of the roaches and *terrified* of the instruments." So I just let it pass.

Dr. *McDermott*: A slang term for the penis is "tool," and an instrument, naturally, is a tool. If you really want to stretch things.

Dr. *Console*: You don't have to stretch things at all. All you have to do is read the many papers which have been written on symbolism to see how all this has developed. From the earliest times, anything which was used in agriculture to till the soil, to do something to the soil, an instrument, a tool, a stick . . . anything that was used and placed into Mother Earth, became the symbolic equivalent of the penis. So there are probably more words in the unconscious that are equated with the genitals than with anything else in our language.

> Dr. *Console*: Terrified of the instruments.
>
> *Patient*: I am, yes . . . you know. If he uses his hands inside of me, I'm all right. But if he uses an instrument, I'm finished. One time I fainted three times while being examined. When I was having an IUD inserted. It shouldn't have to hurt so much.

Dr. *Console*: That's what's cute about the English language. . . . *"One* time I fainted *three* times." In having an IUD inserted.

Dr. *McDermott*: I wonder if it could have been the Dalcon-Shield. That has a buglike shape (*group laughter*).

Dr. *Console*: I don't think the shape is important. She knows that an IUD is an "intrauterine device" . . . and she knows that the doctor is going to put something into her uterus through her cervix. In other words, the doctor is going to do what?

Dr. *Rubin*: Penetrate her!

Dr. *Zimmer*: Very deeply.

Dr. *Console*: Very deeply!

Dr. *Zimmer*: Deeper than just the vagina.

Dr. *Console*: Yes. So one time she fainted three times, it was so bad.

Dr. Console: When you say "He uses an instrument"—what do you think of? What instrument?

Patient: Well, they use a spectrum, I think it's called. And— they use long Qtips. Those are the instruments I know they're using.

Dr. Console: Now she defines the instruments that are so terrifying to her. They use a "spectrum," and I don't think that we should make much of the fact that it is called a speculum rather than a spectrum. It's an interesting slip because both connote a looking into. She obviously is referring to a vaginal speculum and a long Qtip. These are the instruments. Do you have any thoughts about that?

Dr. Zimmer: Well, there might be some realistic problem with the speculum because there are women who find it distressing to have one inserted. But really, there is nothing that should be horrible about a Qtip. It shouldn't be physically painful to have one inserted.

Dr. Console: All right. You offer the idea that there might be some reality in the matter of the speculum, which is a metal instrument, but you indicate that this is in marked contrast to a Qtip, which is a sliver of wood with a little cotton on the end. Again, she has made an equation for us. She has put the two objects together. So, what are you suggesting?

Dr. Zimmer: That she finds the idea of anything being inserted into her terrifying.

Dr. Console: OK. You're suggesting that despite the reality, her equating the Qtip with the metal instrument means that it is an *idea* rather than a fact that is so distressing to her. She is dealing with a psychic reality. Her psychic reality states that anything inserted into her is going to hurt—even if it's only a Qtip. She is not aware that to insert a Qtip to take a cervical smear is completely painless since the cervix has few or no nerve endings. Factually, this is not painful. But it is to her.

Patient: Those are the instruments I know they're using. You know.

Dr. Console: You think that a long Qtip . . .

Patient: Yes—a *very* long Qtip. They dilate me and open me up. And it hurts. It seriously hurts. It hurts inside. I don't know, I talked to my doctor and he seems to think that there's nothing wrong in there. I guess it's psychological.

Dr. Console: She asked her doctor, who said that there's nothing wrong in there. It's a Qtip and it's only a touch. He can't possibly be aware of what's going on in this woman's mind.

Patient: I guess it's psychological. But I feel it.

Dr. Console: Now it's not very clear whether she's saying that this is what the doctor told her or not . . . "it's psychological." But in many instances, a doctor will tell this to a patient, and it is rarely done in the service of reassuring the patient. Unfortunately it is often said with something else in mind. Any ideas?
Dr. Vis: That it is not real.
Dr. Console: That it's not real, yes . . .
Dr. McDermott: He's probably saying, "Leave me alone. This is a problem that isn't in my field. I don't want to hear about it."
Dr. Console: All right. How else might we put this?
Dr. Vis: I think it carries the implication that it's psychological and that the patient, by conscious effort, can overcome it.
Dr. Console: Yes, in part. "Since it's psychological you can forget it." What else might he be implying?
Dr. Marcus: It's a criticism of the patient who may think that he's telling her that she's crazy.
Dr. Console: Yes. Unfortunately, when a doctor says to a patient, "You shouldn't be having this experience because what I'm doing is painless and doesn't cause such a reaction—your reaction is a psychological one" . . . the implication is that the patient is some kind of a nut. This is frequently what the patient hears. That she's being told that she's not a member of the human race and that she's crazy.

Patient: I guess it's psychological. But I feel it, you know. I feel that hurt.

Dr. Console: In effect, she is straightening the doctor out. "I guess it's psychological, but I *feel* the hurt." To her, it's *real*. I am again referring to her psychic reality.

> Dr. Console: Did you question whether there's something physically wrong there?
> Patient: Yes, I did ask my doctor. One gynecologist said to me one time that I was small.
> Dr. Console: Who had said this—the doctor?
> Patient: The gynecologist.

Dr. Console: Any thoughts about this?

Dr. Zimmer: She's going back a little bit. She's giving an anatomical reason for this.

Dr. Console: She's giving an anatomical reason that was given to her by a gynecologist. He, of course, had not heard all that this young woman has told us. His saying she is small helps set up a situation in which any kind of intrusion is going to hurt. Why do gynecologists occasionally say this? They examine a young woman who's very likely tense, and she tightens up. He says, "You're small." What is his intention here?

Dr. McDermott: He might be telling her that it's not his fault. That other women don't have the same pain and it's not because he's clumsy.

Dr. Console: Well, I don't think that he thinks of himself as clumsy in performing this maneuver. I don't think he feels he has to defend himself here. It's something else.

Dr. Bond: Certain women might want to hear that they're small. It can be viewed as being more acceptable.

Dr. Console: Very definitely. Can you take it a step further?

Dr. Clarke: It may imply that they are virginal.

Dr. Console: That's probably the reassurance he thinks he's giving by saying, "You're small." It's almost as though he's saying to her, "I can tell that you're a nice girl. You haven't been around much."

Dr. Kent: I've had patients who've asked me while I was doing a pelvic examination, "Am I tight?" I wonder if that could be the same kind of thing.

Dr. Console: Well, let's see. Why were they asking you that?

Dr. Kent: I'm not sure. Most of them were women who had had children and they wanted to know this. I think they wanted to know if they were still sexually attractive.

Dr. Console: Exactly.

Dr. Kent: Is it the same thing as wanting to be virginal?

Dr. Console: It's in the same direction, of not wanting to be sullied ... to be unused. It is not at all uncommon for a gynecologist to joke with his patient about this. He has a middled-aged woman, a multipara who has a great deal of relaxation in the perineum. She may even have a cystocoele or a rectocoele. In suggesting that he do the customary procedure, the repair, he kind of winks and says, "Your husband will be pleased because we'll tighten things up. We'll make you small again." So, being small is a very desirable state here. You will find that a woman who has had several children may complain that the husband is starting to run around with other women because she's so loose and there's no pleasure anymore.

We see this from the other side, in the man who comes in and tells us that he has a great deal of difficulty because his penis is so small. It's difficult to convey to people that we are dealing with a potential space and that there rarely is a vagina so large or a penis so small that they cannot accommodate each other. This must be your fundamental assumption because you are *not* dealing with the *fact* of a penis being too small or a vagina being too large. You are in the psychic realm and not in the physical, anatomical realm at all. You are dealing with a patient's psychic reality ... a fantasy.

Patient: The gynecologist. You know, and other doctors said that I wasn't. So I can't explain it.

Dr. Console: But you still think you might be and when they put a speculum in and dilate you ...

Patient: Yes. They can't do that to me. They can't do it to me. I go crazy.

Dr. Console: "They can't do it ... I go crazy." Despite the fact that she's been reassured by other doctors that she's not too small, she still wants to tell us that she is. In other words, she is telling us that in the anticipation of having the speculum inserted she becomes so upset that she develops "lockjaw". It's like the patient who "can't" open his mouth when he goes to the dentist. She becomes so overwhelmed and so threatened that everything in her tightens up.

Dr. Rubinstein: It illustrates the power of a fantasy. It also demonstrates the capacity of a patient to concretize a well-meaning physician's casual statement.

> *Dr. Console*: You won't *let* them do it.
> *Patient*: I won't let them do it. I try to let them but it's very hard.
> *Dr. Console*: What do you think is the trouble? You've had it all this time. You've had occasion to really think about it. What ideas do you have?

Dr. Console: This is a question that I frequently ask a patient. Now, this woman has been talking for about thirty minutes and has told us a great deal about her feelings. We're talking about her problem with the pain and so on, and she's obviously thought about it. What am I essentially looking for by asking this question?

Dr. Alper: Some insight.

Dr. Console: I think that would be expecting a great deal. That's a real hope—to get some insight.

Dr. Farber: To see some capacity for self-examination.

Dr. Console: Well, I've already imputed that to her and have asked her what she thinks.

Dr. Vis: Maybe you're looking for psychological-mindedness.

Dr. Console: It's difficult to expect her to be able to put all of these things together. It would be very unusual. No, I'm looking for her explanation . . . her *fantasy* about this. How has she explained it to herself?

> *Patient*: I don't know. I'm very confused about it. I'm not . . . you know, I'm not terribly shy or inhibited.

Dr. Console: All right. So what we get is her confusion. But this does not mean for a moment that she does not entertain a fantasy. It simply means that this is an initial interview and that she's not ready to talk about what she really thinks. And now she's introducing a contrast because she's suggesting that she's not prim and prudish concerning sex. In so doing, she is, in a sense, contradicting herself.

> *Patient:* ... as far as sex goes. I'm not terribly shy of it or anything like that ... I don't think.
> *Dr. Console:* Well, you say, "I'm not terribly shy of it," yet with your husband you tighten up and freeze.
> *Patient:* Yeah—but I mean as far as ...
> *Dr. Console:* He's unable to penetrate you ...
> *Patient:* Yes, I know (*laughs*).
> *Dr. Console:* How does this go with, "It's all right, I'm not shy"?
> *Patient:* I don't know. It's just that ... I'm not shy about it. We've talked about it. I don't feel that things are dirty. I don't think that homosexuality is dirty, or things like that. These things *don't* disgust me. I think the whole thing is very normal.
> *Dr. Console:* To talk about it?
> *Patient:* Right. To do it too. Anything I do doesn't bother me. ... It's just the *penetration* that bothers me.

Dr. Console: So she's gotten quite specific. Dr. Farber, your face lit up with some insight just now.

Dr. Farber: The very fact that she mentions homosexuality may mean that it's a difficult area for her to deal with.

Dr. Console: She is indicating that she accepts all these things. She knows that they exist and volunteers that she has no hang-ups about sex or about doing things. Homosexuality is all right ... but when it comes to penetration, that's another story.

Dr. Clarke: Someone mentioned earlier in the interview that she was threatened ... she's not sure about homosexuality. She's confused about it. I think it's breaking through now. Particularly in view of some of the comments a little while ago about her sexual identity.

Dr. Zimmer: Also, earlier in the interview she said that she feels uncomfortable with women her own age.

Dr. Console: Yes, this is the point that Dr. Clarke was referring to.

It was in response to her statement of feeling uncomfortable with women her own age but not with young men. There were some of you who wondered then about the implications this might have in regard to her sexual identity and possible homosexual problems. And now, some of you seem to feel that this is being reinforced by the blandness with which she indicates that no form of sexuality is dirty to her ... and she spontaneously mentions homosexuality. There's a marked contrast between what she describes in words as this liberal, free attitude about love-making and sexuality ... and the difficulty she has with penetration, which is a painful and threatening thing to her.

Dr. McDermott: The problem is in the area of heterosexual intercourse and yet she brings in the irrelevant ... or seemingly irrelevant fact that she has no concerns about homosexuality. It would probably have been more appropriate for her to mention having no worries about oral sex or something like that, but her mention of homosexuality is way off the mark. We have to wonder why.

Dr. Console: Dr. McDermott is reminding us that a patient cannot introduce an irrelevancy. An irrelevancy is a function of our eyes and ears. As your acuity increases, as you understand more and more of how we function as human beings, your patients will introduce fewer and fewer irrelevancies. Every year I describe to the residents some of my own early experiences. When I started in practice, I used to get the lousiest patients in the world. They spoke in irrelevancies and they gave me all kinds of garbage and none of them ever got down to what was really happening. As time went by, my patients became better and better. They were able to talk "dynamics." Now obviously, it was not a matter of the patients changing. It was really I who finally began to hear and understand what they were saying. And that was the reason the patients got "better."

However, there's a much more important point we have to make here, in the matter of "irrelevancies." There can be no irrelevancies if we believe that psychic functioning follows certain orderly, prescribed, understandable pathways. So that nothing a patient says or does is irrelevant, happenstance or accidental. Even a slip of the tongue is relevant if you really understand that there is a psychic determinism in everything we say or do. What a person says at this moment is in some way connected with the past. It is not a foreign body, nor is it an irrelevant word or an idle thought being brought in from nowhere. This is one of the cornerstones of your becoming a psychiatrist. You must develop the inner persuasion . . . and have not only the intellectual but the emotional conviction as well, that human behavior is psychically determined. Nothing is accidental. Nothing is happenstance. Nothing is irrelevant.

> *Dr. Console*: It's the penetration that bothers you.
> *Patient*: Right. And now it's only momentarily, of course.
> *Dr. Console*: The momentary feeling is still something of a reminder of the way it used to be.
> *Patient*: Right—yes.
> *Dr. Console*: Here again, what kind of thinking have you done about it?
> *Patient*: Maybe I had my temperature taken too often when I was little or something. I don't remember (*laughing*).
> *Dr. Console*: But you think it might have something to do with when you were little?
> *Patient*: Well, I imagine it does. Almost everything's supposed to. Not that I remember it. I've questioned my parents . . . "Have I ever fallen?" Or something like that.

Dr. Console: She now indicates that this indeed has been a source of stress to her and that she has been perplexed. In her attempts to find some answers, she's questioned her parents because she assumes correctly that it started way back, that it has something to do with her childhood. She asked them if she ever fell on something and injured herself. So in a simplistic way, despite her perplexity about this, her questions are in the area of something physical having happened.

> *Patient*: My sister Mary had fallen as a kid and hurt herself. Fallen on a long pointy thing, an object, and hurt herself there.

Dr. Console: She never fell but her sister did, and injured herself *there*. Despite her saying that she was never injured, the fact that her sister was injured in this specific way in the genitals had some impact on the patient. The chances are that when this happened to the little sister, the parents did what?

Dr. Zimmer: Rushed her to the doctor.

Dr. Console: Yes, to find out what kind of an injury she had sustained. If a child falls on a pointed object and injures the vulva, why do the parents take her to the doctor? What are they concerned about?

Dr. Zimmer: Her virginity.

Dr. Console: It happens rarely now, but in my experience as an intern working in an emergency room, occasionally somebody came in with this kind of an accident. Invariably, the mother wanted a certificate . . . a doctor's statement on official stationery, saying that the defloration had occurred accidentally. This is pretty much old-country, European parentage. It's not so common in America now.

So, what were the implications of this to the older girl? She observed the parents' concern and the likelihood is that the sister was rushed to a doctor to insure that nothing terrible had happened. This would have had an enormous impact upon the patient. So, although she denotes that she did not have this experience personally, she had it vicariously . . . just one removed . . . her younger sister. Right there in the family.

Dr. Alper: I just wanted to mention something that I didn't notice earlier in the tape but that I see now. That's the extent to which this woman has her vagina protected as you're talking to her. She has a bag on her lap and her coat wrapped around her. She seems to be continuously guarding against penetration.

Dr. Console: You will observe time and time again, when you have your sumptuous private office, that there will be plenty of room for hanging a coat and you'll have a table or something for putting books and bags and papers on. Despite your having spent money for this elegent table, there will be some women, and some men too, who will come in and insist on keeping these things on their laps. They will insist upon putting up a barrier, thus making penetration difficult if not impossible. You'll have to go through Gray's Anatomy to get in there (*group laughter*). This is an interesting, important and common piece of behavior that Dr. Alper has observed. Now, if a woman comes into your office and does this, what are some of the assumptions you're going to make?

Dr. Alper: It might reflect some anxiety about revealing herself to you. I don't think it necessarily has to be sexually specific.

Dr. Console: Why is it not sexually specific? She's not holding these things on her head (*group laughter*). Isn't it likely that the story you're going to get from a woman sitting in this way, has something to do with frigidity? Has something to do with difficulties with her husband or boyfriend?

> *Patient*: Fallen on a long pointy thing, an object, and hurt herself there.
>
> *Dr. Console*: But you had no such experience?
>
> *Patient*: I didn't myself. I was there when it happened though.
>
> *Dr. Console*: How old were you at the time?
>
> *Patient*: I'm not sure. It's hard to remember.

Dr. Console: I asked her how old she was at the time. Keep this in mind. When a patient reports an incident in childhood, try to establish when it happened. Obviously there's an enormous difference in the impact upon a child whether an incident occurred when she was four years old or when she was eight years old. Often, the patient tends to lump it all together. You're going to see that we are concerned with the development of the ego and the ego state of the person at one age and another. The young child does not have the ego resources to explain strange events, and our concern will be in terms of the potential impact of a given event upon the patient. We can make a more meaningful conjecture about such impact if we know the age of the patient at the time of the incident.

> *Dr. Console*: It probably frightened you to see this happen.
>
> *Patient*: I'm sure it did.

Dr. Console: Did she cry?

Patient: Oh yeah, it was a big thing. I don't remember clearly but it was a big thing.

Dr. Console: So in your own way you've investigated this. You've asked your parents about what happened years ago in trying to account for it.

Patient: Oh yes.

Dr. Kent: This may be spurious. In thinking about kids falling down, I think of them landing on their hands, elbows and knees. It's hard to fall in such a way that the vulva lands on a pointed object. It makes me think that the sister either sat down on one or was thrown on one. I wonder if the patient could have done that to her sister?

Dr. Console: You can wonder about that but I don't think there would be any profit at this point introducing such a conjecture to the patient. It would place her in a defensive posture and probably impair your ability to get the information. Don't forget that when you treat a patient, you're going to have a great deal of time to work together. When you have established a therapeutic alliance . . . when you have what some psychiatrists refer to as *rapport* with the patient . . . then you can go back to some of these things and ask the question. Usually you don't have to go back yourself. The patient will bring up the incident in a different context, at which time you may remember your conjecture and inquire a bit more as to how this came about. But at this point, I think it would be unwise and would impair your ability to get a rounded story. We don't have to know every single detail. This is an initial interview and we're trying to get a global view without pinning down all the specifics.

Dr. Console: In so doing, do your parents know why you are asking these questions? Do they know about the penetration difficulty?

Patient: Oh no, they don't know about that.

Dr. Console: Just some difficulties?

Patient: Well, they know that I have a problem when I get examined. My mother knows about it anyway.

Dr. Console: What about examinations from other doctors and dentists? Does that bother you?

Patient: No . . .

Dr. Console: Another doctor examining you? Listening to your lungs?

Patient: I like it. I feel good when I get an examination and everything's all right.

Dr. Console: So it's this specific sort of an examination that is so upsetting?

Patient: Yes.

Dr. Console: What about your social life now—friends?

Patient: I don't really have any close friends. I never did, you know. Friends have always been around but not that close. In fact, I've had one friend that I was close with, but I don't feel that close that I can ask her anything or discuss certain things with her. And I don't like to discuss things with my mother because she ends up criticizing me.

Dr. Console: So there are things that you would like to discuss with a friend and not with your mother, but you don't have that close a friend?

Patient: Yes.

Dr. Console: And your husband. Does he have friends?

Patient: Yes. He has friends. He has one close friend, Bill. He comes over all the time. You know, he's a good friend. I'm pretty close to him too. You know, as far as I can be.

Dr. Console: You say he comes over alone?

Patient: Yes. He's unmarried. He's a bachelor.

Dr. Console: What am I wondering about? In pursuing the friend's coming over alone?

Dr. Kent: Are you wondering if she, in fantasy or in reality, is having an affair with Bill? I'm wondering that.

Dr. Console: Any other ideas?

Dr. Kent: We've raised the question of homosexuality as it applies to her and perhaps you may have some questions about her husband's difficulties in this same area.

Dr. Console: Yes, this is the area to which I'm alerted. A bachelor friend whom he's known for a long time and who comes over often. You want to check into this gently. Perhaps we'll get

enough of the quality of the relationship so that we don't have to
ask a whole flock of questions.

> *Dr. Console:* Someone your husband has known for a
> relatively long time?
> *Patient:* Oh yes, since he was about sixteen. No, he knew
> him even before that—since grammar school. So, I'm friends
> with him too, of course, for my husband's sake. I can't tell him
> all our business either.
> *Dr. Console:* Well, how do things go between you and your
> husband?
> *Patient:* Pretty well, in general. Except for lately. Because I
> was thinking he was unfaithful and things like that (*laughs*).
> *Dr. Console:* What was making you think this?
> *Patient:* Well, he goes to school . . . two nights a week, and
> he'd come home rather late—twelve o'clock. He gets out
> about eleven and goes for a few drinks with his friend, you
> know, which is fine.

Dr. Console: Whenever you hear, "He comes home late . . . twelve
o'clock, which is fine" . . . translate it into "not fine at all." This is
disturbing to her. So, he's a good friend who apparently is over a
good deal of the time and she reintroduces the thought, at this
point, that perhaps her husband has been unfaithful. As Dr. Kent
mentioned before, there may be something going on in her. What
might this be?
Residents: A projection.
Dr. Console: A projection. She could very well entertain some
fantasies about Bill herself.

> *Patient:* But lately I began feeling that maybe it was not his
> friend. I don't know. He does lie to me at times. I've caught
> him in a few lies.
> *Dr. Console:* What kind of things?
> *Patient:* Mm . . . once he didn't go to class. I found out. I was
> looking in his book to get the name of something and I saw
> that he'd marked down that he didn't go to class one night,
> and he came home late. That was ten o'clock at night. I asked

him about it and he said he was just walking around. That he had to be alone. It's too small an apartment and that he couldn't be alone with me and the baby there. And then, once again that happened. He said that he went to a meeting, but by this time, I knew that he didn't because I can usually pick out when he's not telling the truth. So I went to the meeting myself and I saw that he wasn't there, and he came home and I said, "Did you go to the meeting?" hoping that he'd say, "No I didn't," and he said, "Yes." I pointed out to him that I was there and he wasn't. And then I found something written in his book. Something that said, "Meet Linda at Peter's at eleven P.M." I asked him about it and he told me that a friend of his had written it in as a joke. That just didn't sound reasonable to me. It didn't sound like the guy who was supposed to have written it. He's a very serious guy. Maybe it's possible. I've never really gotten it very clear.

Dr. Console: What might she be doing here? She goes through all these improbable explanations of her husband's behavior and says that it's possible they are true.
Dr. Alper: I think there's an element of denial here.
Dr. Console: Yes, there's a considerable element of denial. A considerable element of giving him the benefit of her doubts, in the service of hoping that she won't have any doubts. She is trying to avoid a conflict and to find peace for herself by accepting a bunch of improbable explanations here. She has grave doubts about her husband's fidelity but the doubts threaten her existence and her relationship. This is a woman who doesn't think very much of herself and is willing to tolerate a great deal rather than demand her rightful due.

Patient: There was a place he had gone to a few weeks before called "Little Peter's." It's a place, you know, with girls dancing. Only a few clothes on (*laughs*) and I guess it was Peter's that was referred to in the book. But sometimes I wonder if maybe it's all in my mind. He says that he's afraid that I'll criticize him, which I rarely do. He does lack a sense of responsibility. He's irresponsible at times. Not anything bad

... he holds his job. He's a good man but he's a little irresponsible at times.

Dr. Console: But ever since you've known him he's been employed?

Patient: Oh yes. Oh yes. Sometimes he takes a day off from work when I feel he could have really gone in.

Dr. Console: With what excuse?

Patient: Well, he didn't feel just right.

Dr. Console: I see.

Patient: So he would take the day off. All the while he probably could have gone in. It's things like that. As far as paying bills goes, I could never have him paying bills, because they would never be paid. You know, he just forgets about them. That's the way he is. A little irresponsible. But I don't criticize him. I pay the bills myself, so I've never criticized him. He just lies to me. Like when he went hunting the first year I met him. He didn't tell me about it until the last minute. Because his exwife used to throw things at him and tell him, "I hope you get shot" ... (*laughs*). Things like that. I already knew about it. It didn't bother me. Fine, all right. He says, "I'm going here, I'm going there." I don't make a big deal over it.

Dr. Console: Well, how many things does he do that don't include you?

Patient: Hunting ... very rarely. He doesn't even do that any more. You'd almost think that it was the challenge that made him go. He doesn't really do that anymore.

Dr. Console: What does she mean when she says that she thinks it was the challlenge that made him go? What do you think she might be referring to here?

Dr. Zimmer: It was sort of a confrontation. He had the power to be able to say, "I'm going whether you like it or not." Her feeling seems to be that since he doesn't go anymore, he went that time just to win the confrontation.

Dr. Console: What might this have been in the service of?

Dr. Zimmer: Asserting his dominance, his masculinity.

Dr. Console: Yes, it sounds very much as though he had to assume this masculine posture.

Patient: He has his friends from work. He doesn't hang around with them too much. Very rarely, once in a while, he goes along with them for a drink. School of course, I can't share with him, but I can now, because I just signed up. So I'm somewhat included in that now. He signed up for a gymnasium, which I was ready to kill him for because we barely see each other as it is. And to sign up for a gymnasium ... I don't know, but there's very little ...

Dr. Console: Is this a private gymnasium?

Patient: Yes ... I was very annoyed about it. At that point I had no real plans for school. I wanted to but I felt that I couldn't, for his sake. So I would write papers and do research for him, stuff like that. If I was doing that sort of thing for myself, I could hardly help him at all. But when he joined the gym, that was it.

Dr. Console: What reason did he give? Why did he want to join the gymnasium?

Patient: He's conscious about his body. All his friends are too. They've all started lifting weights again. They've all decided to lift weights and build up their bodies (*laughs*).

Dr. Console: What is she describing? Lifting weights and improving their bodies.

Dr. McDermott: Her laughing indicates to me that she thinks all this is a bit childish and smacks of masculine competitiveness.

Dr. Console: Yes, I think that she detects the boyish, juvenile quality to this ... the preoccupation with physique. Why is somebody preoccupied with physique? If a man is completely satisfied with his physique, would he be preoccupied with it? Of course not. I would say to you: beware the weight lifter. It's very likely that he has a great many doubts about his masculinity.

Patient: They were all doing it for years and so he decided he was going to join the gym. He's sorry he did it now. He realizes he doesn't have the time to use it. At that time he was excited about it and he joined. I think that it was just plain selfish because I wasn't getting out of the house to do anything that I wanted to do. One night he could watch the

baby and let me get out. Or we could do something together.
It seemed kind of selfish. So that's why I signed up for school.

Dr. Console: On the same nights that he's going?

Patient: Right. I just decided that I was going to do
something for myself . . . something that I wanted to do.

Dr. Console: Look, in light of the fact that you saw this
hypnotist four times, what are your thoughts about
treatment? You do know that it's more than four times?

Patient: What do you mean?

Dr. Console: That you have to come here for a while.

Patient: Yes.

Dr. Console: You have a friend who comes here?

Patient: Yes.

Dr. Console: So that you know that she comes regularly. . . .

Patient: Yes, she's been coming for quite awhile.

Dr. Console: Is that what you expect?

Patient: I hope not. But I guess it's possible.

Dr. Console: You mean that if it was necessary, you would
come for that long.

Patient: I imagine so. I couldn't be sure of what would
happen. But if things were the same as they are now, I would.

Dr. Console: Are there any questions that you want to ask
me about this?

Patient: Well, I've been wondering. In psychological terms,
I've been trying to find out . . .

Dr. Console: What is she asking?

Dr. Iglesias: "Am I crazy?"

Dr. Console: That's the fundamental question, "Am I crazy?"

Patient: . . . in psychological terms, I've been trying to find
out . . .

Dr. Console: What does that mean . . . "in psychological
terms"?

Patient: Am I neurotic, schizophrenic, paranoid? . . .

Dr. Console: What do these words mean to you?

Patient: I know "schizophrenic" is serious. I know "neurotic"
is normal (*group laughter from all the residents*). There are a lot of

people who are neurotic and it's quite curable, I imagine. And paranoid . . . I don't know if I'm paranoid.

Dr. Console: Why paranoid? What does paranoid mean to you?

Patient: Well, you know . . . thinking that people are running around behind my back and not trusting people, you know . . . I'd like to find out.

Dr. Console: Well, I think I can tell you that this is neurotic. I don't think for a moment that you're schizophrenic or anything like that.

Patient: (*smiling*) That's good.

Dr. Console: This is very definitely treatable and I think that you should come and get it straightened out. Now how does your husband feel about this?

Patient: He thinks it's fine. He went for help a while ago.

Dr. Console: When was that? What for?

Patient: I think he went originally because he wanted to get an annulment and that was required. He kept it up for a while. They said he had a "swing personality." He'd swing from his mother's personality to his father's personality. His mother was a wild one. And his father was a nice, gentle man. I sometimes wonder when he's going to swing (*laughs*).

Dr. Console: Have you ever observed anything like that?

Patient: Not in particular. There are times when he's very aggressive and he wants to get things done. There are other times when he's much quieter, you know, and he'll do things that I ask him . . . like go to the store without grumbling. I can see a little bit of a difference but that seems normal to me.

Dr. Console: All right. Dr. Roberts will get in touch with you and set up your appointments.

Patient: Thank you (*The Interview Ends*).

Dr. Console: Now I have absolutely no doubts as to this woman's sanity. There's no indication that she's in any way psychotic. So that when she asked this very fundamental question, namely, "Am I crazy?" I answered it and it was apparent that she was relieved to hear my answer.

This patient was seen in twice weekly treatment for a year afterwards, so we have some follow-up. There are two major points that I would like to make in this connection, to help you see that some of the conjectures we've made on the basis of the initial interview were borne out by subsequent material. This gives us a greater insight into the nature, structure and genetics of this woman's terrible fear of roaches.

She was in treatment for about three months when she reported to the resident treating her that she had seen an old girlfriend whom she had not seen in many years. In the course of their discussion, something occurred which led her to alter some of the things she had told the doctor treating her. This had to do with the fact that she had repeatedly told him that she had no memory of any experience in her early life which related to sexual matters. Her position in therapy had been that until age thirteen or fourteen she was ingenuous and knew nothing of sex. She now described that she had been talking with this friend and indicated to her that one of the new things in her life was the fact that she was in psychiatric treatment. Her friend showed a great deal of interest and asked her how it was going. The patient reiterated her sexual innocence during her early life, saying that she had known nothing. Her friend countered, "What do you mean 'nothing'? Don't you remember Evelyn?" It turned out that Evelyn was an older girl who had informed the patient and her friends about some of the facts of life. In so doing, she had been quite specific in describing how babies were born.

The patient had been informed that babies were born through a process whereby a man puts his penis inside a woman and injects *things* into her. And these things go through *seven layers* to reach a certain place . . . the ovum. And that's how a baby is made. So, this relates to which fear that this patient had?

Residents: Fear of penetration.

Dr. Console: The fear of penetration. So that in a simplistic way, if a child gets the idea that some "things" are injected internally and have to burrow through "seven layers," this does not sound like a great pleasure. This can in fact be enormously threatening.

The other important piece of information came some months later when she was talking to her therapist a little more freely about sexual relations with her husband. With considerable hesitancy and an enormous amount of affect, she related that every time her husband approached her sexually and was about to insert his penis, she momentarily, on each occasion, had a thought. Since he had been married before, perhaps there was still, on his penis, some of the fluid or secretion from the first wife, and this would be injected into her. What has she told us with that fantasy?

Dr. Meyer: I think that she's once again telling us that she thinks very much about the other woman in her husband's life and is very much afraid of contact with another woman. This is tantamount to her saying that she's afraid of homosexual contact.

Dr. Console: So, you will recall that when she wanted to establish that the fear of penetration was incomprehensible to her because she's read these books, and she's very liberal, and homosexuality doesn't bother her and so on, we suggested then that her spontaneously listing as the first idea, her acceptance of homosexuality, was meaningful. I think that Dr. Meyer's statement is quite accurate—that she was in conflict about her desire for the homosexual contact with the other woman ... in this case, her husband's first wife.

Dr. Meyer: Well, the first point that you raised ... about the fear of penetration perhaps stemming from the incident with the girlfriend that she had long since forgotten, doesn't jibe with the second problem, which is a fear of penetration as an expression of a homosexual wish and fear.

Dr. Console: Can't a person dislike apples and oranges?

Dr. Meyer: Well, it makes you think that there's another part to the story. Manifestly, at least at this point, she's afraid of homosexual contact, but there must be something else in addition because her girlfriend didn't forget the story about how babies are made. So, something must have preceded that story in the patient's life, to make her so vulnerable to it that she would *have* to forget it. I'm wondering if there is any data about what happened prior to that incident.

Dr. Console: First of all, you're probably right. This didn't happen in a vacuum. There were undoubtedly antecedents. I regret to say that some of what I wanted most from the treatment of this case was the early data, and this material was for the most part not

obtained by the therapist. Now this again is one of the purposes of
our going through these tapes in this elaborate and microscopic
fashion ... to alert you to the need to get the early and
fundamental material. As we sit here and think about it, it's easy to
say, "Why the hell didn't the therapist get the material?" Well,
you're going to find that it's just grand to sit here in this group and
speculate ... and we may be perfectly right in our conjectures. But
when you are confronted face-to-face with the patient, when no
one else is there and it's all yours, some of your own defenses come
into play. Some of your countertransference feelings enter into
the picture. One of the common ones is the need to hold onto the
patient. You may develop such a feeling when a patient threatens
to leave or indicates a wish to end treatment. You may want to
hold onto the patient. You will be concerned with your
supervisor's response if you "lose" the patient and you will fear
that it was a consequence of an error that you made. Hence, there
is a tendency to lean over backwards and to be "nice." That's the
biggest mistake that you can make, because usually, being "nice"
means avoiding sensitive material. Just remember, in therapy the
golden rule does not hold true. For every good deed which you do,
you will be punished! (group laughter). You may find, for example,
that if your patient starts to cry, your tendency is to let up and feel
that this is so upsetting to him or her that you should abandon that
line of inquiry. And that is invariably a great mistake. In the course
of this year I hope we will have an opportunity to discuss many of
the very difficult situations that will inevitably arise in your
psychotherapeutic work with patients.

   Dr. Cohen: What became of the patient's phobic complaint and
how much of the lesbian tendency was explored?

   Dr. Console: This is unconscious homosexuality, not lesbianism.
That is a very important distinction to keep in mind in our work
with patients. This issue was not explored in nearly the depth it
should have been. This is one of the major areas that beginners
tend to stay away from. I think your having put it as you did ...
"lesbian tendency," suggests the very problem I'm talking about,
and points out the understandable tendency of residents to skirt
this issue. The whole issue of homosexuality is often avoided,
particularly with a male therapist and a male patient, or a female
therapist and a female patient. The entire area becomes too

dangerous and threatening, sometimes even more so for the therapist than for the patient.

As for the phobic complaint . . . it dropped out as a prominent factor because so many other life concerns came up in the treatment. We never really established if the phobia dropped out as a consequence of her having developed some insight or if it did so because of the transference. In other words, because she was in a safe relationship with a man who was good to her, who listened to her and never chided her and who was neither judgmental nor critical of her. At the end of one year the therapist completed the residency and the patient discontinued treatment, at that point much improved.

Dr. Meyer: I know that you said that we could speculate forever and it wouldn't mean very much, but would you care to predict the results if some of these issues had been explored more fully in treatment?

Dr. Console: I think the result would have been very good in that I think she would have been able to deal with the early fantasies of this penetrative invasion of herself . . . of going through the seven layers. Also, her concern about another woman would have been related, as it invariably is, to the original mother-child relationship. You try to help the patient to see that homosexual conflicts, namely ideas or fears about homosexuality, have the most innocent origins in the world . . . for a girl it's the desire to love and to be loved by her mother, and for a boy it's a desire to love and to be loved by his father. Both are perfectly normal.

The prognosis in this case for insight therapy was very, very good. I tried to indicate that by pointing out to you the places in the initial interview where she came up with some insight, by showing how she was able to follow something and make various connections. In an uncritical way, I must say that if she had been in treatment with a more experienced therapist, the result might have been even more dramatic. But at this point in your careers, you're still learning and you will make many mistakes. If you didn't make them, there would be no point to my being here now. In fact, one of the most exciting aspects of our work as psychiatrists is that we never stop learning from our patients and from our reactions to our patients. At least I *hope* we never stop learning.

CHAPTER FOUR

The Polysurgery Woman

Dr. Console: Today we're going to see a new patient. This is a different kind of patient—different, because she is a woman who was hospitalized on a medical ward and not on the psychiatric service. She was seen by a third-year psychiatric resident, who at the time was doing work on the Medical-Psychiatric Liaison Service. This is the group that deals with psychosomatic problems. The resident was impressed with the many admissions this woman had had to the hospital, and felt that there were sufficient psychological factors in her having been here so many times to make him ask if I would see her. So remember, this is not a patient who comes for psychiatric help. She is on the medical service and in a way, it's almost an intrusion on my part to interview her because she didn't ask for it.

(The video tape machine is turned on. Dr. Console and the patient are seen, sitting in their respective chairs. The patient is a black woman who appears to be in her late thirties or early forties. She is dressed in hospital clothing, with a bathrobe and slippers.)

Dr. Console: Will you tell me what the trouble was that brought you to the hospital?
Patient: Well, I had a lot of difficulty, you know, doing anything at home. Like I was weak all the time and tired, and I

was having a lot of trouble breathing—you know—when I'd
run up and down the stairs or when I'd walk half a block. Or
something like that . . . and I couldn't do my work at home.
    Dr. Console: How long has that been going on?
    Patient: What?
    Dr. Console: When did you first notice it?
    Patient: Uh . . . I had been . . . *(coughs)* . . . excuse me . . . feeling
bad off and on . . . um—well, through the years, you know,
during the summer time it got so I . . . like I'd be sitting outside
and suddenly I would fall asleep. You know, just sitting there.
It was embarrassing to me 'cause, you know . . .

    Dr. Console: So in response to the question "Why did you come to
the hospital?" we have this vague, ill-defined description of
symptoms. She felt weak and couldn't get her work done. Do you
have any thoughts about that? Is this any different from your
experience in physical diagnosis where you were assigned a
patient and you asked why he was in the hospital and he said that
he wasn't feeling right? It's unusual for a patient to be able to
quickly and succinctly tell you, "I came into the hospital because I
had a sudden pain in the chest and so on . . ." So, this is not at all
uncharacteristic. Neither is it uncharacteristic in light of the fact
that this is a very novel situation for this woman. She's a patient in
the hospital and the resident has spoken to her. He has explained
to her that one of the senior doctors wants to examine her . . .
interview her . . . and it's going to be done in front of a camera. So
she can understandably be a little uneasy about this. However, in
response to the second question, "How long has this been going
on?" she is not specific either. She refers to some recent events in
which she would be sitting and talking to people and then she
would fall asleep and this is embarrassing. Now, what do you think
of here? What might she be telling us? What might her fantasy be?
Is it embarrassing if you're talking to people and you fall asleep? Of
course. Is this what she's telling us?
    Dr. Kent: Is she afraid that she's going to die?
    Dr. Console: Well, falling asleep might be equated with dying.
    Dr. Kent: It certainly separates her from everyone else.
    Dr. Console: Yes . . . there's the quality that it separates her from
others. Or she feels separated from others.

Dr. Meyer: We know that boredom can be a defense against feelings. If we can get some specific information about when she's falling asleep, we can then speculate further about what feelings she may be defending against.

Dr. Console: All right, then let's see what additional information she gives us.

> *Patient:* . . . everybody else would be talking or walking around . . . like I didn't seem to have any control over staying awake . . . I couldn't hold anything in my stomach . . .
> *Dr. Console:* You say it was embarrassing to you?

Dr. Console: She's given a little elaboration. She's falling asleep. She couldn't stay awake and couldn't hold anything in her stomach. She's becoming, in a way, both more specific and more diffuse. And now she's bringing in a different symptom. What has falling asleep got to do with not being able to hold food in your stomach? Why then do I intervene at this point and say, "You say it was embarrassing?"

Dr. Kent: You're bringing her back to the first complaint and trying to find out more about that.

Dr. Console: Trying to find out more about what?

Dr. Kent: The falling asleep and what's embarrassing about it.

Dr. Console: In a way. Let's say this is a very bright and alert patient. When I ask the question as I have asked it, after she has given these physical symptoms, and I say, "You say it's embarrassing?" what would the alert patient immediately establish?

Dr. Alper: That you're challenging the fact that she really was embarrassed. That you question her embarrassment.

Dr. Meyer: That there's an affective basis for her physical complaints. That you're really interested in looking for the feeling content.

Dr. Console: Let's put it another way . . . you're right . . . but a little differently.

Dr. Cohen: You mentioned the difference between this interview and the diagnostic interview in a medical setting, and this begins to show that difference.

Dr. Console: I think a very alert woman would have said to herself, "Jesus . . . this guy's a psychiatrist. This is not the kind of interview or the kind of question I've been asked by other doctors."

Dr. Rubinstein: You're not going to sit there with her and go through a review of systems . . . head, eyes, ears, nose, throat and so on.

Dr. Console: I'm going to focus on the affective quality here. The embarrassment.

Dr. Meyer: In a sense, you're just picking up on her voluntary information. She offers the fact that she felt embarrassed without having to be asked about it.

Dr. Console: Yes . . . except that she started to move away from it, by saying that she couldn't hold anything in her stomach and so on. As Dr. Rubinstein suggests, she might voluntarily go into a review of systems, that her feet hurt and she gets dizzy, this, that, and the other thing . . . and I want to focus the interview. And so I ask her about her *embarrassment*.

Dr. Iglesias: About her embarrassment. Something occurred to me. Why is this so embarrassing to her? At her age, she might fear that people would think that she drinks. If she was younger, she might fear that other people would think that she uses drugs.

Dr. Console: You say if she were younger, she might be imputing to others some suspicion that she uses drugs. Well, how old do you think she is?

Dr. Iglesias: Late thirties.

Dr. Console: Maybe they think that she kind of nips on the side. OK, that's what I'm looking for. That's why I asked about the embarrassment.

> *Patient*: To me because everybody—you know—if you'd be in a crowd or you'd be sitting down somewhere, people looking at you . . . I mean, I don't know . . . I could imagine any kind of thoughts could be going through their heads because people are sitting, nodding . . .

Dr. Console: "I could imagine any kind of thoughts going through their heads." Whose head are the thoughts going through?

Residents: Her head
Dr. Console: Her head.

   Patient: . . . sitting, nodding all the time. Right away you think, you know . . . maybe something was wrong with them. I think maybe I would look twice too.
   Dr. Console: What would you think if someone was sitting and talking and suddenly they fell asleep?
   Patient: Maybe it would mean . . . well, they didn't say it, because everybody knows that I've been sick for a long time. I mean everybody who knows me. So nobody ever said anything. . . .
   Dr. Console: You said you wondered what they would think and if you saw someone, you would think something. What would you think?
   Patient: Well, maybe another time I wouldn't . . . but now with everybody on narcotics and all . . . if you see somebody sitting and drooping all the time, the first thing that comes to your mind—you know . . .
   Dr. Console: Taking dope?
   Patient: Yeah. But a lot of people suffer from different kinds of illnesses where they could be just plain tired.
   Dr. Console: Well, until this thing happened, had you been in good health? How old are you?
   Patient: Forty.
   Dr. Console: Forty. And have you been sick much in your life?
   Patient: Ever since right before graduation . . . I had an emergency appendix operation. . . .

Dr. Console: Now we're getting to the story. Obviously I know that she's been sick a good deal of her life because I was told that she's had a whole flock of admissions to the hospital. She says, "Right before graduation I had an emergency appendix operation." Now, we want to know which graduation she's talking about, don't we? In other words, we want to know if she was thirteen or fourteen years old, or if she was seventeen or eighteen years old. Why would we want to know that?

Dr. Alper: One thought that I have is that if it was the time of graduation from high school, it might have been at a time when she had to become independent. It might have represented a marked change in her social situation. Perhaps going away to college or to work or something like that.

Dr. Meyer: Going along with that line of thinking ... if it occurred earlier, at the time of grade-school graduation, and puberty, it might have been connected with some sexual problems.

Dr. Console: All right. So at least we know that she now has volunteered a beginning, so far as she is concerned, of her illness. She said she's forty and it goes back to graduation, which means that she's talking about twenty or more years of illness.

> *Patient*: And before that I had had a series of, you know—strep throat ... swollen glands. And um—the doctors told my mother that if I had my tonsils and adenoids removed, more than likely I wouldn't have this problem after that. It seemed like ... because I was pretty—you know—like I wouldn't say fat—but—you know—I've always been pretty strong as far as I can remember—you know. Um ... it just seemed like after the appendix operation I just kept continuously, you know, if it wasn't one thing it was something else ... pneumonia several times. ...

Dr. Console: So now she's quite specific. She'd always been pretty strong, although she had these strep throats, and the doctor told her mother that if she had her tonsils and adenoids removed that would take care of it. Nonetheless, she indicates that ever since the appendix operation, it's been one thing after another.

Dr. Kent: Would you care to comment at all on her style of speaking? It seems that there are a lot of "likes" and "you knows." She starts somewhere and comes around full circle and finishes somewhere else. She generally makes sense but I get a frustrated feeling listening to her.

Dr. Console: Yes, I will comment on that. You're going to see many patients with whom you are going to have this feeling of frustration. And among the many things from which I must dissuade you, is the notion that all you have to do is sit down with a patient and say, "OK now, tell me your story"... and he or she just relates it in a well-ordered way. It is rare that people can do this. You must examine yourself and examine your own frustration, and you must come around to the idea that while the books say, "symptoms, onset, etiology and so on"... that's only in the book ... that's not in people. People are going to tell their stories *their* ways. And they're going to tell their stories in the most prejudicial fashion, in the fashion that will put them in the best light possible. So ... patience, patience, patience. And careful listening to everything the patient says. Because there is no such thing as the patient uttering some words which do not have meaning. The amount of meaning that they have will be a function of how much you can see and hear in what they are saying. There's absolutely nothing frustrating about this interview. This is a woman who I know is not going to be able to give me a text-book description. She's going to tell her story in her own way, as she feels it. She is quite defensive. She is quite protective. She said, "Other people might think this or that ... but they don't think badly about me because they know I've been sick for a long time." And yet, she was the one who brought this up. So she's very worried about whether or not other people might think that she's taking dope.

Dr. Meyer: One more point about this. I just get a feeling that we're going to have to sit through an endless story of one hospitalization after another ... she'll just go on and on ... and I thought of her vomiting. Perhaps the function of the vomiting... maybe here in the interview she may vomit a lot of verbiage at you, verbiage that she will repeat over and over again. Maybe this merely illustrates my frustration but that was my fantasy.

Dr. Console: It's only four minutes of the interview.

Dr. Meyer: Yes ... but that's my initial reaction.

Dr. Console: This is four minutes of the interview. She didn't ask for this interview. It was, in a way, thrust upon her by the resident. So ... sit back. If she starts giving you a grocery list of all her operations ... then let's at least get her to give them in a chronological order. Let's find out how old she was when a certain operation took place and what else was going on in her life at that time. Your psychological orientation is going to protect you from getting an interminable story, because you're going to interrupt her and get her to focus on her relationships with people and on her feelings about those relationships.

> *Patient*: ... you know—several operations, things like that.
> *Dr. Console*: You say it was just before graduation. How old were you?
> *Patient*: High school
> *Dr. Console*: High-school graduation ...

Dr. Console: So she denotes the onset as just before graduation from high school, when she was about seventeen. She had an appendix operation then, and after that, "If it wasn't one thing it was something else". Then followed a whole series of operations. Doctors, what do you think?

Dr. Zimmer: Well, she described herself as a very robust ... almost a muscular girl. Then she describes an operation where something is cut out and she suddenly becomes weak and debilitated. My feeling is that there is some sort of fantasy about being castrated.

Dr. Console: Well, I don't know that it is still the custom as it was years ago, when appendix operations were much more frequent, that after removal of the appendix it was placed in a little bottle and shown to the patient. So the patient could see this little structure that had been removed. Now, at the time of this interview this woman was forty years old and the appendectomy occurred about twenty-five years earlier. I'm quite sure that back then she had the experience I'm describing. I know in those days this was Standard Operating Procedure. ... Oh dear! (*group laughter*).

Dr. Meyer: But isn't it true that many appendectomies were performed when there really was no appendicitis? Since the operation occurred in relation to graduating high school, I think we have to wonder if there was any organic pathology at all.

Dr. Console: Your question about appendectomies being done unnecessarily—were you taught that?

Dr. Meyer: That's my impression.

Dr. Console: I think that your impression is correct.

Dr. Rubinstein: I recall being taught as a medical student that if a surgeon is not overoperating by about ten percent on appendicitis, then he's missing some. He should be overoperating on these people.

Dr. Console: Let me say that thirty to thirty-five years ago, they were ripping out appendices at the drop of a hat, for the flimsiest reasons in the world. It is only with the recent establishment of tissue-review committees and so on, that what we used to call "lily-white appendices" are no longer being removed. The treatment is much more conservative now. You go in only when you have the classical signs of appendicitis. So today there are many people walking around with scars in their right lower quadrants that are completely unnecessary. Now, since I am very keenly aware of this fact, I'm going to try, without putting words in the patient's mouth, to establish what this person experienced at that time, because I want to make my own diagnosis about this appendix operation.

Dr. Cohen: I'd like to offer my association. I know it's not her association. . . .

Dr. Console: You can't give hers, you have to give your own (*group laughter*).

Dr. Cohen: . . . since the previous woman . . . the roach lady . . . with *cockroach*, I've been listening to these words a little more carefully. Words such as appen*dix* . . . dix . . . it struck me in the same sort of fashion of being slang for the genitalia.

Dr. Console: Well, I don't know that we have to go that far. I think of Dr. Zimmer's original remarks here, the matter of being put to sleep and then being invaded in this fashion, and something being removed. We don't have to go beyond the notion that the person will have some feeling or idea about the fact that something internal is taken out and is no longer there.

Dr. Rubin: She also mentioned that her tonsils and adenoids were removed. It goes along with the idea of castration . . . or of something else being removed.

Dr. Console: I'm not clear if she actually had them taken out. The doctor told the mother that she wouldn't have colds if she had them removed. And here too we've had this enormous shift. When I was an intern, every Tuesday and Thursday afternoon was T and

A day. In those days, a kid had colds and was brought to the doctor who would look in the throat and recommend a tonsillectomy. This was done routinely, and regrettably it was done to children at the ages of four, five and six and it is again an experience in which the child is rendered unconscious. To start with, he's scared stiff ... in those days the child was told he was being taken to a clinic where he would be given ice cream, because after the operation that's what he was given. But usually nothing was told the child about the procedure itself and he was rendered unconscious against his will. When he woke up, his throat was sore and here too, he was shown two little objects in the bottle that had been taken out of him.

> *Dr. Console*: High school graduation, so you were seventeen or eighteen years old.
> *Patient*: Uh-huh.
> *Dr. Console*: And you had an appendix operation, you say? Do you remember? What were your feelings? What happened?
> *Patient*: What did I feel?
> *Dr. Console*: Yes.
> *Patient*: I guess I was frightened because outside of the tonsils I had never really been sick enough to be in a hospital.
> *Dr. Console*: Then you'd had your tonsils out as a child?
> *Patient*: Yes. But that was only like, um—an overnight thing. I had my tonsils out when I was fourteen I think.
> *Dr. Console*: About fourteen.

> *Dr. Console*: So her T and A was not done as a child. It was done at puberty ... at about fourteen. She has a T and A. And then at seventeen she has an appendectomy.

> *Patient*: Something like that. And ... I guess I was a little upset too because graduation is a time where you want to ... I mean it's a big thing in your life. You don't want to miss out on anything and after the appendix operation the doctor had told my mother I had a heart murmur—you know—like I

couldn't work too much. And also . . . you know, you used to have to learn to swim in order to graduate. And we had an instructor. She didn't get in the pool. We'd just go in. She was a very large woman. They had a long pole with a hook on the end and she'd push us around and she pushed me down in the pool and I went down to the bottom and that's all I remember. I know that for a long time I couldn't hear . . . something was wrong with my ear. Anyway, I got excused from gym and things like that . . . I remember being given an elevator pass. Anyway, my marks were good enough . . . I didn't have any problems because you had to take regents exams. . . .

Dr. Console: Now, Dr. Cohen, she has given us some of her associations. And the associations to the question about the appendix operation are interesting. "I was scared. The doctor said I had a heart murmur." She was made into a cardiac invalid. She was given an elevator pass. When I went to high school I remember that there was both envy and compassion for the kids who had elevator passes. It meant that you were special and didn't have to climb stairs but it also meant that there was something wrong with you. Her further associations are to the swimming teacher who has this long pole with a hook . . . reminded me of my days in burlesque (*group laughter*). . . . And she was pushed in and went to the bottom. So that her associations to the specific question about the appendix are a host of seemingly extraneous memories . . . all happening around the same time . . . and all involving something bad.

> *Patient:* . . . and I got excused from some of those.
> *Dr. Console:* Because your marks were good.
> *Patient:* Yeah . . . my marks were pretty good. I never really . . . we never played hooky or anything like that. My mother was a stickler . . . she was strict. Anyway it never entered my mind to want to stay out of school. I didn't mind going to school.
> *Dr. Console:* Can you remember just how you got sick with the appendix operation?

Dr. Console: I'm a persistent son of a bitch. I've got to get this story. Despite my asking about the regent exams and all that, I do want to come back to it.

    Patient: Um . . . I'm having a lot of trouble remembering it. I had a lot of problems with . . . like when you have your period.
. . .

    Dr. Console: What do you think about that? In a way, I'm pressuring her to give me the story of the onset of whatever it was that led to the appendix operation. And we've been all over the lot . . . from the swimming pool to the elevator . . . frightened . . . regents . . . and now . . . "I had trouble with my periods." What do you think about that?

    Dr. Farber: Ovarian cyst? Pain in either quadrant?

    Dr Console: A cyst . . . from what? What do seventeen-year-old girls have pain in the lower abdomen from? Connected with periods? If it has an acute onset, it's probably a rupture of a Graafian follicle with a couple of drops of blood that can cause some peritoneal irritation. She doesn't know all of this, but she does know that she was having trouble with her periods.

    Patient: . . . severe cramps . . . my mother's old-fashioned. We never went to any doctors because I've had a lot of trouble with sprained ankles and things like that. I was a tomboy. Everybody goes through a stage like that. Not a long period of time. I've had my share of trying to copy somebody else. I had been having a lot of trouble. I had pain so bad that I just couldn't stand it and I remember my teacher sending me to the school nurse. I had such a high fever and was throwing up, they told me they were going to call the hospital. They explained to me that I would have to go to a hospital, that my appendix was . . . what do you call it . . . ruptured. I knew I was scared. I was really frightened. I know . . . my mother was working at the time and my sisters and brothers were all in school. I remember them bringing me to the hospital and the next thing I know, the police went to my mother's door, which frightened her, and explained that they had to do this operation. That was that. After that . . . I was able to work.

Dr. Console: So she says that she had trouble with her periods and described the cramps, the vomiting and the high fever. Does that sound like appendicitis? We can have very serious questions in our minds as to whether she indeed had acute appendicitis.

Dr. Alper: She's mentioned her mother three times. We're getting a picture of her. Mother was old-fashioned, strict. She never would play hooky because of her mother's strictness. Mother was working at the time. So I'm wondering how much of this revolved around dependency needs centering on the mother.

Dr. Console: Yes, the relationship with the mother is definitely brought in at this critical point. With considerable emphasis.

> *Patient:* I worked in a doctor's office.
> *Dr. Console:* How long did you work there?
> *Patient:* Oh . . . about two years. He was a radiologist. I got the job through somebody else. Somebody else had had it and they got sick and they didn't come back. I was working in a cleaners one time but I got sick from inhaling those fumes.
> *Dr. Console:* So you never had a job for a long, long time?
> *Patient:* Not more than two years.
> *Dr. Console:* After the appendix, you had other operations? What other operations did you have?
> *Patient:* I think after the appendix I had an ovary removed . . . a cyst, I think. And then in between that . . . I think I had pneumonia twice and I had a chronic thing with the bladder . . . an infection. After that I had a bowel obstruction.
> *Dr. Console:* A bowel obstruction?
> *Patient:* And they removed some of that. Not too long after that I had an intestinal obstruction.
> *Dr. Console:* Did you have an operation for that?
> *Patient:* For both.
> *Dr. Console:* Both.
> *Patient:* And then I had a couple of scrapings because I was hemorrhaging quite a lot and then after the last scraping,

when I came back downstairs they . . . the surgeon, whoever he was, said I had . . . I don't know what I had but I'd have to go back to surgery and they gave me a complete hysterectomy.

Dr. Console: Did you notice the language there . . . "They *gave me* a complete hysterectomy."

Patient: I think before that I had spent six weeks in the hospital with peritonitis. The hysterectomy was the last operation. In between, I was hospitalized for about two months with anemia . . . headaches.

Dr. Console: How long have you been in the hospital this time?

Patient: Well I just went home. I spent about seven weeks here and I went home. I was there for about three weeks and I came back last Friday.

Dr. Console: So what's the picture? How much time has this woman spent in hospitals? From age seventeen to the present? Look at the recent events. She's been in the hospital for a number of weeks, was sent home and just came back. So she spends a very significant portion of her life in hospitals. The question we have to ask ourselves is: why? Why does she spend so much time in the hospital? Why does she have all of these surgical procedures done to her? Why, after there's very little left to remove, does she then develop anemia, which brings her back to the hospital? What kind of conjectures can we make about her life? What is there in her life that makes her spend so much time in a hospital? Do you picture her happily married, with children and a family? With all kinds of outside interests?

Dr. Rubin: Not at all. You picture her as someone who depends on and enjoys a great deal of the secondary gain and attention that she gets in the hospital. There may be things happening at home that she'd like to get away from.

Dr. Console: Yes. And while I haven't seen it, I can assure you that this woman has a chart that's about ten inches thick. And we do have to wonder why. Why does she spend so much time in the hospital, and why has she had so many surgical procedures? And,

"The last time they gave me a complete hysterectomy" ... not a partial ... a *complete* one ... the whole business!

Dr. Rubinstein: What makes it even more striking is the fact that this is a forty-year-old woman. She's not in her fifties or sixties ... she's forty!

Dr. Console: Twenty-three years of her life have been involved in a series of major surgical interventions into her anatomy. I don't remember whether it comes out in the tape, but she's left out a number of times that she was hospitalized for removal of adhesions. With this amount of surgery you would expect a fair amount of scarring and so on. But again, the very simple question you must ask when you hear this is why?

I would also like to denote this shift from surgical to medical problems after all the operations have been performed. Anemia and weakness, dizziness ... the usual kind of diffuse complaint. This is always baffling and frustrating to doctors. It's not in the textbook. It's often a confusing picture ... difficulty in breathing with perfectly good cardiac reserve and no emphysema, and the doctors begin to feel baffled. After a while, the doctors' feelings of confusion and puzzlement turn to annoyance. "Why is she bothering us with all these complaints?"

Patient: I spent about seven weeks in here and I was home for about three and a half weeks and I came in last Friday.

Dr. Console: Last Friday. Because of the weakness that you were talking about?

Patient: Yeah. I couldn't breathe ... I was having trouble breathing.

Dr. Console: Do you have family of your own? Are you married?

Patient: No, but I have a son.

Dr. Console: You have a son. How old is your son?

Patient: Twelve.

Dr. Console: Twelve. How is he? Is he in good health?

Patient: No. He has cerebral palsy.

Dr. Console: Oh, I see. What about your mother and father, brothers and sisters, are they in good health?

Patient: My mother's sick now but she's seventy-two.

Dr. Console: You said she's an old-fashioned lady.
Patient: Extremely so.
Dr. Console: Very strict?
Patient: Yeah . . . maybe now she's not as strict, but she was very strict when we were growing up. In a way I resented it. Now, as I've gotten older, I'm glad because I never got into any trouble outside of my son being born. But I'm not the first one it's ever happened to and she's been good to him, and now there's nothing that she wouldn't do for him. They're all real good to him. And to me too. In our family, everybody went to school . . . all my sisters and brothers. You know . . . I have a brother who's a doctor.

Dr. Console: We have the additional information now that she is unmarried but does have a child and he has cerebral palsy. In talking about her mother, she indicates that while the mother was very strict, she's relaxed and loosened up now and is very good to the child. Does anyone have any idea as to what this might represent?

Dr. Meyer: She says that the mother is very nice to the child and of course the child is sick. Now she's becoming sick, possibly with the wish that her mother would be nice to her.

Dr. Rubin: I thought of that too. One implication for her as an adult is that if she acts like a sick child, maybe the mother will be good to her.

Dr. Console: It will be a fairly common experience for you to be confronted with a woman who has a child born out of wedlock and the child is then looked after by the grandmother, by the girl's mother. In terms of some of our theoretical constructs, what might this exemplify?

Dr. Iglesias: A very hostile act on the part of the daughter toward her mother.

Dr. Console: Where's the hostility? That she brings her a baby?

Dr. Iglesias: The mother has to take care of the child.

Dr. Console: The mother takes care of the child and is good to him.

Dr. Iglesias: But it can be viewed as the patient having dumped the child onto her own mother.

Dr. Console: Well, this is part of the question I'm asking. Is it really a dumping of the child onto the grandmother?

Dr. Chassen: In a sense, if a woman has a child and gives it to her mother, there's an oedipal kind of thing. . . .

Dr. Console: What kind of oedipal thing is there?

Dr. Chassen: The woman is having a child in reality, and in fantasy she may be having the child with her father. Then, in giving it to her mother, she makes it the mother's child and by extension, it becomes the father's also.

Dr. Console: The child born out of wedlock is, in fantasy, often born out of union with the father. Now the fantasy is that the mother is going to raise hell . . . she's going to say, "What kind of thing have you done?" Rather than a dumping of the child, it suggests more that the girl makes up for her oedipal sin by presenting the baby to her mother. It's a gift giving . . . a present. You will find this very commonly. People who work in adoption agencies . . . at least the more sensitive ones . . . become aware of the frequency with which the man who impregnated the girl is a stranger passing in the night. He just serves this purpose . . . to impregnate; and the deep fantasy on the part of the woman is that it is her father. Thus the child is given to the mother to make up for the incestuous sin.

Dr. Chassen: The other thought that I had is that the child is deformed and that the patient could see this as being retribution for her sins . . . visited upon the child.

Dr. Console: Well, we don't know specifically when this diagnosis was made. Was it apparent at birth? But the cerebral palsy is of course one more unfortunate thing that this poor woman has had to bear. It's as though the fates conspired to put her in the position of always having trouble.

Patient: . . . I have a brother who's a doctor. He has his degree.

Dr. Console: Is this an older brother?

Patient: Yes, an older brother. My younger brothers all have good jobs and families.

Dr. Console: All of them at least went through high school?

Patient: Yes . . . I did too.

132 THE FIRST ENCOUNTER

Dr. Console: What do you think about that? This was apparently a family in which education and occupational aspirations were at a high level and a good many of them were fulfilled. I was checking to establish that every one of them went through high school and she says, "I did too."

Dr. Alper: When she said that, she seemed to have the feeling that you would think that she did not go to high school. This probably is a projection of her own feelings about herself . . . her own inadequacies.

Dr. Console: Yes. I think that it is an expression of her own feelings of inadequacy. She has suggested that the rest of her family is successful. They are all married and have families and she's the only one without this. She has to say . . . "I went through high school too. Don't think ill of me." All this despite the fact that she had long since established that she had gone to high school.

> *Patient*: I always wanted to study law.
> *Dr. Console*: Why law?
> *Patient*: I don't know . . . I was always interested in law. Well, the whole family is very musical. I like that too. At one time I thought that maybe I could make a go of that, because one thing that my brothers and sisters didn't do and that I did, was study the piano and ballet until I wasn't able to do it anymore. I can't say that I didn't have the opportunity to do what I wanted.
> *Dr. Console*: How many brothers and sisters do you have?
> *Patient*: I have two brothers and three sisters.
> *Dr. Console*: And where are you in the family? How many older and younger than you?
> *Patient*: I have two younger than me. I was a twin.

Dr. Console: "I have two younger than me. I was a twin."

Dr. Iglesias: Where's the other twin?

Dr. Console: Where indeed is the twin? " I *was* a twin" . . . would suggest what?

Dr. Iglesias: That the twin is dead.

Dr. Console: And if the twin is dead, what further does that suggest?

Dr. Clarke: She's dead too. If she's a twin and her twin is dead . . . she's living but she's also dead.

Dr. Console: All right, that's one way of putting it. You suggest that the fact that the twin is dead has had some influence on her thinking, feeling and her performing.

Dr. Kent: One of the important things to determine is the age at which the twin died.

Dr. Console: Why is this important?

Dr. Kent: Depending upon when it happened, it would have a great deal of meaning in terms of how she felt and thought. It could really influence her fantasies. If the twin died an hour after birth, that's one thing, but if it died at six years of age . . . that's something much different. I wonder if one of her fantasies may be that she murdered her twin . . . or was in some way responsible for her death?

Dr. Console: Or was in some way responsible. So we're sure going to try and find out when this happened. Now let me make one more point in this matter. She said, "I *was* a twin," and we assume that the twin is dead. You are confronted with what is known as *the guilt of the survivor*. Whenever there are twins and one of them dies, even if it's an hour after birth, at some point later in life, the information is given the survivor that he or she was a twin and that the other one died. What question does the child ask when given this information?

Dr. Clarke: "Why did he die?"

Dr. Console: Yes, but that's only half of it.

Dr. Rubin: "Why didn't I die?"

Dr. Console: Exactly! "How come I survived?"

Dr. Marcus: Another important thing would be the sex of the twin and along with that . . . whether it was an identical or fraternal twin.

Dr. Console: This too is going to be of considerable consequence. Let me say that one of the things in life over which a person has no control is to be born a twin. In most of our experiences in life we are, to an enormously greater degree than we ever realize, responsible for our own behavior and for what happens to us. Being a twin is one of the exceptions. And very often it turns out to be an important exception.

Patient: ... I was a twin (*pause*). She's dead.
Dr. Console: When did she die?
Patient: She died when we were two—diphtheria.

Dr. Console: I'm sure Dr. Clarke will appreciate the meaning of her comment, "She died when *we* were two." So now, Dr. Kent, two years old.

Dr. Kent: I'm trying to remember what I've learned about child development (*group laughter*). I think that there's enough going on in a two-year-old to be very much aware of himself as a separate entity from his twin, as well as from the mother and important outsiders. Definitely there is a sense of self and of the twin, as well as the strong bond between the two that would have existed. I think that there would also be enough development in each twin for some jealousy and competition to begin. I'm not sure how it's experienced in a two-year-old but I'm sure that it's there.

Dr. Console: Yes. You would have to assume that this woman, at the age of two, was aware of an important loss. I don't think there's any question about that. This is not a situation where the twin died after, let's say, one week of life, and the person grew up and was later told that she was a twin. That would have a different quality. At age two, the other person existed for her. She was real. Now you talk about separation-individuation and so on. Here you have to temper your observations just a bit, because this is precisely one of the things that I referred to when I mentioned that it may be an unfortunate fate to be born a twin. Separation-individuation is made much more difficult by being one of a pair of twins because of the strong identification with each other. This is what Dr. Clarke was alluding to before.

It is also regrettable that parents often foster the difficulty of separation-individuation for the twins. And how do they do this? By dressing them alike, by having a double carriage with both the children in it, and all of that. It makes the task of feeling oneself to be a separate and distinct entity much more difficult.

Patient: ... diphtheria.
Dr. Console: Two ... of diphtheria (*pause*). Do you remember anything about that?

Patient: About her?

Dr. Console: Yes . . . (*pause*). Do you remember . . . what were you told about her as you grew up?

Patient: What was I told about her? I don't think anything really too much.

Dr. Console: Well, somebody told you that you had been one of a set of twins.

Patient: I don't know . . . my mother . . . well, she always said that, well, maybe it's some old wives' tale. . . .

Dr. Console: Now be prepared. When a patient is going to say something and prefaces it with the remark, "I don't know; it's ridiculous" . . . "it's a cockeyed idea" . . . or as here . . . "maybe it's an old wives' tale" . . . be prepared to attach enormous significance to what he is now trying to pass off as something relatively inconsequential.

Patient: . . . some old wives' tale, well anyway, she always said that if it came down to having a cold or whatever have you, I'd always seem to get double the amount. . . .

Dr. Clarke: Well, what one twin gets the other would always seem to get.

Dr. Console: I would imagine this to be very true in the matter of childhood communicable diseases. The chances are that both would get measles and so on. However, in the situation with this woman, one of the twins is no longer there! So what is she saying in effect? Despite the fact that the other one isn't alive, she gets it for both of them. She gets *double*!

Dr. Vis: This again points out the difficulty in establishing one's own identity when one is a twin.

Dr. Marcus: It would be one thing if they were six years old and one died accidently. It's something else to know that the reason her sister died was diphtheria, which is much like a cold. The patient just stated that she would get colds frequently. This makes her life story even more ironic. She must really question, "Why did I survive?"

Dr. Console: Indeed she must question, "Why did I survive?" But the fact is that she *did* survive. In light of the feelings that you are

Dr. Console: Inndeed she must question, "Why did I survive?" But the fact is that she 2did11 survive. Inn light of the feelings that you are suggesting, what then does she go through?

Dr. Chassen: My fantasy is that she feels that her twin got the diphtheria that she would have had . . . that the other died for her.

Dr. Console: If that is the fantasy, that the twin died in order that she might survive, what would a predominant feeling in her be?

Dr. Chassen: Guilt.

Dr. Console: Guilt! And in the face of guilt, what would she have to do?

Dr. Vis: She has to be punished. Suffer.

Dr. Console: Yes . . . suffer. Make up for it. Be punished! All of the things you're saying.

Dr. Meyer: This also sheds a different light on the significance of giving her baby to the mother. Perhaps there was the fantasy of giving back the other sibling.

Dr. Console: A replacement! It very definitely introduces this as a possibility. That in the face of her guilt, in addition to whatever oedipal reasons there were, there was the fact of one twin having died . . . "and I'll give you one to take its place."

Dr. McDermott: One other possibility would be that she sees her lost twin as being there as a phantom. She experiences her own cold and her twin's at the same time. So in a sense, she hasn't completely lost her twin.

Dr. Console: Well, you mention that she is experiencing her twin's illnesses as well as her own. Why am I sitting with this woman and talking to her?

Dr. Zimmer: This sheds light on the fact that she's been ill so much of her life.

Dr. Console: Yes. This woman is being interviewed because of polysurgery. Because of the number of illnesses and operations she has had.

Dr. Rubinstein: I think it comes out a bit later, but many of the illnesses were ones that the doctors couldn't figure out.

Dr. Farber: If she had introjected this twin, couldn't the surgery represent attempts to remove the introjected object? To cut it out of her?

Dr. Console: It's conceivable. But that's getting pretty fancy. My own feeling at this point has to do with the amount of guilt that she must have experienced in having the two-year-old twin sister die while she survived.

Dr. Farber: What about the loss of the companionship also?

Dr. Console: Well, I would be cautious about extolling the virtues of companionship in twins. There is probably a volcano of resentment and hostility in addition to a special bond and a sense of companionship. You see, despite the fact that a woman has two breasts, the chances are that she could not nurse the two children simultaneously. As soon as she picks up one to nurse it, the other is being rejected. And if she puts one's shoes on before the other's, the other feels as though he's being discriminated against. I mention these things only to temper your inclination to see the good aspect to it . . . the companionship.

Patient: I'd always seem to get double the amount. . . . One twin would get enough for the both of them. That was what the doctor always told her.

Dr. Console: She started off with an "old wives' tale" . . . her mother mentioned it. Now there's official sanction given. . . . The doctor always told the mother that this would happen. So her chances of escaping this fate become smaller and smaller, and she's trapped.

Dr. Kent: I wonder if the idea of having everything double came from the doctor . . . if that somehow influenced her choice of the means by which she's got to suffer. There are lots of ways that people can manage to mess up their lives and suffer. There can be difficulties in relationships with others, troubles with jobs, school, and so on. But she's having problems with her body . . . medical things. She seems to suffer medically rather than socially.

Dr. Console: I think that she also suffers socially. We have no indication of there being anything in her life other than hospitals and operations. So she suffers in many ways.

Patient: And the doctor asked me the other day, were we exactly alike? I was talking to my mother and we weren't. Um ... we weren't what you would call identical twins. She looked more like my grandmother. We have Indian blood in the family and they said that she looked more Indian than me. She had straight black hair ... you know. Nobody ever really talked about it too much when we got older. ...

Dr. Console: Now, what has been added with this information? That they were not identical twins. They were different. The one difference that she denotes was that the twin had straight black hair.

Dr. Bond: I would think that the dead twin was the more favored of the two. This was back a number of years and the child with the straight hair possessed what was then more desirable in a black family.

Dr. Console: I think that this is probably so. Of all the things somebody could mention in denoting an alleged difference between the twins ... to say that she had straight black hair. ...

Dr. Bond: This is even more significant if one child had really thick, straight and lovely hair ... that needed more combing and brushing. The mother would undoubtedly spend more time with her.

Dr. Console: I think that this is correct. Not too many years ago, this made a considerable difference in the feelings of many black people. Straight hair was more desirable. For the patient to denote that the sister had straight black hair is enormously significant. So the business of companionship is not really the big issue ... here we can see the envy that she must have felt. The sister had the straight black hair and she didn't. She would have been very resentful and hostile about that. With her sister's death, the patient's angry wishes toward her were realized.

Dr. Console: So that when you got sick, you were really twice as sick as anybody else would be?

Patient: I never thought about it but now that you ask me, I remember my mother saying that.

Dr. Console: In my making this comment to her, do you feel that I was leading the patient?

Dr. Chassen: No. She had virtually said what you did in the preceding sentence. You were only putting it into different words.

Dr. Console: Yes. I feel that she has already said this and I want to make the distinction between a clarification which uses what the patient has said and gives it back in a clearer form, and an interpretation. I am not introducing a new idea. I am not suggesting to her something that she does not, at some level, feel or have an awareness of. There is a partial confirmation of this in her remark, "Now that you ask me, I remember my mother saying that." We're dealing with an enormously important factor in this woman's thinking and feeling, and one that has influenced her entire life. What is that?

Dr. Rubin: Everything's going to be doubled.

Dr. Console: It's going to be twice as much, twice as severe, twice as bad. Because whatever it is, she's having it for herself and for her twin sister.

Dr. Kent: Couldn't this ever work in the reverse? That she could get twice as much happiness or pleasure, or does it always have to be that she has to suffer twice as much?

Dr. Console: Well, I think that, as in all of medicine, we must be very wary of the words *always* and *never*. But for her, it would be predominantly a matter of suffering. This is so because the major response to the loss of a twin sibling has to be one of guilt. As we have discussed before, the whole matter of a person's having to ask *why?* ... "Why the other half, rather than myself? Why did I survive?" If we want to go deeper, there is also the fantasy that she killed the twin. This is similar to the common fantasy that the only child has that he or she destroyed everything else that may have been in that womb, prior to and after his or her having been there. This is a very deeply unconscious fantasy of the only child: that he is responsible for the destruction of all other children or pregnancies ... whether he knows that the mother had other pregnancies or not.

There is a reinforcement of this feeling, where the mother unfortunately finds a need to explain to a child that she was pregnant, either before or after him, and that she lost that child. She had a spontaneous abortion or something of that nature. The mother may give added impetus and *fact* to the only child's fantasy that he is responsible. So, there are some special factors inherent in the treatment of an only child and in the treatment of a twin.

Dr. Cohen: You wouldn't feel that it's wrong for the mother to inform the child of a lost baby if the pregnancy went to term, would you?

Dr. Console: No. There would be nothing wrong in the mother's telling the child what is already apparent to him. However, to tell the child about a pregnancy that went for eight weeks or three months, is telling him something that he need not know, something which was not apparent to him, and something that will reinforce the fundamental fantasy that he killed everybody else because he wanted to be the only one.

> *Patient*: There wasn't really any kind of serious illness in the family that I can remember. They were all pretty healthy.
> *Dr. Console*: *You* had a lot of illness.
> *Patient*: Yeah. I guess that happens. Nobody can pick and choose. It just happens.

Dr. Console: Now here, she makes the statement that there hasn't been a lot of illness in the family. I point out to her that *she's* had a lot of illness and she minimizes it by saying, "Nobody can pick and choose." However, I don't feel that I've succeeded in making my point clear to her, namely, that she's had a lot of illness and seems to be making up for the twin and maybe even for some other people as well. So she says, "I guess that happens . . . nobody can pick and choose." I think this is a very significant remark. Who asked about picking and choosing? Why should she volunteer this kind of information? I don't think that in the normal course of conversation, a person would make this remark about illness: "Nobody can pick and choose."

> *Patient*: If it wasn't me, it would be somebody else.

Dr. Console: There is the confirmation of our speculations. Who's the somebody else?

Residents: The twin.
Dr. Console: I think that this is implicit in what she is saying.

Patient: I don't um . . . I don't feel, um . . .
Dr. Console: You say, "If it wasn't me it would be somebody else." Who else could it be?
Patient: Well, if I wasn't the one that always got sick and all, maybe it would have been one of my sisters or brothers. But I don't wish it on them.

Dr. Console: "Were it not me, it would have been *one* of my sisters or brothers." Then the gratuitous remark, "But I don't wish it on them."

Dr. Console: Maybe if your twin sister had lived, she would have had half the sickness you've had.
Patient: She might have been healthy, who knows? I mean, getting diphtheria doesn't mean that she would have been ill all her life. You could never tell. We might have been as different as night and day. I mean, that's the way things are. I can't say that we were close. We were two years old . . . how close could we be?
Dr. Console: Your father . . . he's been in good health?
Patient: My father's dead.
Dr. Console: When did he die?
Patient: I don't remember.
Dr. Console: How old were you?
Patient: I don't know . . . I know my sister was still small. He died of pneumonia.
Dr. Console: You don't remember much about him?
Patient: I don't remember that much about him.
Dr. Console: How old is your youngest sister?
Patient: About thirty. We don't discuss ages in our family.
Dr. Console: You don't?
Patient (laughing): No. . . .
Dr. Console (smiling): What's bad about ages?
Patient: Everybody thinks I'm the baby. Unless I tell them otherwise, they think I'm the baby.

Dr. Console: Despite the fact that she has a sister about ten years younger than she is, people tend to think of her as the baby of the family. Where do people get this impression from?

Dr. Iglesias: From her.

Dr. Console: This would be something that we might speculate about. If one were to continue to treat this woman, it would be worthwhile finding out about her need to give the impression that she is the baby. We can have some thoughts about it but we would want the confirmation in her own words . . . from her own story.

> *Dr. Console*: Why is that?
>
> *Patient*: I don't know. Maybe up until I had this problem where I had all my teeth taken out or something like that, I guess I was luckier than all of them. And since I've been sick, my mother and I have gotten closer.
>
> *Dr. Console*: Since you've been sick you've gotten closer to your mother?
>
> *Patient*: Yes.

Dr. Farber: Being the youngest is being the most dependent. The one with the most privileges. Being in a sick position is being in a helpless, dependent position and fosters leaning on others. It serves a purpose.

Dr. Console: She describes it as almost happenstance. It occurs in the face of all the illness that she got closer to her mother. Now coming as it does, after her mentioning being considered the baby, it seems quite clear that there is a considerable need on her part to put herself in this helpless, dependent and loved position. And all this comes in the order of our hearing that her brothers and sisters all finished high school and for the most part have families and have been much more successful in life than she has been. This is perhaps one of the things that is left to her . . . to be the sick, dependent baby, who now gets closer and closer to the mother.

Dr. Cohen: I was struck by her making mention of having had her teeth removed. The image I had in my mind was that of the gumming, toothless infant.

Dr. Console: When you see a young person who has full dentures, begin to speculate in your own mind about the defensive quality of having one's teeth removed ... at a relatively young age. This woman is forty years old and this happened some time ago. Ignore, for the moment, all the physiology and pathology. I believe that those physiological changes sometimes take place in response to a need. What would the person be defending against?

Dr. Zimmer: Aggression.

Dr. Console: Absolutely. It's a way of controlling aggression. Over the years, I've repeatedly been able to observe that many, many passive and unaggressive people have a full set of dentures ... at an early age. Many other people have observed this too. Pay attention to the story of having teeth pulled out early. It's often defensive against any kind of aggression. It's an overwhelming reaction formation.

Dr. Console: You've always lived with her?

Patient: Yeah ... up until recently. I live by myself now ... for the last two or three years. But when my son was small I lived with her.

Dr. Console: And now you live by yourself?

Patient: Uh-huh.

Dr. Console: Near your mother?

Patient: No ... but I see her.

Dr. Console: Do you see the other members of your family ... brothers and sisters?

Patient: The one that's a teacher, I don't see him because he travels a lot with his wife. But the others I see, and when I don't see them we call each other ... several times during the week. And they come here to see me.

Dr. Console: What have the doctors here told you about your sickness?

Patient: Up until now, they haven't told me too much of anything, because when somebody asks me, "What did the doctors say" ... I can't tell them. I get angry with them a lot of times and say to them, "You never say what it is." How can you be sick for so long? I don't like guessing at what I might have. All I know is that I'm anemic. . . . I have a doctor on the outside and he's pretty straightforward but he doesn't really know as much as they do about me here, because I've been coming here for so many years. I know I suffer from adhesions and I have gallstones ... things like that I know. But this anemia problem ... I'm not building up a store of iron like a normal person's body should. It'll be a problem giving me enough blood to build up enough stored iron so I'll feel better. It might take a while.

Dr. Console: You say that you suffer from adhesions. What does that mean to you?

Patient: A lot of pain. My stomach swells. You know, sometimes I can actually see the skin being pulled and it's quite painful to me.

Dr. Console: The chances are inordinately remote, and as far as I'm concerned a sheer impossibility, that she can observe her abdomen and see adhesions. But as is customary in these situations, when somebody complains of abdominal distress after a couple of operations, the explanation given is that there are adhesions. Now the adhesions that she fantasizes are attached to the skin. When the doctor tells her that she has adhesions, he's talking about the peritoneum and so on. But she can *see* these adhesions. The fact that she can see them validates for her the fact that there really is something there. But she can't see her anemia. She has to take their word for that.

Patient: But I've had it for so long that I try to overlook it. And then I developed arthritis. But a lot of people have that. It's no big thing. And there isn't too much you can do about it anyway. So outside of that ... I'm healthy.

Dr. Console: When did you have your teeth out?

Patient: It's been more than eight years now. I can't keep my dentures in because my mouth gets swollen and sore all the time. They're supposed to try to make me new teeth but they can't do it because my mouth won't heal. Every time they try to stretch it, the skin splits and it bleeds. It's kind of painful, but my teeth don't bother me too much.

Dr. Console: I took her back to the matter of her teeth. It's more than eight years ago, so she was about thirty-two when she had them removed. Now, over a period of eight years she's been unable to have dentures fitted. She gets sores and ulcerations. What might this suggest?

Dr. Marcus: She doesn't want teeth. She doesn't want to be able to bite.

Dr. Console: I think so. This is in keeping with her earlier statement about everyone thinking that she's a baby.

Dr. Rubinstein: My fantasy is that perhaps she has a great deal of bruxism at night . . . bruising her gums and making it difficult to be fitted for dentures. This too is oral agression.

Dr. Console: Yes. When you hear a story about teeth-grinding or bruxism at night, there too, look for very early oral-aggressive manifestations.

Dr. Bond: There also is a lack of interest in being attractive to men. A young person with no teeth is not going to be very attractive to the opposite sex.

Dr. Console: Yes, she isn't interested in making herself attractive to the opposite sex, but she indeed wants to be attractive to her mother and to people who will think of her as a poor, helpless creature. She wants to be attractive to the world, in terms of helplessness . . . of being a baby . . . of being deprived and deficient, and in so doing, virtually to compel the environment to feel sorry and to look after her.

Dr. Cohen: One of the things that was striking to me is that despite our mentioning her use of this as a defense against the aggression, I don't feel much pity toward her. I feel a little anger toward her. She irritates me.

Dr. Console: Unfortunately, your feelings are shared by many people. General medical and surgical people will tend to make short shrift of such a person.

Dr. Rubinstein: In this context, we have to wonder at what point an element of surgical sadism comes into play. This is a woman who gets cut up pretty often. We could question how much of a vindictive element might be involved on the part of the surgeons toward her. . . . There's a mutual playing out of some conflict.

Dr. Console: She puts herself in this obviously masochistic posture and then whoever is dealing with her is converted by her into a sadist.

Dr. Marcus: After she mentions this incredible list of illnesses, she then says, "Aside from that, I'm healthy." And it was the same with her teeth. She details all these difficulties for years in getting dentures, and then says that it doesn't bother her.

Dr. Console: I think this may be partly what Dr. Cohen is responding to. He finds it offensive that a person is willing to be in this position and not do something about it. Perhaps his therapeutic zeal is burning away and he is being frustrated by the patient. "Why don't you want to get better? Why don't you want to get teeth? Why don't you stop all this complaining?" She doesn't want to . . . and for good reasons. Some of these have already come out and others will become clearer as we proceed.

Dr. Iglesias: Couldn't the teeth . . . the dentures, sitting in the glass of water by the bedside, represent for her, the twin . . . looking at her. This could be the retaliation of the twin.

Dr. Console: Well, that's pretty speculative. But certainly a common expression of this in cartoons is the situation where the clacking teeth are chasing somebody (*group laughter*). The threatening, aggressive component of just the teeth themselves . . . clack . . . clack . . . clack. And remember, so far in this interview this woman hasn't expressed any real anger, aside from some vague dissatisfaction with the doctors who haven't told her much. So, for this woman, anything that might represent anger or aggression would have to be denied or removed.

> *Dr. Console*: Would you say that you've been a happy person in your life?
>
> *Patient*: I think so. I mean, even without doing it intentionally, sometimes I tend to be a comedian. I always come up with something funny without meaning to.
>
> *Dr. Console*: Do your friends enjoy that when you come up with something funny?
>
> *Patient*: Yeah, because I don't really try. Sometimes I don't mean to say things and they come out in a funny way. I like to laugh. It's better to laugh than to cry all the time.

Dr. Console: Do you do much crying?

Patient: No. I get aggravated sometimes when I'm trying to make somebody understand something; if I have to keep telling somebody something all the time. But I don't spend a whole lot of time crying. I read a lot. I like television and crochet.

Dr. Console: You say you get mad when you try to explain something to somebody. Do you feel that way about the doctors? That you can't explain things to them?

Patient: Sometimes. It's aggravating to try to say, "I'm hurting here." And then they come to the side of the bed and they talk and everything and say, "She's got a pain here and she's got a pain there." They act like they don't believe that it's real. But I know the difference between something you dream up and reality. I know when I'm hurting.

Dr. Console: What is she saying? This of course comes in the general context of a complaint about doctors.

Dr. Iglesias: She's not making it up. "I'm not making up these stories about my pain. It's real. I'm not crazy. Why did they refer me to a psychiatrist?"

Dr. Console: Well, she was not referred to a psychiatrist. She was merely asked by the resident if she would like to talk to one of the older staff members. "Psychiatrist" was not specified. But I'm pointing to a more general attitude, one shared by many patients that you will see. While it relates to the general concept of psychiatry, make the assumption in this situation that she is not aware that this is a psychiatric interview.

Dr. Rubin: She's saying that the doctors on the ward, wherever, don't believe her. It's almost as though they're calling her a liar. There's nothing there, yet she still complains about pain. "It's all in your head" is what she must hear them saying.

Dr. Marcus: This is the kind of patient that the people on the medical service call a *crock*.

Dr. Console: Yes, this is the kind of patient that the medical service . . . we . . . particularly in our youth, burdened with a ward full of patients, call a crock. She's always complaining. In the beginning of our medical experience, she's the kind of patient who isn't terribly interesting because there are no fantastic findings, the X-ray doesn't show much, and so on. She is not what the book says people should be when they are sick. The important point about her, I think, is her response to this general tendency of physicians. In their frustration with the patient who complains, and in the face of no findings, they will tell the patient, "It's your nerves" or "It's your imagination." They think that they are doing the patient a service in saying that the difficulty or complaint is psychogenic. However, the patient hears this as a suggestion that he is making it up, faking, malingering, that he is a liar. . . . And the patient must get the feeling of being ignored. "I know when I have pain . . . I know I have pain. The doctor doesn't know what it is. If I have pain then there is something wrong with me. And it is not imagination." Many people simply cannot make the step necessary to understand that they have pain and that it may be a consequence of psychogenic factors . . . of conflict. Hence, they hear the doctors telling them that their pain, in a sense, doesn't exist. Often, after a physician has been seeing the patient for a length of time, he sends the patient to a psychiatrist. But he usually sends the patient out of a sense of frustration. It's, "Go and see a psychiatrist." Not only is this a last resort, but it also suggests the idea that "You're some kind of a nut and I can't really take care of you, so go and see a 'head shrinker'. This is for him." The patient cannot be greatly impressed with that kind of referral and that kind of advice. It is not approached in such a way as to indicate that the patient has a conflict that is surfacing and giving him symptoms. This woman has described an emptiness in her life. What is there? She says she likes to read, watch television and crochet. That's an interesting combination, but to me it adds up to there not being a helluva lot for her.

Dr. Farber: The very fact that she emphasizes that she's hurting and that something must be wrong might lead one to the suspicion that she might have an inkling that something psychological is going on. Sometimes people react very strongly when a sensitive subject is brought up.

Dr. Console: Yes, I think there's validity to what you say and that this could be put in the area of the patient's protesting too much. And protesting with a certain vehemence . . . "I know when it's

real. I know the difference between reality and imagination."
There's a suggestion that at some level she may be aware that the
pain arises from sources other than organic ones.

> *Patient*: And if I say that I'm hurting, don't give me a whole
> song and dance. Either you're going to try to find out what's
> wrong and rectify it or you're not. I don't plan on laying up
> there . . . in here for another seven weeks. Because I don't
> have to. When I was home, I didn't have to . . . I was anemic,
> it's true, but I didn't have to lay there and suffer. The doctor
> should have given me something to ease my pain so I didn't
> have to be suffering all the time. But what's the point in
> laying in the hospital, when you and the doctor can't
> compromise and come to some kind of understanding? Don't
> talk to the wall, talk to me. I'm intelligent enough. I'll talk to
> you if you talk to me.
> *Dr. Console*: And you have a right to know.
> *Patient*: Yes . . . who are you going to tell if you don't tell me?
> Now my family was here over the weekend to try to talk to
> the doctor but they never saw one. And they're quite upset
> and they're very angry and they don't want me to stay in the
> hospital because they feel like I'm being used. They said, "You
> just spent seven weeks in there". Before that, two months in
> another hospital. Before that, six weeks in another hospital. I
> wasn't home six months out of this past year.

Dr. Console: Do you have any thoughts about this portion? Notice
that she says that her family complained. Her family.

Dr. McDermott: Her affect was quite intense while she was
describing this. She attributed the feelings to her family but the
affect was hers.

Dr. Console: So you're suggesting that *she* is the one who feels that
she has spent too much time in the hospital, but that she's
expressing it in terms of the family complaining about this. Is that
what you mean?

Dr. McDermott: I think that what she's complaining about is that
she's spent a great deal of time in the hospital and hasn't received
what she hoped for.

Dr. Farber: I think that the family is putting pressure on her to come home. I think that she wanted a doctor to tell them that something is really wrong and that she needs to stay in the hospital. She was angry at the doctors for not being available to do this.

Dr. Waldemar: There is also a great deal of secondary gain. It's very clear to me that she's happy that the family is involved to this extent. If the doctor could be there to discuss her illness with the family, she would be much more satisfied and would be getting what she seeks.

Dr. Console: But again, to come to the issue of wanting or not wanting to be in a hospital. She has said that her family has complained about her being in the hospital too much. Do you feel that this is her complaint as well? Does she feel that she has been hospitalized too long and wants to get out?

Dr. Iglesias: She must feel that her family is being critical of her staying in the hospital.

Dr. Console: That is one implication of her description of the family's displeasure with her remaining in the hospital. It may be that she is feeling their impatience with *her* . . . not just with the doctors. *She* is not doing enough to effect her discharge.

> *Patient*: . . . and what did I accomplish? They sent me home bleeding inside. My blood count was something like twenty-three. How was I supposed to take care of a sick child and myself too? And these things, they don't tell me. When they sent me home they said, "You're all right."

Dr. Console: "How was I supposed to take care of a sick child and myself . . . in this condition? Did I belong at home in this condition? Or did I belong some place where they would take care of this condition. Where they would take care of *me*?"

> *Patient*: Why lie to me? I won't feel sorry for myself. I want to know my limitations. So if I am not well, I know what to do and what not to do. How to take care of myself. I want to live a

long time. I want to be able to see my child get so that he can care for himself. He's doing very well now. He's an independent child. He doesn't spend time crying and whining and what not. But with me being sick like I am, I'm very short-tempered with him. And I yell at him a lot . . . for just walking across the floor. A lot of times I have such terrible headaches.

Dr. Console: It shouldn't surprise us hat she characterizes her child as quite independent. Why is there great likelihood that, despite his physical disability, he is able to shift for himself?

Dr. Farber: His mother is hardly ever at home.

Dr. Console: Yes. His independence is largely a function of her absence. . . . She's in the hospital all the time.

Patient: The headaches give me terrible pain. I can't stand the least little bit of noise. And I don't like being like that with him because we're very close. I don't want him to hate me.

Dr. Console: Do you ever talk about these things with your physician brother?

Patient: I've talked with him about my son. Yeah . . . some of the things, like this business of me being irritable and cranky. He said that he could understand it too because if I don't know what's going on with me . . . I'm only really guessing, if I'm in pain and there's nobody there to help me. A lot of times I can't even get up in the morning. I'm worried about my friends seeing me all the time, laying here sick. I hate for everyone to see that.

Dr. Console: So let's take this one point. She can't get up in the morning. Her child would have to get breakfast for himself. This is the kind of self-reliance that he had to develop in order to survive.

Patient: Then I wonder who's going to take care of my boy. He's got to go to the doctor. He needs shoes. Who's going to take him? All these things worry me. I mean you get so much inside and who is there to talk to? I don't ever really have anybody to talk to.

Dr. *Console*: What about the boy's father? Do you see the boy's father?

Patient: No.

Dr. *Console*: Did you have a long relationship with him?

Patient: I went with him a long time, yeah. But I haven't seen him since my son was born. When he found out that the boy was sick, he just took off.

Dr. *Console*: Have you ever been in love with any other man?

Patient: No, not really.

Dr. *Console*: Just one man.

Patient: Yup. That's just the way I am. I've thought about others. It's not that I haven't met anybody else. I just haven't found anybody that I could become interested in. I don't go out too much.

Dr. *Console*: You don't miss things?

Patient: At times. But I guess I like to be alone a lot too.

Dr. *Console*: There has only been one man in her life. A man who abandoned her after the child was born. She does not indicate much interest in other men. So in terms of a lifetime, here too is a void of substantial proportions. She's alone.

Dr. *Waldemar*: This woman is very masochistic. Do you think there's any possibility that she managed to make the one man in her life go away? It seems like an ideal way for her to continue punishing herself.

Dr. *Console*: We just don't have that information. She certainly has spent a great deal of her time punishing herself. But I don't think we can view this situation as one that she engineered as a self-punitive measure. As she describes it, the man, when he saw that the child was defective, just took off. This is one of those unfortunate tragedies in life. It certainly must have had an impact on her. It must have had a great impact on the manner in which she looks upon men. I don't think that she looks very kindly upon them if this was the only experience she had with a man.

Patient: I don't like a lot of crowds and all. I have friends who, when I feel like company, come over. Or I go see them. Otherwise ... I'm with my boy. I don't encourage a lot of company. I've been invited to a few things but I haven't gone.

Dr. Console: Why not? You're invited. Why don't you go?

Patient: I'm kind of shy too. I always have been. But lately I just haven't felt up to going any place. Not really. I have too many problems with my son. He has convulsions . . . and asthma. That's something we both have. So I'm constantly running back and forth to the hospital, staying up nights, making sure he don't choke to death and things like that. It wasn't easy.

Dr. Console: She makes it clear that because of her condition lately, it's been difficult to get out, but it was always a difficult thing for her to do. She was always kind of shy. She likes being alone. We would have to conclude from this information that her interpersonal relations are quite limited.

Patient: Like I said, I could do it on my own so I did it.

Dr. Console: You have asthma too?

Patient: It bothers me most in the summertime.

Dr. Console: What's it like? What happens?

Patient: The muscles in your neck pull and sometimes you feel like you just can't get any air and you feel pulled. I really try not to get too excited because once it happened while I was in a recovery room after an ulcer operation. Well, I didn't know anything about that, I just know I had it. And then another time I know, I was upset about something and the next thing I know I couldn't breathe. It took quite a lot of injections and medicine and stuff to make it stop. I had to take all my drapes down and get rid of the animal I had, and it got a lot better after that. The doctor said it has a lot to do with something in the air. Because when I go outside I can't breathe.

Dr. Console: Outside.

Patient: Yeah, if I go out to the store or something like that, I have to go back in. I can't get any air.

Dr. Console: Did you ever hear of this kind of asthma? Where you can't go outside and have to stay *indoors*?

Dr. Console: What could be in the air, outside?

Patient: I don't know what it could be. I just know I wheeze a lot. I sound like a teakettle. Sometimes I wake up at night with it. But it doesn't bother me that much now. I haven't had it since I've been in the hospital.

Dr. Console: But you've been a pretty happy person?

Patient: I think so. I don't think I've been very morbid . . . very sad.

Dr. Console: Even with all your sicknesses you haven't been morbid.

Patient: I don't feel that I have. I try to be pretty cheerful. There's no point in crying about it. It just happens. All I want is to get better. To know what it's like to get up and not be hurting or have headaches, or you know, can't eat. Things like that. Be able to do the things I used to do. I'm not a fanatic about cleaning the house and things like that but I like my son's clothes to be just so. And I feel the same way about myself. But when you don't have that get-up-and-go where you can do anything, it bothers me.

Dr. Console: So if you got well, you would then have a lot of energy to do all this cleaning and take care of your son's clothes.

Patient: And get out and get a job and, you know, see things, do things. I want to . . . maybe travel somewhere, do something. I don't want to just sit in a rut.

Dr. Console: What about my question to her, "If you got well then you'd have the energy to clean the house and clothes and so on?" What was I pointing to?

Dr. Bond: If she gets well she'll have to be a normal, adult mother . . . a woman.

Dr. Console: Yes . . . and notice that after that she adds "to travel." What traveling might this woman be able to do? What is the patient really describing?

Dr. Vis: A fantasy.

Dr. Console: A fantasy. A very sad fantasy. If she got well, she still would not have the ability to travel.

Dr. Bond: She seems very depressed. Or maybe it's me.

Dr. Console: Yes . . . I think it's you (*group laughter*). I think it's all of us. This is a very sad . . . a very tragic picture. But she tells us that she's a happy-go-lucky person. She does enjoy and find pleasures. And I think she's right. She does. What's one of those pleasures?

Dr. Waldemar: Being in the hospital.

Dr. Console: Absolutely! One of those pleasures is being in the hospital and being taken care of. To be somebody. And the traveling that she has done is from hospital to hospital.

> *Patient*: I look forward to the day when I can do that.
>
> *Dr. Console*: You say that you're a shy person.
>
> *Patient*: Well, I have to come out of my shell sometime, you know. I just can't talk to everybody. Like if I go somewhere, I sit in a chair and I stay there. If someone doesn't talk to me, I'm not going to talk to them. I'm at a loss for words. I can't talk on the telephone or anything like that because I don't have anything to say. Maybe if you asked me about something I read or something I did, I could tell you about it, but as for talking about the latest dance step and all that . . . I can't.
>
> *Dr. Console*: You know, you've been talking to me for a good thirty-five minutes.
>
> *Patient*: You're easy to talk to.
>
> *Dr. Console*: How is that?
>
> *Patient*: I don't know. The other doctor . . . Dr. Sverd, he talks very soft. He listens too.

Dr. Console: She has been talking about her shyness and her inability to carry on a conversation . . . even on the telephone. Inability to carry on a conversation almost anywhere. I pointed out to her that she'd been sitting there talking to me for thirty-five minutes.

Dr. Rubin: Most of the medical doctors on the ward aren't listening to her anymore. They're not interested. Your merely listening, in what she must see as an empathic manner, has obviously affected her in a positive way. The other doctors must say, "Oh . . . she's here again."

Patient: . . . the other doctor . . . Dr. Sverd, he talks very soft. He listens too. That's the biggest thing.

Dr. Console: That's the biggest thing.
Patient: For me . . . he listens.

Dr. Console: After having made this tape, I've occasionally had the fantasy of showing it to internists, surgeons, gynecologists, and so on. I would like to impress upon them the importance of listening to a patient. People often pay lip service to this idea but the usual posture is, "I'm too busy." There's an office full of patients and they can't sit and listen. It is not infrequent that a patient starts to give a history and the physician cuts him off and guides him into his area of expertise. "I don't have the time to listen to what else might be going on with you." I will also tell you that it has always been my practice, and I hope it will be yours, that when I see a patient who is confined to a hospital bed, the first thing I do is grab a chair from somewhere, draw the chair up to the bedside and sit down, and in so doing indicate that I am there to talk with and listen to the patient. That I do not have one foot in and one foot out the door. That I will spend a reasonable amount of time permitting the patient to unburden himself or herself of whatever is bothersome.

Patient: For me . . . he listens. I said what I wanted to say.
Dr. Console: And what about the other doctors?
Patient: They don't listen. They're always going. One foot is always out the door while you're talking. I think it's very rude. If they're too busy to talk, then what's the point in me even trying to say anything? I mean, I'm friendly with a lot of the nurses here because *they* listen.

Dr. Console: We discussed at some length the question of whether she wants to be in the hospital or out of the hospital. In which direction would this make you lean?
Dr. Farber: In the direction of wanting to be in the hospital. At least she has people to talk with. Also, from my own experience . . . it is true that nurses listen to patients. The nurses are present on the ward all day and often know much more than the intern or resident about what's going on with a particular patient.

Dr. Console: Well, when I was younger and made consultations at different hospitals, I would get a request from the physician to see a particular patient and do an evaluation because of some problem. I would read the chart, the history and physical ... then I would very carefully go over the nurses' notes. After that I would talk with the nurses and only then would I see the patient. I usually obtained the most valuable information from the nurses. Because the nurses are there all day long and talk with the patient. The patient tends to tell the nurse things that he knows the doctor is not going to be interested in. These are often the things you will want to know.

> *Patient: They* listen. They come in when they don't have to and say, "How do you feel? How are you doing?" Those two sentences mean a lot to me. But to be just sitting there like a lump on a log. That's for the birds.
> *Dr. Console*: How's the food?

Dr. Console: What am I pursuing here? What kind of stupid question is that, "How's the food?"

Dr. Rubin: You're focusing on that part of the oral gratification she gets from being in the hospital, her oral-dependent needs and how they're satisfied.

Dr. Console: I believe very firmly that it goes way beyond the concept of oral gratification. Indeed, that is important ... that someone feeds you, but this is the difference between the mother who props the child up with a pillow and leaves him with a bottle propped up on another pillow ... and the mother who does more than that. The propped-up child is getting substantial physiological, oral gratification ... he's being fed. But this is vastly different from the mother who is holding the child and giving it its bottle ... talking to it, cooing, smiling, hugging and loving it. This is what I mean when I say that this goes beyond the concept, strictly speaking, of orality ... that the nurses bring in a tray and give her food. It's more than food. That's why I asked the question, "How about the food?" It's an asinine question. In an institution ... a hospital ... how's the food? It's crummy! It's tiresome. It's the same thing over and over again. But it also is an opportunity for human contact.

> *Dr. Console*: How's the food?
> *Patient(laughs)*: It'll do. That's all I can say ... it'll do. I remember when it was better here. I remember when it was much better. I mean there are certain things I like, you know. I don't get them. I like liver. I like spaghetti. Things like that and they don't have it.
> *Dr. Console*: They don't have it.
> *Patient*: The only thing I really get enjoyment out of is drinking my coffee. Cause it's mine, not theirs (*laughs*). I'm not particularly—picky. I like to eat. I like to cook. And here I can't do those things. Nobody really restricts me. Before, when I'd get up at night and say that I'm hungry, somebody would go make me some toast and coffee or some tea or something like that. They're pretty nice to me. I don't have any complaints. . . .

Dr. Console: Do you think that by this eating in the middle of the night, she's primarily looking for calories? No, of course not. It's more in the area of companionship and human contact. The food is crummy. Things that she likes they don't have, but this isn't really said in a critical fashion. Is she saying, "I can't wait to get the hell out of here so I can go home and have the liver and spaghetti that I like and that they don't serve here?" Of course not.

> *Patient*: I don't have any complaints about being treated bad. Like I said, I've known mostly everybody in the hospital for a long period of time. Like they'll say, "What, are you back again?" (*smiling*). It's a big joke.

Dr. Iglesias: It has the connotation of, "I'll see you next time," whenever she leaves the hospital.
Dr. Console: Yes . . . it sort of has the quality of "until next time," doesn't it? When she's admitted, what do the people say?
Dr. Iglesias: "Welcome back."

Dr. Console: She implies it. She says they say, "Oh, you're back again," and we laugh. This is quite different from the situation of a chronic alcoholic who is admitted periodically to dry out and who is tolerated with the feeling, "Oh no, that guy is back again." The nuisance quality, the displeasure . . . it's lacking in regard to this woman's description of the readmissions. "We laugh." . . . It almost has the quality of a homecoming.

> *Patient*: What else can I say.
> *Dr. Console*: They laugh too?
> *Patient (smiling)*: Sure. Why not?
> *Dr. Console (smiling)*: You're back again, huh?
> *Patient (smiling)*: Yeah. What can I say. I didn't plan it. It just happened.
> *Dr. Console*: What did you say about ulcers earlier?
> *Patient*: Yes. I had an ulcer operation. I didn't mention that?
> *Dr. Console*: No.
> *Patient*: It's hard to keep up with it all *(laughing)*. I'd like to forget about them. If they didn't hurt I wouldn't even remember them. You know, I get . . . what do you call them again, keloids. I got another one growing up here from a bone marrow. I have a tendency to do that. They just hurt. But that's neither here nor there because I had it for a while. It doesn't really bother me too much.

Dr. Console: She's describing the keloids and she says that they don't really bother her that much. What is she really saying?

Dr. Marcus: "They bother me but that's the price you pay for being a hospital patient." She's saying that she's had so many procedures and operations that this is to be expected.

Dr. Console: You're suggesting then that they do bother her but that she's covering it over.

Dr. Marcus: Yes.

Dr. Chassen: I think that she enjoys having them. It's sort of like an albatross that she can wear around her neck. It's almost an expiation to have a deformity.

Dr. Console: I think that what she's saying, though, goes beyond the keloids.

Dr. Zimmer: She's talking about being used to pain in general.

Dr. Console: Used to it in what sense?

Dr. Zimmer: I think it's gotten to the point where she's deriving gratification from the pain.

Dr. Console: Firstly, do keloids hurt? I never knew that.

Dr. Vis: I think her point is that chronic illness doesn't bother her. She has been having illnesses for so many years that there's almost nothing that bothers her.

Dr. Console: That's exactly what she's saying. She's not saying, "I've grown accustomed to it" but rather she's saying that this is a way of life. This brings her to the hospital and the nurses say, "Oh, you're back again," and they all laugh. They come at night. It's a home for her. It is a haven from the impoverished life that this woman has described.

Patient: The ulcer operation I had when I was working in that cleaners. I started to have trouble with my stomach. And then I had never even heard of ulcers. The doctor said that it really was unusual for someone that young to have them that bad. And I neither drank nor smoked. And I don't drink now. I always used to think that people who drank a lot were the people with all the problems but it's not true.

Dr. Console: How might we interpret her internal response to the doctor having told her that it was unusual to have ulcers so early? So young?

Dr. Alper: Well, it seems from what she said afterwards, that she neither drank nor smoked, that in some way the doctor was putting some of the responsibility on her. As though she had caused or wanted to have the ulcers. She's defending herself by saying that she didn't drink or smoke.

Dr. Vis: She seems to have the feeling that she's somewhat unique. It gives her a sense of importance.

Dr. Console: I think that is so. She's not really being defensive here. She says, in effect, "Look how different and unique it is. I didn't drink and I didn't smoke." There is the quality of importance ... uniqueness. In *one* area ... "I am something special."

Patient: I always used to think that people who drank a lot were the people with all the problems but it's not true.

Dr. Console: Even people who don't drink have problems.

Patient: Right. The ulcers were pretty painful. Something I don't even like to remember. It really was very uncomfortable and even after I had them out . . . that's really when all this trouble with the anemia started. And I've never really been, you know, together since. I just seem to be getting one thing on top of another. I just hope that there'll be a time when I'm completely free of all of this.

Dr. Console: Do you worry about anything?

Patient: I'm looking for an apartment. I'm worried about that.

Dr. Marcus: Looking for an apartment is something that means taking responsibility. You have to be active and aggressive in doing so.

Dr. Redley: Saying that "I'm looking for an apartment" means also, "I've got to leave the hospital."

Dr. Bond: Well, looking for an apartment is a minor problem compared to what she's been going through.

Dr. Console: Yes. We've been talking about all her troubles . . . her operations. She has just finished telling us that perhaps it was after the ulcer that everything deteriorated and that maybe the time will come when she's rid of all this. In response to my asking her if she worries about anything, she replies, "I have to look for an apartment."

Dr. Vis: This again demonstrates how comfortable she feels with her chronic illnesses.

Dr. Console: How does it demonstrate that?

Dr. Vis: That she doesn't worry about her somatic complaints. She focuses on an outside event . . . one of relative unimportance.

Dr. Console: That's a very nice way to put it. My question to her really was, "What about conflict? What about worries? What about internal feelings?" And all she mentions is that she's looking for an apartment. This is her big worry? In the face of all of this illness and all of this hospitalization?

Patient: I'm looking for an apartment. I'm worried about that. That bothers me tremendously. Because I've gotten robbed several times. I actually caught a man coming in the window and that keeps me nervous. Well, you know, trying to live on a budget that the city provides isn't too easy either. You worry about eating, clothes, stuff like that. I really don't care too much because we really don't go out that much. And my son . . . I give to him. I try to keep him dressed nice . . . the best I can. Outside of that, I think about what kind of life I'm going to have but I don't dwell on it. The only thing that's really on my mind is how to find a decent place to live.

Dr. Console: You said earlier that your mother was somewhat old-fashioned and somewhat strict. Though you resented it at the time, now you can appreciate that maybe what she was doing was the right thing. So that you've always tried to do the right thing too. Do you think about having done any things that were wrong? Have you done any wrong things in your life?

Patient: Any wrong things? Outside of being pregnant . . . no. I don't think so. When I was growing up, there wasn't really anything bad to be doing.

Dr. Console: There wasn't?

Patient: Not to me anyway. Not us. My mother was a pretty strict Baptist. We were all raised strict and we always lived by all the rules. And I didn't hate going to school at all.

Dr. Console: Any thoughts about my question and her response? I am trying to explore her awareness of guilt. Her response was that there never was much chance of doing anything wrong. How does that strike you?

Dr. Kent: She amplifies it by saying that her mother was a strict Baptist and that they lived by the rules. There were lots of opportunities for guilt.

Dr. Alper: I hear her saying that she needed the rigidity, the structure, to keep her from doing wrong. She may have had impulses or wishes but the structure protected her from having to deal with the realization of them.

Dr. Console: What other possibility is there in the matter of her not doing anything wrong? Mind you, she says that the only thing she did wrong was to get pregnant.

Dr. Rubin: Her being ill most of the time could very well be a device she uses to protect herself against having wishes to do something wrong.

Dr. Console: All right. So you suggest that she has a defense. Since age seventeen, when she had an appendectomy and all kinds of trouble after that, it's as though there hasn't been much opportunity for wrongdoing. Now, a defense . . . against what? You must always be able to keep in mind what a patient is defending against.

Dr. Alper: One thing that we know about her is that her twin died at a very young age. She may feel some responsibility about that death and may of course feel very guilty. So she may need all these illnesses to prevent herself from doing something terribly wrong to somebody else.

Dr. Console: Any other thoughts?

Dr. Meyer: Well, we also speculated that the child who died may have been the favored child. The mother may have had some angry feelings toward the patient for having lived on. The patient would also be angry at the mother. Possibly the constriction that the patient describes is a product of that hostility. In your question, you made a statement about the values of the mother and how they were taken on by the daughter, and that identification may be a defense against the angry feelings toward the mother.

Dr. Console: Are there any other explanations for what you've described as this constriction?

Dr. Farber: Her description of her mother is a very cold one. I suspect that she spent a great deal of time questioning whether her mother loved her. I can imagine the anger that she must have felt. It's pretty lonely to think that perhaps one's mother doesn't care very much.

Dr. Console: Which might have led to what feeling about herself?

Dr. Farber: A feeling of low self-esteem.

Dr. Console: She didn't think herself attractive, worthy, capable of a relationship with a man. And when it did happen, it took a very unfortunate course, with an unfortunate object choice. The man impregnated her and left her. That was at age thirty and I believe that before that time, her sexual experience was minimal or nonexistent. I believe she always considered herself to be unattractive and unworthy. She couldn't conceive that anybody would care enough about her to establish some kind of relationship. So she avoided relationships.

> *Patient*: I went to school with my brothers. And believe me, they kept an eye on us. I guess that when I got out on my own I believed the first bit of hogwash somebody gave me, that's all. That's the way I feel anyway. I didn't really get a chance to meet a variety of people. I can't see anywhere along the line, where I really had an opportunity to do anything wrong. You know? Not really.
>
> *Dr. Console*: Well, as you look back, do you find anything that you feel sorry about?
>
> *Patient*: The only thing that maybe I'm sorry about is that I'm not able to be what I wanted to be. Maybe I just wish I had the chance again. Maybe I would do things a little differently, I don't know. I don't feel that that much of my life has gone by where I can't still do something. If you can't be a lawyer, you can always work in a law office or something to that effect. Maybe teach music to children. I think about those things but I don't think there's anything I could change, because I couldn't change my mother's views ... or the way she thought about things. They haven't changed in seventy-two years and she's not about to change them now.

Dr. Console: So my question, "Are you sorry about anything?" was in pursuit of what? I'm still looking for some area of conflict. Some area of what kind of distress?

Dr. Farber: Psychic distress.

Dr. Console: Psychic distress. Some evidence somewhere of some kind of psychic distress. Where has all the distress been?

Dr. Farber: Somatic.

Dr. Console: The distress has been somatic all the way. "And I've got all the scars to prove it!" But other than a minimal suggestion in the last few minutes, the whole quality of an inner self that causes some kind of turmoil in a person, that gives rise to questions and to conflicts, to doubts and indecisions ... is practically nowhere to be found. She has somatized. Everything is expressed in organic, physiologic pathology.

> *Dr. Console*: You said you've been in different hospitals. You were at Kings County for the appendix. What other hospitals have you been in?
> *Patient (pause, thinking)*: Brooklyn Eye and Ear, Brooklyn Jewish, Cumberland, lots of others.
> *Dr. Console*: Have the doctors said anything about discharging you?
> *Patient*: What, now?

Dr. Console: It becomes quite clear that she has indeed made the rounds of several hospitals. But I stopped the tape at this point to demonstrate something else.

Dr. Rubin: She seemed very surprised that you might think that she's ready to leave. She doesn't want to leave at all. It seems that the mere thought of it upsets her.

Dr. Console: Yes. Her response to the question is a mixture of surprise and remorse, as Dr. Rubin implies. She is quite comfortable where she is.

> *Dr. Console*: Have the doctors said anything about discharging you?
> *Patient*: What, now?
> *Dr. Console*: Yes.
> *Patient*: I wish they would.
> *Dr. Console*: You feel ready to go out?
> *Patient*: No, but I'm bored.

Dr. Console: "I wish they would." Is she ready to go out? "No, but I'm bored."

Dr. Kent: I think that her, "I wish they would," really means, "I hope they don't."

Dr. Console: Then what would make her say, "I wish they would"?

Dr. Kent: It's hard to admit that you want to be in a hospital.

Dr. Vis: I think that unconsciously she recognizes her need to stay in the hospital. She is using denial to deal with this. She thinks that she wants to leave the hospital but the doctors haven't given her permission to do so yet.

Dr. Console: Do you have the feeling that this woman is alert, intelligent, perceptive and that at some level she may be aware that this is the right answer? She is supposed to say, "I wish they would." Except she's not ready for it. Again, none of these are wasted words. Whatever your patient says to you is psychically determined. It has a place in the individual's psychic economy. It serves some function. It accomplishes some purpose . . . some goal. I think at one level this is a matter of her doing the correct thing. She wishes they would discharge her, but she's not ready yet.

> *Dr. Console*: You feel ready to go out?
>
> *Patient*: No, but I'm bored.
>
> *Dr. Console*: Nothing's happening here.
>
> *Patient*: That's right. I don't feel like I'm getting any stronger. The nurse told me yesterday that it would take a while before they accomplish anything. The doctor said yesterday that they gotta take tests and keep track of my blood count. I know it doesn't happen overnight. But that doesn't stop me from wishing. I know you just can't feel better overnight, unless there's some way for them to pour a lot of blood in me and they said they don't want to give me any transfusions. I have the feeling that that would help but it wouldn't solve my problem.

Dr. Console: She makes it very clear that if they transfused her it wouldn't really solve the problem. It wouldn't help very much. What's a transfusion? It's a one-shot thing. You fill up your tank and you drive out. But she doesn't want that. She says, "That wouldn't solve my problem. I know it'll take a long time. They told me I have to have these tests." She says, "I'm bored," but I would suggest that she is not bored at all. If she was really bored she would probably have wanted a transfusion so she could get the hell out of the hospital.

> *Patient*: I have the feeling that that would help but it wouldn't solve my problem because I bleed internally and it starts on its own and stops on its own and they haven't found the source of the bleeding yet. So that's one problem that I do want solved before I leave here.
> *Dr. Console*: Have you had any thoughts about the fact that these things happen and the doctors don't seem to be able to pick it up? That you baffle them so?
> *Patient*: I heard that too. I've heard *them* say that. That they really don't know what to do.

Dr. Console: What does that add up to?

Dr. Iglesias: She's different. She's special.

Dr. Console: She's unique. She's special. The doctors don't know what to do.

Dr. Waldemar: She doesn't seem to be overconcerned.

Dr. Console: That's right. She does not say this with any depression. She doesn't convey any concern at all.

Dr. Cohen: I've been observing the way she sits and I think it is striking. She's slouched down in the chair with her legs spread wide apart . . . in an open, receptive sort of way.

Dr. Console: I must confess an unwillingness to see it quite that way. Rather, I would see her posture as a partial validation of what we are talking about. Namely, that she has an illness which baffles the doctors. With that there is no expression of any regret, remorse or depression, but rather there is a peaceful and relaxed quality. It is as though someone else saying this might have been sitting rigidly, with knees together and would look worried and concerned. She is wide open in that sense rather than in a sexual sense.

Dr. Rubinstein: I think that this also confirms some other speculations about her. I think that she's enjoying this talk, likes the attention, and is feeling relaxed. Very much at ease . . . maybe too much so. Her posture demonstrates that.

Dr. Console: Yes, I think I've mentioned to you that when I began doing these tapes, I was concerned about the effect of cameras upon any interview. I was quickly cured of the idea that this was going to be a serious interference, because very few of the people seemed to be concerned about them. Particularly so with this woman, who seemed so relaxed during the interview.

> *Patient*: I heard that too. I've heard *them* say that. That they really don't know what to do. But, if they don't . . . I don't. It bothers me because I figure that if they don't know what to do, how are they ever going to help me? And this in and out of the hospital business is just tearing my life up. I mean I can't ever get something started and finish it. It's just a constant in and out. I never know when I'm going to be home or when I'm going to be in here. When I went home, I didn't expect to come back here. I just thought I would have to be followed in the clinic and that would be that. One of the doctors said in the clinic downstairs . . . I have a lot of confidence in him. You know, he's pretty straight and certainly I figured if anything could be done, he could do it, but he said that my stomach problem . . . I had better get used to the idea that I'll have to live with it. They can't do much about that. The gallstones . . . they try to keep under control as best they can but the anemia is the big thing that needs to be taken care of. So when he said that I would have to come in, there was nothing I could really say. I didn't want to but he said they couldn't treat me outside any longer because they wouldn't be responsible. I was scared. Let me put it that way. You know, getting dizzy and falling in the house or something, and nobody could be there.

Dr. Console: Do you have any feelings about what she had told us in this segment?

Dr. Farber: I think that even though she gets a great deal of satisfaction from the feeling that she is unique, there is an inner realization that the doctors are not treating her correctly. That they're tearing up her life. They're not really getting at her real problem, which is emotional.

Dr. Console: Your feeling is that she thinks this?

Dr. Farber: In an inner sense, yes.

Dr. Console: I would have to say ... way inner.

Dr. Farber: Her statement, "They're tearing up my life" ... there's something to that.

Dr. Console: Yes. They sure have torn up her body.

Dr. Farber: With no results.

Dr. Console: I think there have been quite a few results. Again though, I think that a fair portion of this segment is her taking the posture that a sick person should want to get well. To not want to be in the hospital. But she's been there so many times and for so long that it all adds up to the idea, again, that the hospital is really a haven for her. Fundamentally, she enjoys being there. There is little else to her life. The hospital means people who care to some degree ... people who do things for her. I think that her mentioning waking up in the middle of the night and the nurse making toast and tea for her is something that would not happen at home. There's no one there to do that.

Dr. Console: All right. Thank you very much for coming down. I'll talk with Dr. Sverd.

Patient: I was scared for nothing.

Dr. Console: You were scared for nothing. What were you scared of? What did you think?

Patient (laughing): I don't know. I had a lot of second thoughts about doing this. I told them really that I don't have anything that I want to hide. He said maybe ...

Dr. Console: Something would come out?

Patient: Yeah. I thought that maybe the doctors upstairs had told him to psychoanalyze me and that when I told them I'm hurting and begged them to believe me, they'd think that I was loose upstairs. *The Interview Ends*

Dr. Console: So, we've now seen this forty-year-old woman who has given us a significant amount of information about herself in about fifty-eight minutes' time. How about an overall impression from all of you?

Dr. Chassen: I have a question. Somehow, my fantasy about how the tape would end was that you would mention psychiatric treatment to her. That you would try to convince her that she needed treatment. I'm wondering how you go about helping someone who is resisting and who doesn't seem to be psychologically minded.

Dr. Rubinstein: Do you think she would benefit from treatment?

Dr. Chassen: I think she might.

Dr. Console: What would you want to accomplish? What would your goal be?

Dr. Chassen: To help her stop somatizing.

Dr. Console: Using what devices?

Dr. Cohen: Substitute verbalizing for somatizing.

Dr. Console: That sounds good (*group laughter*). But how do we do it? How amenable is this woman to the things we have been talking about? How accessible to her is the idea that her life on the outside is grim, and her life in the hospital affords her gratification, pleasure, status and importance?

Dr. Rubinstein: And expiation.

Dr. Console: How accessible is all this to her?

Dr. Iglesias: Very little.

Dr. Console: So we ought to make the point immediately that in the course of the next three years, I'm going to try to teach you the best psychotherapeutic technique that I can. In that process, I hope you all learn that it is not a technique that is applied willy-nilly to everybody that comes along. In other words, you will not put a cast on a patient's ulna when he has a fractured tibia. This will be one of the more difficult aspects of your learning . . . the assessment of how much can be done. What would be a reasonable goal for this person? What would be overly ambitious and virtually impossible to accomplish?

I believe that to try to get this patient to deal with her deep-seated, unconscious fantasies would be overzealous and unrealistic. However, I think a great deal *can* be done for this woman. It can be done first by establishing a relationship with her. Suppose I could select patients and see them for years afterwards. I would establish a relationship with this woman, which would mean that after a relatively short time she would develop a very positive transference. She would develop the feeling that I was someone who knew what I was doing and who was very much interested in her welfare. I would probably see her on a weekly basis for many years. During this time I would hope to wean her away from her dependence on all the doctors who have operated on her and done all these procedures ... and help her to live with a bit more comfort, within the limits that have been imposed by her lifetime's experience. This woman is eminently treatable, but the treatment would have to be at a relatively superficial level. This does not mean that you would be concerned with superficial dynamics, but rather that by your awareness of her deep-seated dynamics, you could give her, in the proper doses, the kind of medicine that she really needs—attention and support.

Now, I just want to remind you that when we began this tape and had covered the first two or three minutes, a few of you made some negative comments about this woman. One of you was very disenchanted with her style of speaking and commented that she talked in circles and that listening to her was a frustrating experience. Another of you stated, "I just get the feeling that we're going to have to sit through an endless story of one hospitalization after another. She'll vomit a lot of verbiage. Verbiage that she will repeat over and over again." He mentioned that he too was frustrated in listening to this woman.

So two of you responded with a feeling of frustration. How do I put this question now ... was this feeling justified?

Dr. Alper I think it was. I think that she's got an interesting way of expressing aggression. She's going to make you sit there and listen to her story for as long as it takes her to tell it. Your role is to sit and wait and listen ... even if you're uncomfortable.

Dr. Console: Is that what happened?

Dr. Alper: Well, I think she did expect to tell her story in her own way. ...

Dr. Console: Was it an endless story of vomiting verbiage at me?

Dr. Alper: No. I don't think it was that.

Dr. Console: That's the point I'm asking about. I'm asking if that frustration was valid in light of our having seen the entire tape.

Dr. Meyer: One of those statements came from me. I recall making it (*group laughter*). At the time, I was anticipating that that was going to happen. Perhaps this was because of many of the interviews that I had done during my internship. I don't think it was justified.

Dr. Console: No . . . it *was* justified, at *that* point. If we were going to stop the tape or the interview there . . . it was justified. But in light of what comes afterwards, we have to reorient ourselves. What I'm saying is, look into this sudden feeling you may get of frustration. But then give the patient a chance to tell the story and pick up on the story. As we can see with this woman, it did not wind up as an endless and repetitive vomiting of verbiage, for which it did indeed have the potential. Rather, it turned out to be a rich, instructive and fascinating story of this woman's illness and the way she has dealt with it.

Dr. Meyer: I think that sometimes those initial feelings can set the tone for the rest of the interview. Had somebody maintained the initial feeling that I did, the interview would have turned out to be a disaster.

Dr. Console: Probably.

Dr. Cohen: I think that from a number of viewpoints, *she* is a disaster, even though the interview itself went very well. We learned a tremendous amount from this woman and it was exciting. But from the viewpoint of a taxpayer . . . from the viewpoint of a physician who is going to cut this woman open again . . . it's disastrous.

Dr. Rubinstein: I think your point is well taken. There's a disastrous element to the way this woman's life has evolved.

Dr. Cohen: I'm just wondering why you didn't mention treatment to her if you felt that she needed treatment, whatever kind.

Dr. Console: As I said, I feel she could definitely profit from treatment. However, not only must we consider the type of treatment, but there is also the question of when and how to introduce the idea. She wound up the interview with concerns about being "psychoanalyzed" and being "loose upstairs." That would have hardly been the time to mention to her that she should receive psychotherapy. She would have reacted very adversely at that point. It is a matter of your understanding what's happening and picking the time to mention such an idea.

Dr. Rubinstein: A number of you have commented that this is the type of patient whom the medical and surgical people tend to make short shrift of. She would be called a *crock* on a ward, and would be the patient whom the doctors ignore. But I think that this tape demonstrates that you don't have to let that situation prevail. By listening, you can elicit a great deal of information and avoid an endless cataloguing of symptoms and hospitalizations. You can, without bludgeoning the patient, avoid a review of systems approach, and help the patient tell a rich story, which you can then use at the proper time in the proper way, to help her. Something can be done to help her . . . rather than just cutting and cutting, which *is* a disaster.

Dr. Console: Yes . . . this woman has had a tragic and empty life. This leads me to another point that I want to mention. There was one time during the tape where all of you were very silent . . . you weren't saying anything. Dr. Bond then said that the woman was depressed and added, "Maybe I'm depressed." I tried to make the point then that it was not only Dr. Bond who was depressed . . . we were *all* a little depressed listening to the emptiness of this woman's life. And you would have to be aware of her capacity to elicit such feelings of frustration and depression within you if you were ever going to be of help to her. Psychotherapy would have to *begin* with this realization on your part, otherwise the counter-transference feelings would very quickly bring the treatment to a halt, or to an interminable and unproductive stalemate.

CHAPTER FIVE

The Merchant Mariner

(The video tape machine is turned on. The patient and Dr. Console are seen sitting in their chairs. The patient is a white man in his forties, casually dressed.)

Dr. Console: What is it that brings you to the clinic?
Patient: I came because I had cracked up. I was hallucinating and had the DT's a while ago and I wanted to straighten some things out. I went through the DT's before, a few years ago, when I was in Los Angeles . . . about two and a half years ago. I was in jail and in the hospital. I was in pretty bad shape. It was a strange experience.
Dr. Console: So two and a half years ago was the first time you ever had any such experience?
Patient: Yes.
Dr. Console: Any kind of strange experience? DT's is one kind of strange experience. You said you had cracked up, hallucinated.
Patient: Uh-huh.
Dr. Console: So, was that the first time you had such an experience? The DT's two years ago?
Patient: Right.

Dr. Console: Any impressions? What's my emphasis with this man?
Dr. Iglesias: The emphasis is on psychotic symptoms.
Dr. Console: Yes . . . the emphasis is on "strange" experiences. And of course this may mean psychosis. I have the feeling from what he has said that I must try to establish the nature of the first strange experience. Now it is very common that you will ask this

of such a patient and he will say, "What do you mean? What kind of strange experience?" Obviously, you don't want to describe the experience you're looking for. You want the patient to describe it and you don't want to tell him what you want to hear. So I characteristically say something like, "Anything that seems strange to you." Naturally I try to get, as best I can in the patient's words, his memory of something unusual . . . something different and strange happening to him. With the psychotic patient it would not be unusual for the chief complaint to contain the information that he or she had experienced a vision, a voice, or something of that order.

> *Dr. Console*: Can you tell me about what happened two and a half years ago? How old are you?
> *Patient*: Well . . . this is nineteen-seventy-four, so I'll be forty-two in November.

Dr. Console: He had mentioned all these things happening two and a half years ago in Los Angeles and I wanted to take him back to that point and find out more specifically what had happened at that time. With this, I asked him how old he was and what about his response? "This is nineteen-seventy-four, so I'll be forty-two in November."

Dr. Iglesias: He has to use a frame of reference in order to answer the question.

Dr. Console: He feels the need to establish this frame of reference. He has to know the year we are in at the moment so he can then figure out how old he is. Is this what most people do when they're asked how old they are? No . . . they just tell you. What does this suggest to you?

Drr. Iglesias: In view of his having already mentioned that he had had the DT's, I'm thinking of the possibility of organicity.

Dr. Cnnsole: Organicity because he needs a point of reference to figure out how old he is?

Dr. Vis: If there was an organic problem, you would have to wonder how he is able to figure his age out at all. I view his not remembering his age as his placing little emphasis on age. It's not important to him. This may be a clue that there is something a little different in his relationship to the external world.

Dr. Redley: To me he looks younger than his age. He looks as though it's difficult for him to say that he's forty-two. As though he is reluctant to admit his age . . . he doesn't want to be forty-two.

Dr. Console: He has white hair. He's prematurely grayish.

Dr. Redley: I thought it was blond hair (*group laughter*).

Dr. Clarke: I get the feeling that this man is going to screen what he's going to tell you . . . he'll be quite guarded.

Dr. Console: Screening and being guarded suggest the operation of some defenses. He's already told us that he "cracked up," he had DT's, was in jail and in the hospital. He doesn't seem to be on guard to me.

> *Dr. Console:* Forty-two in November.
>
> *Patient:* Right.
>
> *Dr. Console:* You were in Los Ageles for how long?
>
> *Patient:* Throughout nineteen-seventy-one.
>
> *Dr. Console:* What was it that you were doing there?
>
> *Patient:* I had just got off the ship. I retired in nineteen-seventy-one. I was a seaman in the merchant marines for twenty years.

Dr. Console: What about the speculation that there may be some organicity here?

Dr. Iglesias: He seems intact enough. It just seemed to me that his method of answering the question about his age was a concrete and possibly organic one.

Dr. Console: Perhaps. But at this point there are large portions of his memory that are intact. He seems to have good recall. So, he was in Los Angeles because he had just gotten off the ship. For twenty years he had been in the merchant marines. Does this tell you anything?

Dr. Bond: There may be a fear of getting older now that he's retiring. He had been involved in a masculine sort of career.

Dr. Drucker: It sounds as though he must have had enough stability to stay at a job for this period of time.

Dr. Dulay: I would be thinking about drugs and alcohol, since he was in the service for so long a period.

Dr. Alper: It suggests that he may have been a rootless man. He may not have had much family or friends or any particular home.

It sounds like he's drifted for twenty years. He's been at sea for long periods of time.

Dr. Marcus: Yes. There's a sense of nomadism. Even if he did have a family, he was out to sea for prolonged periods of time. . . . There's an isolated quality to it.

Dr. Console: In view of these thoughts, what about the idea that the patient may have been stable . . . that it took stability to hold down a job for twenty years?

Dr. Waldemar: Someone who spends twenty years at sea is not someone who has the usual goals in life. He's not someone who takes pleasure in acquiring things, keeping close ties to family and so on.

Dr. Vis: We have to speculate that he has a great need to lead this kind of life, a need to stay away from closeness.

Dr. Drucker: This type of work may be such that it allows a person with profound emotional problems to still hold a job. It reminds me of the night shift at the post office.

Dr. Console: That's a very reasonable conjecture. So a great deal of stability is not required. This type of job allows for a great deal of pathology. And indeed the post office is a prime example of that sort of thing. So also is the rootless and isolated quality of the life of a merchant mariner.

> *Patient*: I was in Los Angeles. I got myself an apartment. I was going to AA. You want the whole story?
> *Dr. Console*: Yes . . . of course.
> *Patient*: Well . . .

Dr. Console: He had left the ship and was in Los Angeles and was going to AA. So the retirement that he mentioned may have been a forced retirement, in the service of his trying to deal with alcohol.

> *Patient*: Well . . . I was going to AA meetings. I was going for four and a half months and I had retired and had gotten a new apartment. I had one beer in the icebox. One day, some strange feelings came over me and I figured that maybe a beer would help me. I felt that one beer couldn't hurt. Annd it was about two o'clock in the morning and just one beer . . . I

couldn't get any more. And I took that beer and before I knew it I didn't know what happened. I was out drinking and I was full of resentments and hate, and things like that had come up from nowhere and I passed out. And the next afternoon I woke up. I woke up in my apartment. Next, I was walking down the street with no shoes on in Los Angeles. I figured, "Well, I might as well walk around like the rest of the hippies." I was dressed . . . I had a nice suit and a shirt. And I was headed right back to the bar that I was in. The cops picked me up. I was giving some guy a match on the corner and the cops picked me up. They were picking up people. Then I was in jail in the "drunk tank" with about thirty other guys. I thought it was all funny. It was all a joke, you know?

Dr. Meer: He seems to view things as happening from the outside. There was a beer in the refrigerator and then everything happened to him. It doesn't sound as though he feels that he had any responsibility for his actions.

Dr. Console: Well, he said that it was about two o'clock in the morning and he was having some "strange" feelings. He was a member of AA. He knows that he's not supposed to drink. He tells himself, "One beer . . . How much can it hurt? One beer." So, I'm not sure that he perceives these things as coming from the outside. After that he finds himself drinking and so on. He's carried away by it but he makes very clear that there was deliberation and considerable thought in the matter of whether or not he should drink that one beer. I'm not sure that he feels that these events were visited upon him from the outside.

Dr. Chhassen: He talked about the "strange feelings" that preceded his taking the beer. We have to find out what these feelings were.

Dr. Console: We'll try.

Dr. Meyer: He said, "I only wanted one beer." But for some reason, after that he got quite drunk. There's the question of what his impulse control is like.

Dr. Console: It has the quality typical of the alcoholic. "Just this one" . . . overlooking the fact that with someone who's had these problems, there's no such a thing as just one drink.

Dr. Allper; First, we get the implication that he wasn't drinking very much for these four and a half months, that he had been refraining. Yet he had the strange experiences that he mentioned. He drank the beer, it seems, to relieve himself of these experiences and apparently they got worse. He said that he then felt that he was full of hate and resentment and he apparently got into some sort of trouble. Then he woke up in his apartment, didn't mention that he'd started drinking again, but there was some bizarre behavior that occurred after this. He was walking around with a suit on and no shoes. It all makes me think of the various stories that I've heard in the emergency room here. The pathology that is present in this man is really unrelated to his drinking. His drinking may have exacerbated the problem.

Dr. Console: Absolutely! While it was true that the Los Angeles police department was enormously hostile to the "hippies," I doubt seriously that a man standing on a street corner, giving another man a light, and not wearing shoes, would have been arrested. Something else must have been going on. He must have been behaving in quite a disorderly fashion.

Dr. Vis: His affect seems to be quite constricted. Even though he is talking about all these events, there is not much affect at all.

Dr. Console: Well, is it true that there's no affect at all? He doesn't seem to be terribly anxious. Is there a flatness here?

Dr. Kent: I don't think so. He asked you if you wanted the whole story and he then sort of wound himself up and began to tell his story.

Dr. Console: Yes. I don't think it's accurate to say that his story is without affect. I think there is affect. As I perceive it, it is one of pleasure, but there's not any great range or lability. He tells his story in a rather routine way, as though this is not the first time. As though it's something he's accustomed to telling.

Dr. Vis: It's possible that he's seen many psychiatrists over a long period of time and that he's repeated the same story over and over. It may not be very anxiety-provoking for him and he tells it in a matter-of-fact way.

Dr. Console: Well, we know that he's been hospitalized, so that indeed he has seen some psychiatrists in the past.

Patient: I didn't really do anything. And then the booze wore off ... I must have had at least six bottles ... and then I started hallucinating. I thought that everybody was going to kill me there and I got really fearful. They took me out of there and they put me in solitary. I was in a cell by myself. I was still hallucinating and I remember the cops taking me out of jail. They took me to the hospital. I didn't even know what I was doing at this hospital. I walked away and began wandering around Los Angeles and ended up drinking more in a bar somewhere. I had a beer. I was drinking so fast ... my mind was working so fast. Some friends took me home and I was still hallucinating. I was stopping up the sink. I was putting garbage in the refrigerator. I was turning around the pictures. Everything was all wrong. They took me to a psychiatrist ...

Dr. Console: What do you think of his description of these events?

Dr. McDermott: He was turning his world upside down and inside out, putting the garbage in the refrigerator and turning the pictures around to face the wall. Maybe that's the way he felt—as though he was inside out, mixed up and upside down.

Dr. Console: And he's trying to right things in some way.

Dr. Marcus: There's a vivid quality to his talk about these hallucinations. It makes me think that maybe it's related to the alcohol. But we have to wonder ... he was dry for four and a half months beforehand. What were these strange feelings that he had before he started drinking and that he had when the alcohol began to wear off? It doesn't seem to have been a withdrawal reaction. It seems to have been more related to a psychotic process. Also, I'm struck by the episode in jail. Conditions in such a place are not the most propitious for someone who has problems relating to people. Dirty, intimate ... with thirty other men in the same cell.

Dr. Iglesias: We have to wonder further about the nature and quality of these hallucinations. He hasn't described them as visual or whatever. No story about feeling things crawling on his skin or anything like that.

Dr. Console: All right, so up until now he hasn't given us the classical story of the onset of an episode of delirium tremens, with the possible exception of his experience when he was in the drunk tank, where he thought that people wanted to kill him.

Dr. Kent: I'd like to take a flyer at this point and try to draw a few things together. He talked first about being in the merchant marines, which is an isolated life that involves being exclusively around other men for long periods of time. The only detail that he offered so far about his so-called hallucinations, was that he felt that other people were going to kill him. The paranoia raises the question of homosexuality. He was in a drunk tank with thirty other men and it was at that point specifically when he began to feel that other people, probably men, wanted to kill him. He described his thoughts racing through his mind and I wonder if he was in some kind of a panic state.

Dr. Console: Let me tell you that when you hear one portion of the triad, you must think of the rest of the triad: alcohol, paranoia, and homosexuality. If you hear any one of them, at least think about the other two. I think this is what you're doing. These three things often go together. Alcohol may very well lead to homosexual impulses . . . and then to paranoia, in the susceptible person.

Patient: They took me to a psychiatrist. I went to see him in a hospital. I thought I was sitting in some whorehouse. I saw my friend out there in the hall, I saw the Coca-Cola machine, and it was a strange thing. He was asking me questions and I was answering all the questions. They put me in the hospital. I was in the hospital for five days. Then, after they let me out of the hospital, I was still on drugs. For a while everything was quiet and peaceful but I still had these strange feelings. So I went back to the bar and I began drinking again. I seen myself getting worse, to the point where I could hardly walk. I couldn't function properly. I could run down the block but I couldn't walk. It was a strain to walk down the block and I had to run. Everything I did was a strain. My friends couldn't take care of me and they lent me the money and put me on a plane and sent me back to New York.

Dr. Marcus: I think this man is in a panic. He feels more comfortable running down the street than he does walking. He was probably quite comfortable when they put him on a plane and sent him to New York.

Dr. Console: Yes. Don't you get the feeling that he's enjoying the interview situation? Is he trying to cover things up? Is he withholding?

Dr. Waldemar: No ... the impression he gives is, "A funny thing happened to me."

Dr. Console: Yes ... "On my way here, a few funny things happened to me" (*group laughter*). Now, all of this is being said by him with affect. You might have questions about the appropriateness of the affect with which he presents his story. But there's plenty of affect here. As though all of this was a big joke. The quality is inappropriate ... he's enjoying telling the story.

Dr. Meyer: It's pretty clear that he is or was psychotic. We don't know if it's an organic psychosis or if it's functional. You have to wonder if he isn't lying about being dry for that four-month period of time, because he talked about being disoriented and confused as well being paranoid and frightened. So I really wonder if this isn't a case of DT's mixed in with an acute schizophrenic reaction.

Dr. Console: Yes ... you have a perfect right to wonder about that. A schizophrenic person is not immune to other illnesses.

Patient: I was still a nervous wreck on the plane. I couldn't get any sleep. I got back to New York. My mother put me in bed and kept me on tranquilizers. She gave me three a day. I was in bed probably for a month and she cut me down little by little. At this time I couldn't stand up in the shower. I could hardly stand up. You know I'd get in the shower, I'd be so tired I'd have to sit down. I hung around. I was sitting around and going to AA. I had to go to AA because at this time I was remembering my hallucinations. I had seen so much fear in the hallucinations, I saw so many deaths. Like I was killed in the hallucinations and everything. There were bugs crawling down my throat. All this kind of stuff and everything. For a while I didn't really want to live. But after a while things

changed and I got back into working and things like that. For a
little over two years things were going all right. I was even
thinking of going to school to learn engineering but then I
quit my job. There were things bothering me. I was playing
the horses and drinking. I didn't know what was bothering
me. I was staying home trying to figure it all out. I lost maybe
fifty or sixty pounds. Then I just cracked up.

Dr. Meyer: Losing fifty or sixty pounds is quite extreme. It almost
sounds as though he was a derelict.

Dr. Console: Well, he was doing a good deal of drinking and
probably not eating.

Dr. Meyer: I think there's another triad here: alcoholism,
gambling, and promiscuity. He seems to be almost describing that
triad.

Dr. Console: Well, when they took him to the hospital in Los
Angeles and he was waiting to see the psychiatrist, he said that he
thought he was in a whore house. But what about the last portion,
in which he says that he had this job and things weren't going so
well for him. So he was at home trying to sort things out and
figure out what was what and then he "cracked-up." What does
this suggest? What might he be describing?

Dr. Drucker: It sounds as though his reaction to stress is to stay
home. His reaction to the job leads to a psychotic break.

Dr. Console: He's definitely describing a psychotic break. He's
describing the fairly usual situation that you will hear many, many
times in practice. You'll see a youngster who a few months ago was
in college and is now at home. The family brings him to you and
tells you that he's been staying in his room by himself, not going to
classes, and then something bizarre occurred. A rather typical
psychotic episode of a schizophrenic quality. This man isolated
himself and did this figuring by himself and then had a break. So
your idea that there could very well be something else going on
along with the alcoholism is quite right.

Now, about the second triad.... namely, that of alcohol,
gambling, and promiscuity. While there is some validity and no
doubt a certain frequency in the occurrence of this particular triad,
it does not have the causal interrelationship that exists in the one

that I just described. I think that you'll see many alcoholics who never laid a bet, nor a woman, and these things do not go together as fundamentally and with the same dynamic relationship that exists in the first triad.

> *Patient*: I was doing a lot of meditation. I got very involved with the workings of the subconscious mind. I don't know if you've read metaphysics and things like that but I was really doing some heavy studying. . . .

Dr. Console: Do you recognize anything here? He says that in the midst of this turmoil, he went into some heavy study and reading. He wonders whether I've ever read metaphysics. Is there a familiar ring to this for you?

Dr. Drucker: One of the things I've seen and read is that schizophrenics often become involved with pseudointellectual concepts. On examination, these so-called profound concerns usually turn out to be fairly superficial.

Dr. Console: You're suggesting then that this is not an uncommon finding at all. That people with serious disturbances in their psychic functioning become involved in a quest for some kind of an explanation . . . an answer. And they read all kinds of very complicated and esoteric material, that often, as you've indicated, is beyond them.

Dr. McDermott: I've had a few patients who've read extensively in philosophy and psychiatry. My impression is that the more disturbed ones tend to read more philosophy.

Dr. Console: Well, my experience with psychotic patients isn't extensive enough to enable me to say that the sicker ones tend to read more philosophy. However, I would put the reading of philosophy, psychiatry, psychology and higher mathematics in the area of the patient making an attempt at restitution—an attempt at finding some answer because he feels himself falling apart inside. Things are crumbling within him and he's trying to put them together.

Dr. McDermott: Do you make anything out of his asking you whether you've read metaphysics?

Dr. Coonsole: I think this is a common thing. It's an attempt to establish a shared understanding. "If you've read this stuff then you'll know what I'm talking about." It may also have the suggestion of an inner awareness that his reading is bizarre . . . he could be checking reality with you. If *you've* read this stuff then maybe it's not so bad.

> *Patient*: . . . I sort of became conscious of a higher order of existence. I became conscious of a higher power. I seen harmony . . . I seen peace . . . I seen beauty and all these things. There was no fear. I didn't have any fear at all. But . . . people couldn't understand me.

Dr. Console: So, the reading did have some effect upon him. W at effect did it have?

Dr. Drucker: I'm not sure I heard him correctly but I thought he said he was conscious of or was in contact with "higher powers." The reading seemed to reinforce the delusional material, as though he began to feel that he was a part of the metaphysical world.

Dr. Console: There was a communication with a higher power and this gave him the meaning of truth and beauty. This too is characteristic of seriously disturbed patients. They will talk of these overwhelmingly global concepts . . . truth . . . beauty. There is almost a poetic quality to their preoccupations and concerns with the ineffable. What it is that he really understood at this point is still beyond us. However, it is in the service of doing something about what he feels is happening inside himself.

Dr. Rubinstein: I think this segment confirms Dr. Console's statement before, that much of this is a restitutive attempt on the patient's part, because what he's really talking about is a crystallized piece of psychotic insight.

Dr. Console: He's actually said that he's found an inner peace that other people don't understand.

> *Patient*: But . . . people couldn't understand me. I was seeing such beautiful things. Then, it got to the point where I couldn't sleep because I was aware that when you fall asleep

you come into contact with your subconscious mind. I didn't want to lose contact with my conscious mind and I was staying awake for days and days. I knew that I was in real trouble. At this point I went to AA to get some help. I laid myself down in the middle of the floor and I guess everybody there thought that I really needed help. So they picked me up and took me to the hospital.

Dr. Console: Anything about this description?

Dr. Drucker: He seems to be describing pressure of thoughts. I've seen this often. There are so many thoughts sifting through the mind and the pressure to get them out is overwhelming. This can lead to very bizarre behavior.

Dr. Console; Well, he describes the ordinary person who falls asleep as being then involved with subconscious thoughts. But he couldn't let go of his conscious thoughts. So he wasn't sleeping and he attempted to do something about this. He went to AA and stretched out in the middle of the floor. This conforms to your description of doing a bizarre thing. But he puts it into words . . . that he wanted to get some help . . . to draw attention to the fact that something terrible was happening inside him. And the people at the AA center responded appropriately in recognizing that the man was seriously ill. They took him to the hospital.

> *Patient*: I was really in bad shape. I got a needle in the arm. At about five in the morning I wound up at Kings County. A straitjacket. I started to hallucinate the same DT's that I had in Los Angeles.
>
> *Dr. Console*: The same DT's. What sort of hallucinations?
>
> *Patient*: Well, I saw myself getting killed with swords and everything like that.
>
> *Dr. Console*: You were getting killed with swords . . . and bugs crawling down your throat?
>
> *Patient*: No . . . There were no bugs this time. It was the same thing again . . . I had to go through those deaths again this time. Only . . . they were more violent deaths. You know what I mean? Like being buried alive and things like that. At

this time I was in Kings County. I was in a deep drug state
from all the medication they gave me. Things got better after
a while. I got along pretty well with all the people on the ward.
You know ... sharing cigarettes and stuff like that.

Dr. Console: What happened twenty years ago that you got
into the merchant marines? How do you get into the
merchant marines? You were originally from New York?

Patient: Right ... from New York.

Dr. Console: So you were a young Irish kid from New York.
Eighteen, nineteen years old. How the hell did you get into
the merchant marines?

Patient: Well, all my friends were going into the merchant
marines. It was a matter of whether you were drafted or not.
It was either going to Korea in the army, or going into the
merchant marines.

Dr. Console: So this was nineteen-fifty-one, nineteen-fifty-
two?

Patient: Uh ... nineteen-fifty-one ... right.

Dr. Console: Nineteen-fifty-one

Patient: Yeah ... most of the kids in the neighborhood were
joining up.

Dr. Console: What had been going on before that? Until the
age of twenty. Tell me about your family.

Patient: Oh ... my family? All right. My mother ... well, my
real mother ... she died. A car accident. A drunken driver and
she died. That was in ... nineteen-forty-three. ...

Dr. Console: Here's a very important point. His original mother
died in a car accident, a drunken driver. Now, you are going to
make a very serious error if you do not inquire into the details of
this accident. There is a famous paper by Phyllis Greenacre* in
which she describes some of her experiences with "re-analysis."
Dr. Greenacre had a vast experience with the re-analysis of people
who had previously been in analysis for some years ... usually
four or five years ... and nothing seemed to be happening. Hence,

*P. Greenacre: Re-evaluation of the process of working through. Int. J. Psa. 37:439-444,
1956.

a change was made. I recall her telling of an interview she had with a young man who had been in analysis for four years and it had gone nowhere. He had come to see her in consultation, with the knowledge and consent of the doctor who was treating him. He had come to find out, if possible, why nothing was happening, and what could be done. Dr. Greenacre took an introductory history and in this session, the patient told how, when he was age twenty-one, his mother died in a car accident. Dr. Greenacre asked for the details of the accident. The details were that he was driving the car and his mother was seated alongside him. He ran into something and his mother went through the windshield and was killed. This question had never been asked in the previous analysis. So that, the first analyst regrettably was unaware of the true circumstances of the mother's death. He did know that the mother had died a traumatic death in an automobile accident, but he did not know the other circumstance. In other words, he did not know that this boy felt responsible for his mother's death . . . that he felt he had killed his mother. So, when I hear this man say that his mother died in a car accident . . . was hit by a drunken driver . . . I want to find out a little more about that event.

> *Patient*: . . . That was in nineteen-forty-three.
> *Dr. Console*: A drunken driver hit her?
> *Patient*: Yeah . . . she was on her way to change some gift I had bought for my uncle, you know. And uh—she said it was too expensive. I was a kid at the time. She went out to change it and she got hit by a car on her way back. You know? That was the finish of her.

Dr. Console: Is this a significant piece of information?

Dr. Vis: Of course it is! She was returning the gift that he had bought because it was too expensive. The implication is that he was responsible for her death.

Dr. Console: Notice how blandly he tries to deal with this. He had bought a gift for his uncle. She had said that it was too expensive and she was returning it, and on her way back she was hit by a car and "that was the finish of her."

Dr. Console: You were how old at the time?

Patient: I was eleven then. It was nineteen-forty-three, so I was eleven, right? She had always hated the Irish . . . because my father was never home. She had a lot of resentment toward the Irish. My father was never home at this time. He remarried and the woman I had mentioned before is really my stepmother. She had two kids and he had two kids. They got on together. I love my stepmother . . . she's a beautiful woman. There's no trouble now . . . they stay together. I have three sisters now and she raised them all. They're all married and they all have kids and everything else like that. There are no divorces in the family or anything like that.

Dr. Console: You have three sisters now? How old are they?

Patient: Fran is two years older than me. The other one is three years older. Then there's me. Then there's Dorothy who's a year younger. She's got six kids. Fran's got four and the other one has three.

Dr. Console: You never married?

Patient: Oh . . . I did get married in nineteen-fifty-nine.

Dr. Console: Nineteen-fifty-nine.

Patient: Yeah. I met a girl. She was a drinker. I was a drinker. I met her in a bar in Boston and we got married. She had a broken marriage already. We went to New York, then to Baltimore and finally to California. After that I shipped out. When I came back she said, "This isn't for me. I'm not going to sit around and wait." She couldn't take married life. She liked the barroom life and everything. So I said, "OK, it's your decision," and we split up. As a matter of fact I'm just getting divorced from her now.

Dr. Console: Your father was a drinker?

Patient: My father drank up until . . . well, he still drinks today. You know, Christmas, New Years. He worked in the liquor industry. He was a salesman and used to be able to get a lot of stuff for free.

Dr. Console: What was his work when you were a kid?

Patient: Salesman. And uh—I don't think he drank too much. I seen him come home drunk once. I seen the fights in

the house, you know with my first mother.
    Dr. Console: What were the fights about?

Dr. Console: What about my question at this point? "What were the fights about?" He's talking about the father sometimes coming home drunk and he indicates that the relationship was not very good. The mother didn't like the Irish. She had married an Irishman, but she was critical of the Irish and there was distress in the house. And my question is, "What were the fights about?" Now, in terms of the triad, what can we anticipate about these quarrels . . . what were they about?

Dr. Kent: I'm wondering if we'll hear that the fights were about sex, in that the father must have felt he couldn't get any love from her and the mother must have felt that he didn't really care for her. That he would rather spend his time with the guys at the bar, with his friends.

Dr. Vis: Stretching the point a little bit further . . . he might have accused her of infidelity.

Dr. Console: This is probably the most common thing that you will hear. The man comes home drunk and accuses his wife of having an interest in another man who was there while he was gone. That's the paranoid and homosexual component. Fundamentally, his interest is in the other man who allegedly was there.

    Dr. Console: What were the fights about?
    Patient: I really don't remember, but I think it was because he was always out of the house . . . gambling. As far as his relationship with the kids . . . I don't remember him ever taking us anywhere. He got married at sixteen. My mother was sixteen. I guess he was too busy working and when he wasn't working he was out gambling or whatever the hell he was doing. I guess that's one of the reasons I went to sea. I could never figure how people would want a family. All I ever seen was fightin' and things like that.

Dr. Console: So there we have a very clear expression of how parents are often models for children. All he ever saw in married life was fighting and arguing and stress and strife, and after all of that why would he want to get married? He went to sea instead. Now earlier he had said that it had to do with the Korean War and that his friends were doing it. That's fine on the surface. But now he's given us a somewhat deeper reason. He had long since decided that there was no pleasure and no real point in getting married and raising kids. He had never been raised himself. His father had never taken him anywhere or done anything with him. These are more of the reasons why people behave the way they do. Deeper reasons rather than the more superficial and seemingly common-sense ones . . . "Well, everybody else was going to sea so I went along." No. He had more reasons than that.

Dr. Rubin: His own married life was quite strange.

Dr. Console: Yes. You would have to wonder what the woman wanted, marrying a man who was a seaman. What kind of closeness was she looking for? A check once a month, a letter? Some of these voyages could be as long as six months.

> *Patient*: Almost everyone I knew who went to sea had a broken marriage. Maybe ninety percent of the guys in the merchant marines had lousy marriages. So I guess I fell into the same thing.

Dr. Console: So again, a rather facile explanation of all this. "Ninety percent of the other men had this difficulty and I guess I fell into it also." Well, this isn't falling into anything at all. This is "falling into" things that are responsive to inner needs. It is not accidental. It is not happenstance. It appears so only on the surface and once we get beyond the surface we can appreciate some of the reasons for the person's behavior.

> *Dr. Console*: What about school as a youngster?
>
> *Patient*: Well, I went for two years to high school. I quit at fifteen. And I never went to continuation school or anything like that. And where did I work? I worked in a factory. I worked in a laundry when I was fourteen, in the summertime. And at eighteen I went to sea. I was out in California and I joined up. One of the guys did his best to discourage me

right at the beginning. He said, "Quit now, on your first ship. I've been going to sea for twelve years. I'm broke. I haven't got a dime and you'll be the same way if you don't quit right now." So I ended up the same way. I didn't know the value of money then. I would go to sea and spend the money on a good time. Go ashore and give it away or throw it away. Then you come back on the ship and you eat and you sleep.

Dr. Console: So, this is where the expression "spending money like a drunken sailor" comes from. He's describing it very, very well. On his first trip a man warns him to get out. "Quit now, I've been to sea for twelve years and I haven't got a dime." Our patient realizes that he's been to sea for twenty years and he hasn't got a dime. But he had lots of fun during this period. He liked the guys. This was the companionship that was important to him.

Dr. Drucker: I'm wondering about the little interchange a while back, about the auto accident where his mother died. You didn't seem to follow up on the information. I'm wondering why. Do you feel that he wasn't ready for it at that time?

Dr. Console: You have to be patient. I know that I have an hour and will get back to this point. I felt no need to push him to explore it at this moment. Here we have a man who describes an incident of this magnitude, occurring when he was eleven years old, and he passes it off so blandly . . . "That was the finish of her." And then his father got together with this other womanm Notice that when I ask him about his natural sister, he mentions her and also mentions the stepsisters. He makes an immediate integration . . . he pulls a family together out of this. This was one of his needs. But he still indicates no affective response as he tells the story of his mother's death. I know that there's dynamite here . . . but I have time.

Dr. Kent: It's been about thirty years since her death. Is there the possibility that it was all so long ago that the emotion has worn off?

Dr. Console: I would think not. There should still be something there. It would still be accompanied by some indication of a sense of loss, of remorse . . . if not a direct sense of guilt.

Dr. McDermott: What if he had told it many times over the years to many psychiatrists? Would that make it less filled with affect?

Dr. Console: I don't think so. No amount of telling is going to desensitize the person to the meaning of an event like that.

Dr. Console: What kind of ships did you work on?

Patient: I worked on freighters mostly. I was on one tanker. I liked mostly these ships that sailed around the world, because they'd hit like twenty-six ports. Out of a hundred ten days at sea, maybe fifty-five of the days would be in various ports. The rest was sea time. I got to know all the ports, the bars and all of that. I was a refrigeration engineer. That was pretty good because you didn't have to stay in the engine room. You could go up on deck and walk around. And when they did load booze, they'd give you slips for all the booze, but you could still take a few cases. I'd have enough booze in my room for a trip around the world. So I didn't have to be ashore to tie one on. I could be carried onto the ship and then I'd still have enough to drink until the next port.

Dr. Console: So, he gives us a description of the work that he did. He had a certain freedom. In loading the ship, he could steal a few cases of booze and would always have enough around to keep himself at alcoholic peace for many days at sea, and then in a somewhat more vigorous alcoholic state when he was in port.

Patient: I would spend so much time drinking while we were at sea that I'd have to go ashore to recuperate. I used to go ashore and the girlfriends I used to have had to put me to bed. And I played a lot of poker. I was a confirmed poker player. I used to win, just about every trip too. I had maybe, in all the trips I took, one or two trips where I really lost . . . the other times I almost always won. I had one year where I really lost a lot. At this time I was smoking a lot of pot and playing poker and drinking. And I lost a couple of . . . I didn't really lose, because I made it up later.

Dr. Console: You said that you came into port and that you had such a good amount of booze stashed away on your ship that by the time you got into port the girls would have to put you to bed. . . .

Patient: Yeah . . .

Dr. Console: When you went to shore you didn't go ashore with the intention of having the girl put you to bed . . . the intention was to kind of get in bed with her . . . wasn't it?

Patient: Oh yes . . . sure, but I needed rest too, you know? I'd go ashore and sometimes I'd get a shower and a shave and a massage. After a trip where I'd be playing poker and drinking sometimes for days on end . . . I'd be in pretty rough shape sometimes . . . after staying up all night particularly. . . .

Dr. Console: What have I pointed out to him?

Dr. Rubin: It sounds like he wasn't going ashore to have sexual relations with the women, but that he was more interested in being taken care of. Either that, or he really preferred to be with the boys on the ship.

Dr. Console: Why would that be?

Dr. Meyer: Because he's anxious about having sexual relations with women.

Dr. Console: Yes. It could be put that sexual relations with women is not a primary concern to him. It's not necessarily a goal for him.

Dr. Console: Were you able, under those circumstances, to have intercourse?

Patient: Oh sure . . . I didn't have no trouble . . . no! (*laughs*) (*pause here*).

Dr. Console: If you had your choice in the matter of shipping out, which did you prefer, freighter or passenger ship?

Patient: Oh, freighter.

Dr. Console: Why was that?

Patient: Well, you're more confined on a passenger ship. There's not as much space to walk around in. Some of the chief engineers and all are stricter, you know. On a freighter, you miss a watch or something like that and you make it up with the other guy. On a passenger ship you would automatically get fired for something like that. They don't put up with a lot of nonsense. It's just better on a freighter . . .

you don't have too many guys, it's not crowded and everything else like that. On passenger ships you got a different type of crew. Everybody's looking to make a buck and to impress the passengers. It's a different type of trip altogether.

Dr. Console: It's really difficult at times to refrain from injecting a personal note or inquiring along a certain line that reflects one's own interests and experiences. My question to him about his preference, a passenger ship or a freighter, really results from the fact that for six months, between the end of my internship and the beginning of my residency, I was a ship's doctor aboard a passenger ship. I knew that his answer would be "a freighter" because I got to know some of these people and they made it clear to me that it was irksome to them to be on a passenger ship because the rules were stricter. On a freighter, with only the other crew members around, you could be the biggest slob in the world and nobody would bother you. Beyond that, this man makes it clear that contact with passengers was threatening and that he preferred the relatively isolated environs of the freighter. Obviously, passengers are of both sexes. Some of the crewmen would prefer the passenger ship because there was the myth that in the summertime, many of the passengers were "repressed" school teachers and the sea air relieved many of their repressions. The crew members liked to feel that they would be able to accommodate these newly "liberated" women. But the majority of these men are exactly as this man describes. Again, some of this is a result of my own life's experience and I'm sort of checking it all out to see if it fits with what I know.

Patient: Freighters were more comfortable. It used to be a brotherhood. I got used to them. We all were buddies. We used to complain a lot.
Dr. Console: Well, all of you were buddies and all of you used to complain about life at sea, but nonetheless you kept shipping out.
Patient: Yeah ... we kept shipping out. Looking forward always, to the next port, you know? I always couldn't wait to

get to this port or that port. "Wait till we get to Spain," you know. The good ports were the ones that were the cheapest places for booze and where the girls were cheap. That would be a good port. Like Barcelona was a good port. They were all good ports before they became so expensive. Like in Japan you can't even go ashore and have a good time anymore. It'd cost you a lot of money, you know? So . . . I didn't have no value for money, you know. I'd just go ashore and throw away everything I had. I figured what's the use of savin' money, you know. Because when I'd get back I'd gamble. I'd usually go to the race track when I'd get back. I'd go until I'd be busted. If you're gonna go with the horses, what's the difference where you spend your money? One time I thought I had a money problem instead of a drinking problem. I thought that the reasons for my troubles were that I was bad with money. I don't count my money. I don't have to worry about it.

Dr. Console: If you don't count it.

Patient(*(laughs)*): If I don't count it, I don't have to worry about it. I actually made two trips around the world, which was in seven months, and I went ashore and spent money all over on booze and cards and girls and everything like that, and you'd ask how much this or that is and they'd say, "This is five thousand yen, or ten thousand yen or ten thousand francs. . . ." Instead of figuring out how much that would be in American money, I'd just pay for it and that would be it. So after the trip was over I figured it out that I spent seven hundred dollars more than I made. That doesn't work. The reason that I spent seven hundred dollars more than I made was because I swung nineteen hundred dollars in a poker game . . . 'cause I used to keep track of my poker winnings. And I only went off the ship with twelve hundred dollars. What can I say . . . it was a sailor's life. It was a drunken life. It was a poker-player's life. It was a horse-player's life, and that's what it was. I lived it to the fullest. If I had twenty dollars in my pocket and they told me there was a sea-going job upstairs, and I had to decide should I take the job or should I go to the racetrack . . . I'd go to the racetrack. I'd figure, "why should I go to sea? I have twenty dollars."

Dr. Console: Do you have any feelings about the philosophy that he's expounding? "Why go to work if you have a few dollars? You can go to the racetrack. Money is nothing." Any thoughts as to what this might derive from?

Dr. Drucker: Well, he certainly doesn't sound like the kind of person who hoards his money . . . the anal, compulsive character. I'm not sure I'm familiar with the sort of character structure that makes for the person who always has to squander.

Dr. McDermott: There are many reasons besides money for which a person may work. He apparently works, or he claims to work, not primarily or exclusively for money, but for what he can get with it. When he has his alcohol and so on, he no longer has to work.

Dr. Console: Well, the question of character certainly is involved. It has little to do, I think, with the "anal" character, but more with the "oral" character.

Dr. Drucker: The retention or the spending?

Dr. Console: The behavior in general.

Dr. Meyer: I was thinking that this behavior can derive from a number of things within him. There may be a great deal of anxiety for him when he has to deal with people in a situation where there may be some permanence or lasting relationships. Also, he seems to me to be a man who is chronically depressed and who seeks excitement in his life to make him feel something.

Dr. Console: Well, I would ask you this question: is it your conception that the baby at the breast worries about where the next meal is coming from?

Dr. Meyer: No.

Dr. Console: Is there such a great difference between what this man is describing, and the baby's attitude toward being fed? He gets it, his belly is full, and he's satisfied until the next time, and then something's put in the mouth and he's satisfied again. There's a very primitive and oral quality to this man's description of his attitudes about money . . . the no saving. That brings in some "anal" qualities to be sure . . . but I think that, fundamentally, we're dealing with a severely regressed oral character.

Dr. Rubinstein: I think that, striking as this squandering and incorporative behavior is, it's the incapacity to delay that is most prominent. He cannot delay gratification.

Dr. Console: Yes . . . there is the quality of, "I want it and I want it now. What kind of nonsense is it to put off or delay?" To tolerate some frustration in the service of a more advanced goal is clearly beyond him.

Dr. Marcus: He even mentioned that when he was impulsively spending his money he stopped trying to figure out how much the foreign currency was worth. He just spent it. He didn't want to be aware of the fact that he was spending the money,

Dr. Rubinstein: His comment about this is very interesting. He said that if you don't count your money, you don't have to worry about it. He tells us that he's an expert at denial.

Dr. Console: Yes. This is a very primitive quality, the denial. "Don't count your money and then you can't really worry about it. You don't know what you've got or how much you had to begin with." It's a magical and primitive solution.

Dr. Cohen: Do you think that this man obtained pleasure from all these activities?

Dr. Console: That's a good question. I think you're asking if he obtains pleasure in a positive sense. I would have to say that the answer to that is probably no. He's obtaining a negative pleasure in running away from something . . . in the avoidance of anxiety. In a fundamental way, this is what unfortunately constitutes the nature of much of the pleasure in this world—the avoidance of anxiety.

Dr. Farber: Could his spending money be symbolic of defecation or of ejaculation? It's almost like he's a seaman spreading his semen (*group laughter*).

Dr. Console: I think that as we go along, we'll see that this is not quite the situation with this man.

> *Patient*: In fact there was a guy there who was three months on the beach in Los Angeles one time, and at this time I think I was eating a piece of rye bread each day . . . that's all. My money was run out and I couldn't pay my rent. And, there was a job at the union hall available and I was ahead of this guy. It was a fireman's job. He says to me, "Patrick, if you

don't take this job . . . if you let me take this job I could let you have some money." He knew that I was ahead of him. So I said, "How much money?" and he said, "A hundred dollars." He was gonna lend me a hundred dollars. So I said, "You can have the job, give me the hundred." You know? It was only a loan. I paid him back. I went to the racetrack with it and I lost. So I finally had to reregister at the hall and take a worse job than that one.

Dr. Console: Was this something you regretted?

Patient: Yeah . . . but I had to do it. You can have only so many "no-shows." If you don't take a job after you register, within ninety days, you have to reregister. Sometimes, if you wait . . . like I would always wait for a refrigeration engineer's job . . . I would always wait until the last minute. Once I waited until the last day and the ship come in late and I didn't get the job and the next day I had to go on the bottom of the list. When you're on the bottom of the list and you're broke, you have to take anything that comes along. So I took the first job on a ship that used to go back and forth to Honolulu. I stayed on there for three months until I got enough money to get off. I was so relieved to get off the ship. They didn't want me to get off because they would have had a tough time replacing me. It was a low-paying job and everything like that.

Dr. Console: How was it low-paying? Wasn't there a union standard?

Patient: Some jobs are lower than others. Then too, it depends on what ship you work on. On certain ships . . . cargo ships, you get overtime after five, when you stay on ship while they're in port. But on these ships, they were at sea all the time, so there was no overtime. And the ports were lousy too. Like Honolulu and San Francisco. The pay was bad and you didn't have the port-time. So I just had to stay on there until I had enough money to get off.

Dr. Console: It's striking that when we started this interview, it very soon became apparent that this was a man who had suffered a severe psychological difficulty. The original description of his behavior with the DT's and the other bizarre experiences certainly had a schizophrenic quality. However, things have now sort of calmed down and the man is talking about his adventures; and he doesn't sound psychotic at this point, does he?

Dr. Cohen: He doesn't sound psychotic and he seems to be enjoying the interview.

Dr. Drucker: His impulse control is really quite poor. Do you think that impulse control as poor as this man's raises your level of suspicion . . . makes you think of psychosis?

Dr. Console: I would be careful about using that as a fundamental indicator or as a differential distinction. You'll see lots and lots of neurotics with poor impulse control and there won't be one aspect of their behavior that would suggest psychosis.

Dr. Rubinstein: I think you'll see quite a bit of this in your adolescent patients and in some hysterical patients who do a lot of acting out. They can have very poor impulse control and yet not be psychotic.

Dr. Console: They'll respond to every imaginable impulse and it can't be considered equivalent to psychosis. I would dissuade you from making that connection.

Dr. Console: So the good ships were the ships that stopped in good ports, had a good bunch of guys on board, and you played cards and drank, and you talked about the women you had in the various ports.

Patient: Yeah . . . sure, that's what it's all about, isn't it? (*laughs*) I missed a ship two times . . . each time about ten years apart. What was it, those crises at the Suez Canal? They were ten years apart. We had to go all the way around Africa on a trip. We had to go from Karachi to Marseilles and ten years later I was on the same ship where we did the same thing again because of this crisis and everything. That was a long trip . . . about twenty-three days. And both times I missed the ship in Europe. I was dried out with nothing to drink. In Karachi you couldn't load up with booze because it was two dollars a bottle for beer. Scotch and everything was very high. I'd spend a good two dollars in Karachi but it wouldn't be enough to last even two or three days at sea.

Dr. Console: So by the time you get to Marseilles . . .

Patient: One or two drinks and you've had it. We were really flying. In fact, one time there was three of us who missed the ship and got to Genoa. And the next time was in Marseilles . . . yeah it was in Marseilles again. This time I was alone. I had actually made it back to the ship in time but I had two hundred dollars in my pocket and I said, "The hell with this, I'm going back into town." I was drinking cognac all the way down the gangway. They were picking up the gangway and I was going down the gangway. There was a gate this way and one that way and I figured, "I gotta get to the bar" . . . and there was a barbed-wire fence there. I just climbed over it and ripped up my hands. I went in the bar. I ordered a drink and I passed out . . . right there. My friend Dave seen me going down the gangway and said, "Wow, I wish I could go with you." He liked playing around too. And, so anyway, I went uptown and I go into this bar and I met this woman there. She was about seventy. And she remembers me from like ten years previously. She remembered me. She said, "Patrick, you missed the ship again." I says, "Who cares." How did she remember me from ten years before that?

Dr. Console: An interesting vignette. There was a ten-year interval where he missed his ship in the same city. A seventy-year-old woman remembered him and said, "You missed the ship again." He wonders, "How did she remember me? It was ten years!" I think that this illustrates how incomprehensible it seemed to him that another person could have that kind of investment . . . that kind of memory. His object relations would permit only a fly-by-night affair.

Dr. Kent: Perhaps it wasn't quite so fly-by-night for him. Perhaps it wasn't too coincidental that he missed the ship twice in the same port, to find himself in the city of Marseilles and to run into this same woman again. Perhaps in some way she was very important to him.

Patient: So, we had a few drinks 'cause this time I had money and the time before I hadn't. Anyway, she helped me get a ticket on the train down to Genoa. It was a nice ride and by the time I got there the ship was just pulling out. So I had to get back on the ship. And one time I took off in Spain too. I liked Spain. I was there a couple of extra days. We'd always get into port at four o'clock in the morning and leave at four o'clock in the afternoon. Spain was like the best port going. You know? I says, "The heck with this. I gotta stay overnight and find out what this place is like at night". You know? I think I stayed an extra three or four days and I got to Milan on my own. From Milan I took the train to Genoa. I can't even think about these things . . . there were so many times.

Dr. Console: What things do you think about when you're by yourself?

Patient: Well, I don't think about the past at all. I stay . . . mostly I spend a lot of time meditating about spiritual values and everything else like that. I'm interested in spiritual laws. Like cause and effect and supply and demand and all this sort of thing. This is what I read, you know? My faith . . . I'm interested in raising my faith and raising my consciousness. This is all past. It doesn't even sound like it's part of me.

Dr. Console: So there's an attempt to obliterate all of the past. To spend his time in meditation and prayer, raising his level of consciousness. Consciousness about the present, but not about himself in the past.

Dr. Console: When you were aboard ship, you talked about all the guys raising hell, playing poker. What was the concern about Greek sailors?

Dr. Console: Again, this is a function of my own experiences. Do you know what a Greek sailor is?

Dr. Kent: I think that refers to a member of the crew who might be homosexual.

Dr. Console: It is specifically a homosexual who submits to or permits anal intercourse.

Patient: I don't know about any Greeks. (*pause*) Oh . . . I guess you don't mean Greek sailors. Are you talking about guys who like boys?
Dr. Console: (*Nods his head*).
Patient: There's some guys who are fruits on a ship . . . if you want to call them fruits.

Dr. Console: So he responds to my lead and says that there are some "fruits" aboard the ship . . . another term for homosexuals. So he is aware that at least part of the population of the ship is overtly homosexual.

Patient: There were a fair number of guys that are "girls," you know. But I never had no trouble with them. They'd mind their own business and I would mind mine.
Dr. Console: They'd kind of stick to themselves?
Patient: No, no . . . we'd treat them with respect. They'd come back to the ship and they'd tell you, "Oh, you should see the boy I had uptown," you know? Stuff like that. "He's my sweetheart," or something like that. And I always accepted them. They do their thing and I do mine. Sometimes I guess they'd fool around. One time I walked into a room and there was some guy who was in bed with a fruit. I didn't realize that he was that way.

Dr. Console: What surprised him?
Dr. Drucker: He didn't think that the other man was homosexual?
Dr. Console: Yes. One of the men was known to be a homosexual but the other guy was allegedly straight. This is the revelation that comes to people, that there are homosexuals who do not advertise or display the fact, and they are indeed like everyone else. This is what surprised him.

Patient: I didn't realize that he was that way. He really surprised me.
Dr. Console: You mean you thought he was a straight guy?

Patient: Well . . . you know, I, uh, I didn't care one way or the other, you know? I've had experiences with boys that were dressed like girls and everything like that. I've had good experiences. Didn't bother me one way or the other. In fact there was one time in Genoa the best-looking girl in the bar was a boy . . . you know? I always used to go for the best-looking girls. I seen this girl and I said, "Wow . . . she's a beauty." I go up to her and say, "What's your name?" and she says, "My name is George." I says, "Well I don't believe it! George!" I says, "Well, you gotta come with me, George." We went from bar to bar drinking and every bar I was in, I had the best-looking girl in the bar. I would say to the other guys, "Well, this is George . . . a guy." I had a relationship with him. And he told me he was from Canada and everything else like that. He was showing me pictures of other girls which were boys. They were working in shows and clubs . . . things like that. And some of them were pretty good. The first experience I had was in Manila. They got long hair and everything like that. I went into this lounge. I was looking for a girl and I ended up with one of them. I got angry this time. It felt strange. I didn't have no relationship. I just felt something was strange. They were all there. They had long hair and looked feminine. I just felt that something was strange there, you know? When they want to get laid, they just swing it up and cover it up. It was a nice bar too. I got mad and went downstairs and said that I wanted my money back. I wanted a girl.

There was a time in Singapore I had a relationship with a boy and I didn't even know it. I didn't even know it until the relationship was all over. This is funny . . . can I say it here?

Dr. Console: Sure.

Patient: I'm in this room with this boy which I thought was a girl, right?

Dr. Console: Uh-huh.

Patient: And I found out that I was putting my finger up his ass because I wanted to put it in the other hole and there was no other hole. Wow . . . was I in shock! This was a boy! I mean these guys are pretty good ... you gotta give'em credit (*laughing and smiling*).

Dr. *Zimmer*: This is the most animated I've seen him in the entire interview. He's having a great time telling you about this. Some of his best memories seem to be with boys who he thought were girls.

Dr. *Cohen*: Female impersonators can be very good ... I guess they can do a good Judy Garland but still, I'm hard pressed. ...

Dr. *Console*: When you get down to it ... (*group laughter*).

Dr. *Cohen*: The "lump" kind of gives things away and yet this man apparently had to go searching it out before he realized he was with another man. You have to wonder.

Dr. *Console*: What would his rationalization be if you confronted him with this? There'd be no point in doing it, but suppose you did.

Dr. *Clarke*: He would say that he was drunk or something like that.

Dr. *Console*: Exactly. He was drunk and she had long hair and looked nice and so on and he just didn't know. In the course of wanting to insert his finger into her vagina, he found out that there were no other orifices to enter.

Dr. *Drucker*: I'm a little puzzled at his inability to see that "she" was a "he." He didn't see that it was a man and I have the feeling that he didn't want to see this. At least at first.

Dr. *Kent*: The thing that struck me most was the incredible denial of the obvious genitalia of the male. I'm assuming that these people were biologically males. They hadn't had sex-change operations.

Dr. *Console*: I think that's an assumption that we have to make. He makes it clear that the technique these people used was to swing the genitalia up and to expose the rectum.

Dr. *McDermott*: If we assume that the patient is ashamed or that he would be ashamed to be considered a homosexual, then this sort of situation is an ideal compromise. It's dark and he was drunk, so how could he tell that it was really a man with whom he was having sexual relations?

Dr. *Console*: I don't really think that this man is ashamed of these activities. As Dr. Zimmer has pointed out, he's really enjoying this interview at this point and is more animated than he's been so far.

Dr. McDermott: He did say that homosexuality was not his thing.

Dr. Console: Everybody does his own thing. You see, I would want to point out to you that with this man's ego disorganization, there goes a polymorphous perversity. A perversity which is essentially a regressive phenomenon, going back to childhood, when any kind of stimulation that resulted in pleasant and gratifying sensations was all right. We can think of this polymorphism persisting in this man. He's making clear that it really makes no difference to him . . . that one hole is like another and he discharges . . . he relieves whatever sexual tension there is . . . and the manner in which it's done is of no great moment to him. It's of no great consequence. You will see this in neurotics as well. They will engage in all sorts of homosexual, heterosexual and autosexual behavior, just for gratification. In this sense, the object is of no consequence. Or we could put it that the object is an "object" rather than a person. I have always regretted the translation of Freud's works in which what should be termed "people" relations was translated literally into the word "object." With some people, as with this man, they are "object" relations . . . in the literal sense. They are not personal relations at all.

Patient: In Singapore, in one of these bars, somebody asked me how you tell the boys from the girls. I told him that the girls were the ugly ones (*laughing*). The girls were really not as good-looking as the boys. And now today, they have breasts. You get a girl in San Francisco . . . you just want to go get a blow-job or something like that. If you get a room and just go to get a blow-job, you wouldn't know if you got a girl or boy because they have big chests and all of that . . . the operations and the hormones. In fact, you get out afterwards and you wonder sometimes. I didn't have too many experiences like this but when I came back from this bar in Singapore I told the guys on the ship, "There's a whorehouse full of boys." You know? I says to the other guys, "Go up to this place." They came back and they said that they couldn't find it. They were bull-shittin', you know?

Dr. Console: So there really isn't much shame at all. The other men apparently felt the need to cover up whatever they did. But he didn't feel that need.

> *Patient*: Even in Japan this sort of thing would happen. Some of the boys would dress like girls and a drunken sailor . . . he couldn't tell, you know?
>
> *Dr. Console*: You mentioned that you knew of this place in Singapore that was full of guys and that you told the other guys on the ship about it. Then they went but when they came back they said that they couldn't find it and you knew they were lying.
>
> *Patient*: Yeah.
>
> *Dr. Console*: It didn't seem to make any difference to you. Why do you suppose they would have lied?
>
> *Patient*: Well, you know, some guys are ashamed of that sort of thing.

Dr. Console: I haven't seen this tape in quite a long time so I had forgotten this part. But I approached the question of shame quite directly with him and indicated the enormous difference in his attitude compared to that of the guys who came back and maintained that they couldn't find the place. He makes it very clear that he wasn't too concerned and didn't feel ashamed.

> *Patient*: I'm not ashamed. It's an experience in life. Life is full of experiences to be lived. In France, I used to know a girl. She used to fix me up with another girl. Not because I wanted the other girl but because *she* wanted the other girl. *She wanted to make love to her.*

Dr. Console: Now he describes a *menage à trois*. And he could probably just as easily describe a *menage à trois* where two men are with a woman. Here it's two women with a man and he's participating, but it could just as easily be the other way.

> *Patient*: So the three of us had a good time. It was a good experience. A lot of times I was with two girls. In Italy too. In

fact I have an erection faster if there's two of them in the room. I don't know why. It just happens. You know?

Dr. Console: You say you would have an erection faster. Do you mean that at times you might have difficulty in getting an erection?

Patient: No, I don't have any difficulties. But I think that if you're with only one girl and everything, that ten minutes later you wouldn't have an erection. With two of them, you want it right away again. That's the way it worked with me.

Dr. Console: When you came back from Los Angeles, your parents picked you up and put you to bed and so on. What was it you were thinking about . . . about this past life? All these good times and so on. . . .

Patient: I wasn't thinking. All I was trying to do was to feel well. That's all I wanted to do. At this time I was shakin' . . . I couldn't even sit in a chair like this. I was just nervous and I was afraid. I would close my eyes. I was remembering the DT's and the hallucinations and things like that. I was trying to put them together but they were hallucinations and you just can't put them together.

Dr. Console: Why would anybody be trying to stab you in these hallucinations?

Patient: Who knows? I haven't tried to figure them out.

Dr. Console: You haven't tried to?

Patient: To me . . . like after a while I was seeing people's crimes. I looked at a guy and I'd see, you know, like I'd see him runnin' over somebody or something else like that. You know.

Dr. Console: Now he's describing his hallucinations and he says that he'd see other people's crimes. What crime? "I would see him running over somebody."

Dr. Alper: This goes back to his mother.

Dr. Console: Have you ever heard of this sort of an hallucination in DT's? As Dr. Alper says, it derives directly from the experience that he passed over so blithely in telling us that he purchased a present for his uncle and his mother thought it was too expensive and took it back to the store. On her way back she was run over by an automobile and killed. And that was the finish of her. The hell that was the finish of her! He's telling us that to this day his guilt haunts him and he hallucinates men committing crimes and the crime is that of running over somebody.

> *Patient*: I'd never see who he was runnin' over. Or, I'd look at a guy . . . I'd see a guy stabbing somebody. I was somehow the victim all the time. You know what I'm talkin' about?
> *Dr. Console*: The question is, do *you* know what you're talking about? You give me an example of seeing somebody and thinking of them as having committed a crime. . . .
> *Patient*: Right. . . .
> *Dr. Console*: The crime is that they'd be running over somebody.
> *Patient*: Right, right. . . .
> *Dr. Console*: Running over somebody . . . is the person being run over a man or a woman?
> *Patient*: It was me.
> *Dr. Console*: It was you?
> *Patient*: Yeah . . . it was always me. So I figured that maybe this is what Jesus seen when he seen people and he seen into their subconscious mind. That he seen their sins and he was able to forgive 'em all. Do you know what I'm talking about? And he probably seen the sins of everybody in their subconscious minds like a picture gallery.
> *Dr. Console*: Could it be *one's own* subconscious mind where one sees a picture gallery of what's inside oneself, rather than what's in the other person?
> *Patient*: Well if you're in contact with the subconscious mind you can see what's within you and within me . . . it's all one. The subconscious mind is the subconscious mind.

Dr. Console: So, what am I trying awfully hard to do?
Dr. Alper: Trying to get him to see the connection.
Dr. Console: Will he be able to?
Dr. Alper: No. Not at all.
Dr. Console: On the first occasion that he said, "Do you know what I'm talking about?" I confronted him, hoping that I could get

him to see the connection. I didn't feel that I could do it the second time he said that. I think it would be a little harsh. You have here some fascinating psychodynamics. Here is really the whole picture of the destruction of this man's life. He led this nomadic, perverted, almost aimless life . . . like in the western movies where the girl says to the guy, "What are we going to do? We can't keep running forever." This man has been running . . . running away from a crime and being punished for the crime. When I asked him if the victim is a man or a woman, he said, "It's me. I'm the one being run over."

Dr. Kent: Is this tied up in any way with his homosexual experiences? I'm struck by his description of the fantasies that he occasionally lives in . . . his hallucinations. . . . He sees a guy running over another person, his being stabbed and penetrated.

Dr. Console: You can make a connection in light of the fact that he is a victim being run over. His mother was the victim of such an accident. She was run over, and in that sense he may be indentifying with his mother. In identifying with her, he becomes a woman and this means of course that he can engage in homosexual activities . . . with another person who is a man.

Dr. McDermott: There's another way in which he was a victim . . . in the loss of his mother. I wonder if he would have been able to make the connection if he had been asked, "Were you ever a victim when you were a child?"

Dr. Console: I doubt it seriously. I think that when he described missing the ship in Marseilles . . . ten years apart he missed the ship in the same port. And this woman remembered him. The woman who said, "Patrick, you missed the ship again." And he was surprised that she had remembered this. Now, he told us that this woman was seventy years old and he was surprised that she remembered. It is not inconceivable that this elderly woman was his mother to him, and they were being reunited. Her remembering him and his surprise could have indicated that he didn't want her to remember the prior incident ten years earlier, as he doesn't want his mother to remember that he caused her death. Now that may sound a little poetic to you but this is the essence of the working of the unconscious. The unconscious is timeless. What's happening today and what happened thirty years ago can be juxtaposed with no space between them.

Dr. Console: I'll tell you what I'm thinking about. I'm thinking about the fact that you said before that when you were eleven years old, you had bought a gift for an uncle and being a kid you had overspent. . . .

Patient: Right. . . .

Dr. Console: And your mother went out to do something for you. If you hadn't bought this gift, she would never have to have gone out. Then she was run over. And now in these hallucinations you see somebody being . . .

Patient: Well, I got hit by a car once. . . .

Dr. Console: Got hit by a car?

Dr. Console: What's he done?

Dr. Clarke: I think he's identifying with the mother and makes it pretty clear in this last statement.

Dr. Console: What's the reason for his interrupting me and saying, "Well, I got hit by a car once"? What's his object in saying this to me? As I mentioned before, I haven't gone over this tape and I didn't remember that I had tried to go into this carefully. I must say I don't know how I could have resisted the temptation, particularly because these tapes are made for a specific purpose . . . for you. I want to bring these things out . . . in the patient's words. I don't want you to believe what I tell you. I want you to see that it's the patient who will tell you these things.

Dr. Vis: I think he's using denial here. At some level he understands that you're interpreting his hallucinations as having to do with his guilt feelings over his mother's death. He's denying this.

Dr. Alper: I think this is making him anxious. He interrupts you and is trying to get the interview onto much safer ground. He doesn't want to deal with this at all.

Dr. Iglesias: He's aware . . . he's made the connection.

Dr. Vis: Not consciously. The connection is unconscious. That's the reason he's feeling anxious.

Dr. Console: I don't think he's aware. In effect he's saying, "You're right . . . I do think about these things, because I was hit by a car." He is defending . . . using denial to be sure. He has adopted an enormously defensive posture. He's saying, "All of what you are telling me is of no consequence. The reason I have these things is because I was hit by a car."

Dr. Iglesias: It's interesting. He joined the merchant marines at age nineteen or twenty and spent this nomadic life all over the world. His vehicle was a ship . . . he spent a great deal of his life inside a ship, floating on water.

Dr. Console: You're suggesting a very deep unconscious motive, which may have some validity. A ship may often represent a woman. We talk about "she." And also, he would spend a lot of his time on the water. If you want to carry it that far, it could represent a living out of an intrauterine fantasy. Such a fantasy would establish the most intimate possible connection with his mother . . . that he is again part of her body.

Dr. Drucker: Would you be concerned, considering how unstable this man is, that these kinds of questions could cause him to decompensate?

Dr. Console: I don't think so. He's quite defended . . . with psychotic defenses to be sure . . . but he's heavily defended. In a way, you would want to exercise more caution with a healthier person. You would be careful about the possibility that you might precipitate a real anxiety attack . . . a panic. This man has had all these homosexual experiences and has made it clear that they don't bother him. The better-put-together person has not had such experiences and whatever homosexual concerns exist, do so in a latent or unconscious way. So, with that patient you would approach these issues by pointing out his dependency upon you before you would approach the homosexual transference—about his loving you and wanting to submit to you. You would proceed very carefully because there, the ill-advised, poorly timed and premature interpretation could precipitate a homosexual panic with potentially disastrous results.

Dr. Console: Got hit by a car?

Patient: Yeah . . . I was dancing across the street. I was stoned. The guy actually stopped in time. He seen that I was drunk and stopped his car. But I just stood there dancing

around in front of his car and he stepped on the gas and went
into me. I went right up on the windshield. He drove me
about half a block. I was screaming at him, "Stop this
goddamm car." After that I went into a bar and had a few
drinks. You know?

Dr. Console: So, what does he tell us, which tends to confirm the
conjecture we have made?

Dr. Drucker: Well, first of all he sounded very defensive, as
though at some deeper level he was aware of some connection.
Secondly, I wonder if he tried to get hit by the car. He said, "I knew
he was coming at me. I was dancing across the street." I wonder if
he wanted, in some way, to repeat for himself what had happened
to his mother? I think that's what you mean when you say that this
is somewhat confirmatory.

Dr. Console: He said in virtually so many words that he invited
and provoked this situation.

Dr. McDermott: He said he was dancing across the street and that
the car actually stopped in time. Having missed that opportunity,
he then made the driver angry enough . . .

Dr. Console: How do you imagine he would have done that?

Dr. McDermott: He may have danced on the bumper or the hood
of the car, or something like that.

Dr. Console: I think he made it clear that he didn't move. He's
dancing across the street, drunk. A driver recognizes that this man
is drunk and steps on his brakes and stops, and waits to let the man
go his way. He very likely just stood there and provoked the driver
. . . asking for it, and the man stepped on the gas.

Dr. Console: When was it you last had a drink?
Patient: July . . . nineteen-seventy-one.
Dr. Console: Do you think you're through with alcohol?
Patient: Oh yes. I can't drink anymore. Alcohol takes me, I
don't take it. I don't know where it's going to take me.

Dr. Console: So here's a man who says that he hasn't had a drink
since July of nineteen-seventy-one and I believe him. He says that
he can't do it because alcohol takes *him*, not that he takes alcohol. It

then does things to him which are beyond his control. Does anyone know where he gets this idea from?

Dr. Farber: Is this from AA?

Dr. Console: Absolutely. This is one of the fundamental tenets of Alcoholics Anonymous. They persuade their people that they have lost control . . . that alcohol controls them. It does so because they are different from the rest of humanity in that they have a special sensitivity to alcohol. This is in their own language of course and I'm sort of rephrasing it. The message is that they must give themselves to a higher power and that only in abstinence is there salvation for them. I think that virtually any psychiatrist who has an alcoholic patient who says "I'm going to join AA . . ." will encourage the man to do so. He will encourage him when the drinking is of such a nature as to render the patient inaccessible to psychotherapy. The psychiatrist will be very content if the patient can stop drinking by going to AA.

Dr. Cohen: Do we have any modality to treat the alcoholic? You mentioned the difficulties involved and the resorting to AA. Can we offer such a patient analytically oriented psychotherapy?

Dr. Console: If he comes for treatment. But alcoholic patients are quite unreliable. Unreliable in the sense that it's very difficult for them to stay in a psychotherapeutic relationship. Again though, I would want you to be at least familiar with the approach that AA takes with its members. It may be useful to you in your work. I think that in some cases it is a somewhat simplistic conception of the conflicts and the vulnerabilities of the alcoholic patient, but there is no denying the fact that a great many alcoholic patients have been helped through AA.

Dr. Console: I'm not clear now. Last month . . . what happened that you found yourself here at the hospital? You were going to your AA meetings pretty regularly?

Patient: Right. I was going to them regular. I was doin' too much studyin' like I said. And I wasn't sleepin'. And then I started havin' the hallucinations.

Dr. Console: And it was your AA counselor . . .

Patient: Yeah . . . he took me to Kings County. Actually what I needed probably was a good night's sleep.

Dr. Console: You're taking Thorazine now?

Patient: No. I'm off it.

Dr. Console: You're off it?

Patient: The doctor had me on a hundred milligrams of Thorazine four times a day and eventually I was supposed to be taking a hundred at night. But I had a bad dream a couple of days ago ... a week ago or so. So I figured I'd get off the hundred milligrams. I don't want no drugs in my system at all.

Dr. Console: You've been feeling pretty good, now.

Patient: Yeah ... I'm feeling pretty good. It's my thinkin' that I have to keep in check. I think feelin' follows your thinkin'. If you think good you feel good. If I feel bad I know I'm thinkin' bad. If I change my thinkin' to good thinkin' then the feelings follow, right?

Dr. Console: This is another aspect of the instructions from Alcoholics Anonymous. They believe quite fervently in the power of positive thinking.

Dr. Waldemar: This reminds me of a couple of alcoholic patients I've seen who were leaving the hospital and had been placed on Thorazine. They insisted that they didn't want to take any drugs at all. Their feelings were that they had depended on one drug, alcohol, and now that they were abstinent, they didn't want any other drug at all. They wanted their minds clear and their bodies pure. This man was meditating and trying to purify his mind. It goes along with this line of thinking.

Dr. Console: Yes, to purify his mind by the proper thinking as opposed to contaminating it. It's almost contradictory on the surface. He suggests that the Thorazine was responsible for the dream or that it poisoned his mind.

Dr. Drucker: It seems like just about every patient ... every schizophrenic patient ... hates Thorazine or Stelazine. I haven't seen this with other disorders. You know, if a diabetic has to take insulin, he may not particularly like it but he continues to take it. Most of these patients, when you ask them, admit that they do feel better when they take the Thorazine or whatever. And then you hear them saying, "The Thorazine caused my bad dreams." It's never stated, "My bad dreams are being helped by the Thorazine." I don't know why there's such an enormous denial and hatred of these drugs by this patient population. It seems to lead to so much therapeutic defeat.

Dr. Console: I think that this is an important observation.

Dr. Drucker: It also seems to me that this class of drug is looked on as something special by the patients. If you ask a cardiac patient to describe his medications, he may know them but he may not know the names and the doses. He'll describe a "water pill" or a "heart pill" and all that. But the psychiatric patients know the names of drugs, they know the number of milligrams each day. I'm not sure I understand the kind of interest that they have.

Dr. Cohen: I wonder if it isn't something more basic than this. I remember a pharmacology lecture in medical school where the lecturer asked how many of us had had occasion to go to a physician within the last year and have a prescription filled. About half the students raised their hands. He then asked how many of us could remember taking the medicine as it was prescribed . . . exactly and for the proper length of time. Hardly anyone raised his hand. This was a group of two hundred future doctors.

Dr. Rubinstein: Well, doctors are the worst patients (*group laughter*).

Dr. Farber: I think that the whole idea of getting patients to take medication in general is important. There are many articles appearing in the journals that deal with this problem. I think this is especially prevalent with the blood-pressure medications. This group of patients seems to be the worst when it comes to not taking the medication as prescribed. Also, diabetics have a great deal of trouble following medical advice.

Dr. Console: What's the most simple explanation of this? What does it represent?

Dr. Vis: Denial?

Dr. Console: Of course. Denial of being ill.

Dr. Rubinstein: I think that there's the additional problem of the magical thinking when we're dealing with severely ill psychotic patients and psychotropic drugs. If a large portion of these people are suspicious and disorganized to begin with, we end up dealing with questions of mind control and the like. You often hear questions about "slowing down my thoughts" . . . or "Will this medicine change me or change my personality?" These issues don't come up with other drugs.

> Dr. Console: How are you eating now?
> Patient: I'm eatin' good. I have bacon and eggs every day.

Dr. Vis: I'm wondering why you didn't say anything to him when he mentioned the idea of thinking good and then feeling good.

Dr. Console: What would you have me say to him at that point?

Dr. Vis: I'm not sure, but I was struck by the fact that you were sitting there and nodding your head up and down in apparent agreement.

Dr. Console: Well, that's characteristic of me. In doing an interview, I usually develop Parkinsonism (group laughter).

Dr. Vis: It might have been an indication to him that you agree with this line of thinking.

Dr. Console: I think that to have questioned this would not only have been a waste of time but in addition might have been a little disturbing to him.

Dr. Waldemar: When you asked him about food were you looking for bizarre eating habits . . . health foods and all that?

Dr. Console: No, not really. I think I was just checking up on whether he had really stopped drinking and was eating a bit more sensibly.

> Dr. Console: What about women?
> Patient: Women . . . I just had a relationship with my girl. We were busted up when I come into the hospital . . . right?

Dr. Console: What do you think about that? "We were busted up when I came into the hospital . . . right?" What about that? You will find that some people speak like this quite commonly.

Dr. Vis: Is he looking for reassurance?

Dr. Console: What kind of reassurance? Can you be a little more specific?

Dr. Vis: I get the feeling that he wants to enlist your support right from the beginning. He's obviously going to launch into a long narrative and he wants to make sure you're following him and that you would agree with him.

Dr. Console: Let me make the question more specific. My interest is in ego functioning. In these terms, what might his question represent?

Dr. Farber: It's a statement about his object relations.

Dr. Console: What I believe this could very well represent is an inner awareness of a kind of ego deficit on his part. He needs another ego to find out if he's saying the correct thing. It is reassurance in a sense, but at an extremely profound level. This is the person who will describe to you that he goes to a party and watches another person. When that person laughs, he laughs. When the other person seems to be sad, so is he. Because, in a sense, he doesn't have the ego strength himself. He has to use an "alter ego" as a base line for himself.

Dr. Vis: I have a patient like this one, who always asks me "right?" I'm never sure how to respond to these questions. I'm wondering if I should answer and continually reassure him.

Dr. Console: Well, you would not respond to this kind of question early in the course of treatment. You would want a good deal more confirmation of the conjecture that the patient's ego state is a somewhat impoverished one. Then, the technique would not be one of confrontation with a patient like this. You would want to help him test reality.

> *Patient:* We were busted up when I come into the hospital . . . right? So when I got out of the hospital . . . uh . . . we got together again. Now this girl always told me, you know, she had an abortion a long time ago . . . right? She says she'll never have another abortion or anything else like that. So I come out of the hospital. She had got pregnant. She thought she wanted to get pregnant at the time. I didn't really care much either way. Oh . . . she's a drinker. She had a drinkin' problem too. You know? She hasn't drank in eight months. Anyway, for some reason she was drinkin' and I had to put her in a medical place to dry out. They pay a hundred and thirty-five dollars to get dried out. It's up in the country. And she came out . . . she was worried about the Thorazine. Oh,

then she didn't think she was gonna get pregnant. She did . . .
she missed her period. You know what I mean? Which made
me feel good. You know, I was surprised to find out I could
have children.

Dr. Console: Does anyone want to comment about his last
statement? "She missed her period, got pregnant and I felt good."
Dr. Drucker: Right after that he said, "I didn't think I could."
Dr. Console: Yes.
Dr. Drucker: He can now feel good in terms of his own sense of
masculinity.
Dr. Console: What are his expectations of having had intercourse
with this woman?
Dr. Drucker: Impotence.
Dr. Console: Not exactly. He said that he's never had any trouble
having intercourse or in getting an erection. I don't think that he
was concerned about impotence, but rather that he would be
sterile. He's surprised, and pleasantly so, when there is evidence
that he is not sterile. How is this different from most men? After
all, if you are married and the time comes when you want to have
children, you or your spouse simply don't use a contraceptive. She
gets pregnant. Is anyone surprised? Not at all. If you're surprised,
there's something going on. This man is surprised. So what might
he be telling us? In terms of his own awareness of the life he has
led?
Dr. Drucker: He may be thinking that the life he has led has made
him sterile. Destroyed his capacity.
Dr. Console: Has depleted him of this capacity. He is surprised
because in the light of his awareness of the dissolute life he has led
. . . drinking and whoring . . . he thought that he had lost this
capacity.

Patient: You know, I was surprised to find out I could have
children . . . after all those years of screwing around and
everything.

Dr. Console So there it is. "After all those years of screwing
around."

Dr. Meyer: Couldn't it be interpreted the other way also? That his life style is the result of the fear that he really couldn't perform adequately as a man and therefore had to run from woman to woman, never really staying long enough to find out if they would become pregnant or not.

Dr. Console: I have the feeling that you're taking a concept and trying to squeeze this man into it. While your speculation is one that might be valid for some patients, what evidence is there on this tape, that this man had this question about himself? Very little really. When this man described his playing poker and staying up all night and then going to port where his girl would put him to bed and look after him, I confronted him on that. At that point in the interview I asked him if he'd ever had difficulty and the answer was a definite no. In his conscious view, he's a capable performer ... very much a man in the matter of being able to have intercourse.

I think that his stating his surprise at being able to impregnate a woman is a result of a host of moral and religious ideas, as well as ideas from childhood which have to do with the admonition the child receives in the matter of masturbation. Kids are told all kinds of things in an effort to get them to stop masturbating. "Your brain will get soft or smaller ... some terrible thing will happen to you." Men—some men—develop the idea that they have been given a quantum of semen and that this is to be conserved and used properly. You must not use it improperly ... abuse it ... and here, years ago, before the sexual revolution and the sexual enlightenment, people did not talk about masturbation ... they talked about "self-abuse." This was one of the colloquialisms for masturbation. So the concept of doing harm to oneself through promiscuity, through repeated sexual experiences, is really what he's talking about. He was surprised that he still had some good "bullets" left.

Patient: So, what happened was that she said somethin' about the Thorazine I was on. She's afraid these are the pills ... the "zine" pills that had ... bad babies were born or somethin' like that. So she decided to have an abortion.

Dr. Console: That's an interesting observation. He was on

Thorazine and she thought that he was on these "zine" pills and that they cause birth defects. What does this suggest about the woman in this case?

Dr. Drucker: Well, certainly, she's not well-educated and it seems as though she was looking for an excuse not to have the baby.

Dr. Console: Well, I think it's fair to expect that she's probably not a college graduate and, for the purposes of our discussion, let's assume that she was looking for an excuse. My interest, however, is in the nature of the excuse. That he's taking Thorazine and it's one of the "zines" and these cause birth defects . . . therefore she sought an abortion.

Dr. Farber: It's a terribly aggressive thing to do. In a sense she says to him, "Your capacity to reproduce, at least a healthy and viable baby, is defective."

Dr. Console: That could very well be true, but as I see it, her concern is not primarily punishment, hostility or retribution directed toward the patient. Rather, I think she is doing this to protect herself. She has some persuasion that because he's taking Thorazine . . . and the "zine" pills cause these things, she doesn't want a defective child. Do you have any feeling that this woman may also be quite disturbed?

Dr. Alper: It's striking, but the only drugs that I can think of that end in z-i-n-e are the antipsychotic agents. Thorazine, Stelazine, Compazine and so on. It makes me think that she probably has some familiarity with these drugs or with people who have been on them. Perhaps she was institutionalized for reasons other than alcoholism. In the patient community there's always a great deal of talk about drugs and many misconceptions about them.

Patient: I didn't want her to go ahead with it but I gave her the money for the abortion and since then she's been in a depressed state. I have to let her alone though because she's alcoholic and at least now she's not drinking and she's doing the best she can for herself, so maybe it's just better that I let her alone. Let it go. So right now we're on the outs. I couldn't reverse her opinion about the abortion, so that was it.

Dr. Console: Are you seeing Dr. Sommers at the clinic?

Patient: No, I'm seeing another doctor. Just once a month.

Dr. Console: Well, thank you very much for coming in to talk.

Patient: It's quite all right. Thank you. *The Interview Ends*

Dr. Drucker: I was struck by the abruptness of the ending. I have trouble ending an interview. Often the time is up and the patient wants to stay. I was just súrprised at how suddenly it all seemed to end.

Dr. Console: I would suggest that when you're seeing a patient on a regular basis, you make a contract with him. In its most fundamental form the contract is that on the two days or so of the week you have arranged, and for the specific period of time that you and the patient will meet, you will be there to try to help the patient deal with his or her problems. When the time is up, the session is over. This is really your contract with the patient. Many patients will unconsciously use all kinds of devices to draw you into some very interesting situations in their desire to extend the hour. You must not permit that to happen. When the time is up, you so indicate.

Now in this situation, your perception of the abruptness is quite valid and legitimate. My basic concern with this man was the elucidation of his unusual hallucinations during the delirium tremens, namely his having seen other people's crimes and his having been run over. I wanted to bring this out in as much detail as I could, to establish that any kind of aberrant, bizarre and seemingly incomprehensible behavior, is fundamentally understandable if we really know what's going on. If we can elucidate the person's fantasy behind it, then the behavior is no longer senseless . . . it makes sense. Another group of residents pointed out to me that I often end the interview by asking the patient if there are any questions he or she would like to ask me. I didn't do that with this man. I learned after I had made this tape that this man had been seen by two residents and that one of them had asked him if there were any questions that he wanted to ask. He said, "Yeah . . . where'd you get that tie?" (*group laughter*). Now, the usual response to that question is, "Am I crazy?" In a variety of forms, this is the most common question that a psychiatric patient will ask you if he's given the opportunity. This man was given such an opportunity and he made a most unpredictable response, one that would make you wonder about his motivation for psychotherapy.

Dr. Drucker: What about the future for this man?

Dr. Console: Yes ... what about the future? What's going to happen to our merchant mariner? There is a slight suggestion of some stability. He talks about this woman with a quality of interest and concern for her. So it may very well be that sixteen years after having married the other woman, he will get a divorce. He's not divorced yet. And perhaps he'll marry this woman.

Dr. Rubinstein: I looked at the patient's chart recently and at the time of this interview, he was living with her. As far as we know, he's never really lived with a woman before ... not even with his first wife. He was at sea. So there's evidence of some stability and relatedness.

Dr. Console: Another thing. People who are quite ill have the uncanny ability of finding others who are just as ill as they are. A relatively healthy individual would find it inordinately difficult to live with a man who is as obviously disorganized as this man is. So that being psychotic does not for a moment preclude the capacity for loving at a particular level and in a certain way. Witness our patient's efforts on behalf of this woman when she started drinking again. There's something taking place between them.

This man could be like the many thousands in this city who are quite disturbed, but who are working and functioning in their own ways. They appear normal as far as the outside world is concerned. But their inner world is chaotic. Remember that this man worked for twenty years in the merchant marines and we hear of nothing other than the drinking, the gambling and the whoring, until he retires after those twenty years. The moment he comes ashore he quits his job and disintegrates. The disintegration may have been in the nature of an acute schizophrenic reaction or it may have been a psychotic exacerbation of a long-standing depression based on a pathological mourning and yearning for his mother. So the life of the merchant mariner was the defense ... it was the structure within which he could operate comfortably. He decompensated when he was ashore and when the demands that society made on him were of a different order than those of the brotherhood of the mariners. This is when he lost his hold on things. Now, he may be in the process of reordering and restructuring his life with this woman. And certainly any psychotherapy that you might conduct with this man would have to take cognizance of the importance for him of this heterosexual relationship, and a very legitimate goal of the psychotherapy would be to help the patient to nurture and maintain this relationship to the degree that he would be able to do so. Indeed, in the deepest sense, it might very well represent his finally achieving a rescuing reunion with his mother, but now in life rather than in death.

Postscript

Soon after the interview with Dr. Console, the merchant mariner stopped attending the clinic and disappeared from sight. He was not heard from again until nearly two years later when he appeared at the Kings County Hospital Psychiatric Emergency Room, desperately in need of treatment. He was accompanied by his stepmother, who detailed many of the events of his life during those two years.

His relationship with the woman with whom he had been living came to an end shortly after his interview with Dr. Console, and the patient had been living alone since then. His apartment was not far from where his father and stepmother lived and he saw them frequently. He had been working as a refrigeration engineer and had been seriously considering enrolling in a trade school so that he could take on a more skilled form of employment. The patient's stepmother stated emphatically that during this two year period he had totally abstained from alcohol. He was attending Alcoholics Anonymous meetings regularly, was a vocal and active participant in this organization, and felt little need for any other form of help. Indeed, according to his stepmother's account, it seemed that the patient had made a good adjustment and was leading a well-regulated and structured life with only occasional difficulties.

Those difficulties, however, were notable, and despite the infrequency with which they arose, they constituted major disruptions in his life. According to his stepmother, every five or six months and for no apparent reason, the patient would begin to act in a seemingly bizarre and incomprehensible manner. He would run frantically to the home of his father and stepmother and beg them to hide him. He seemed confused and dazed at these times and extremely frightened. He would run about the house in a distraught manner, putting food in the trash can and trash in the refrigerator, turning pictures upside-down or turning them around to face the wall, rearranging furniture, loosening light bulbs from their sockets, and peering behind closed doors and into closets.

His stepmother clearly recognized his actions as disturbed, but also realized that they had a private and peculiar logic and purposiveness that she could not understand. She and her husband would return with the patient to his apartment, only to find there the same scene of disarray. It thus became obvious to her that when her stepson was in the throes of these episodes, he was living in a world of "opposites" where, in a disruptive and maladaptive way, he was attempting to "undo" things that had been done, "hide" from imagined pursuers, and "rearrange" his entire world. During these periods his speech would become wild and pressured, and invariably the prevalent theme had to do with "peoples' crimes." Specifically he would state that he could see the sins of *others* and he believed that he was being followed. He would then express the fear that he was about to be stabbed or *overtaken by a vehicle.*

Following each of the first two episodes, his stepmother assumed that his condition was caused by alcohol, an assumption that seemed to be validated by the transient nature of his psychotic symptoms, which abated each time within twenty-four hours. Subsequently, the patient would have vague memories of these frightening events but would vigorously deny having been drinking. The denials were so emphatic and his life style so generally alcohol-free, that his stepmother gradually relinquished her former conviction. During the third psychotic episode she made a point of noting that there was no alcohol on his breath nor any other evidence that he had been drinking.

Any lingering doubts that she had in this regard were fully eliminated by the fourth eruption of psychotic symptoms—which led to the merchant mariner's appearance at the hospital once more. The symptoms were again strikingly similar. There was the same need to rearrange things in a manner which precisely opposed their usual order. He again placed food in the trash can and trash in the refrigerator. He rearranged furniture and turned pictures so that they faced the wall. He talked about the pictures on the wall as being part of a "gallery" through which he could be seen. While the intensity of this episode was slightly greater than those of previous occasions, it was mostly the duration of this disturbance that convinced his stepmother that her stepson's troubles were not due to alcohol and that he required further medical attention.

After four days of unremitting anxiety and uncontrollable and bizarre behavior, the house was in a shambles. He was fearful that he was constantly being watched, and frantically begged his stepmother to give him refuge and not to divulge his whereabouts to anyone. She was now certain that he had not been drinking during this period of time, since she had been tending to him virtually every minute of the day and night. Remembering that he had been ill two years previously and that he had greatly improved with the medication he had been given at the hospital, she asked her husband to go to her stepson's apartment and to return with the entire contents of his medicine cabinet. He did so, and together they sifted through the medications. Recognizing the Thorazine tablets, they administered this medication to the patient. When he was more controllable, they brought him to the hospital where he was seen in the psychiatric emergency room and was immediately admitted for treatment.

Thus, while at first the patient's stepmother suspected that these psychotic episodes were caused by alcohol, she eventually became convinced that the patient's alcoholism, while certainly a long-standing problem, was in no way related to these outbreaks. Alcohol had simply been an anesthetic by which he attempted to gain respite from the pain and guilt in his life. For the merchant mariner was a haunted man. His curse was the death of his mother for which he unconsciously held himself responsible. During the thirty-three years since her death, his life had been consumed by the need to escape the harsh railings of his conscience and the hallucinated sufferings which he endured. His tragic story is a testament to the power and the timelessness of unconscious guilt.

CHAPTER SIX

A Family In Distress

Present at the proceedings is Dr. Adams, a third year resident. Dr. Adams had interviewed the patient on the day prior to the interview that was taped by Dr. Console and has been treating the patient in twice-weekly psychotherapy for the last year and a half.

(The videotape is turned on. The patient and Dr. Console are seen sitting in their respective chairs. The patient is a white man in his mid thirties, well-groomed and sitting comfortably. He is immaculately dressed.)

Dr. Console: Will you tell me why you've come to the clinic?
Patient: Well, I have a son ... eight years old. And, he's presently seeing another psychiatrist ... Dr. Thomas. He's under therapy. He's been under therapy for approximately two to three months.

Dr. Console: Any impressions?
Dr. Iglesias: "Approximately" ... he's not sure how long his son has been in therapy.
Dr. Console: All right. Here's a point. "He's been under therapy" for approximately two to three months.
Dr. Vis: Apparently this man has been referred for treatment by the son's psychiatrist, which leads me to speculate that he might see the problem as one concerning his son rather than himself.
Dr. Console: Yes. But following up on Dr. Iglesias' comment ... what about a man who has a son in treatment and who does not state with precision the length of time that the son has been in treatment? He says ... "approximately two to three months."

Dr. Marcus: I think we can anticipate that throughout the interview there's going to be a certain quality of vagueness or indecisiveness. You might have some difficulty pinning him down to the facts as to what's really going on.

Dr. Console: Yes. You might anticipate that he will be given to approximations rather than specifics.

> *Patient:* He's been under therapy for approximately two to three months. And . . . we have weekly meetings with Dr. Thomas by ourselves . . . to attempt to settle my son's problems and in the meantime possibly finding out why this is happening.

Dr. Console: So there was the "approximately" two or three months and now he's used the word "possibly." So, Dr. Marcus' original feeling about the lack of precision is quite valid. Dr. Vis's speculation that the referral was made by the son's doctor is also borne out.

> *Patient:* Possibly there's something we are doing wrong. And through these meetings Dr. Thomas suggested that one of us should undergo therapy. So . . . I volunteered.

Dr. Zimmer: It seems unlikely that anyone would suggest that "someone" undergo therapy without actually specifying who it was to be. A responsible therapist, at least in my estimation, would have a good idea of who the patient should be. I imagine that this man was told that he was the one who needed therapy and in fact is covering it over by saying that the doctor felt that one of them should be in therapy and . . . "so I volunteered."

Dr. Console: It is quite likely that the doctor suggested that "both of you" . . . should be in treatment. The doctor would be running quite a risk in saying, "You the mother" . . . or "You the father" should go into treatment. What is the risk?

Dr. Vis: He would be putting the blame for any and possibly all difficulties on that one parent.

Dr. Console: Exactly. Now, if we are dealing with a disturbed child, it is entirely reasonable to postulate that both the parents have made some contributions to his difficulties. We can also postulate at this point that the relationship between the parents is not very good. If this is the case, then the matter of the psychiatrist saying, "You go into treatment" ... specifying *one* of the two partners, is fraught with what danger? What would the other one ... the spouse, do for the rest of eternity?

Dr. Zimmer: Keep saying, "It's your fault."

Dr. Console: Absolutely! In one form or another the message would always be, "Don't tell me I'm wrong ... you're the one who's crazy. The doctor said you should go into treatment." So don't do that. If a couple comes to you for a consultation because of marital difficulties ... both of them are making a contribution and your suggestion must be that both go into treatment. Now, when you make the suggestion that they both enter treatment, how do you determine which one of the two you will take?

Dr. Parker: You should not take either one into treatment.

Dr. Console: You do not take either of them! You should refer them to two of your colleagues. For pretty much the same reasons ... or an extension of the reasons we've already mentioned. If you take one into treatment ... you have made a choice. You've seen them both and then chosen one to be your patient. The one who is not chosen will be continuously asking what question?

Dr. Vis: Why not me?

Dr. Console: "Why not me? Why did he pick the other?" And you would have unwittingly thrown a contaminant into the treatment of both. The chosen one may decide, especially if his orientation is masochistic or depressive, that he was chosen because he is the sicker one. Or, if he has some grandiose or narcissistic feelings, he may decide that he's the better of the two. So, when you see a couple, either refer them both and take neither of them, or else see them together if you are experienced in doing marital and family therapy.

Now, what do we want to know about this man's having volunteered for treatment? At some point in the course of the next few minutes of the interview, what question should be asked about his having volunteered?

Dr. Vis: Why did he volunteer?

Dr. Console: Why did he do that? Assuming that the doctor had long since decided that both parents were making a contribution to the son's problems, what made him volunteer?

Dr. Marcus: His choice of words is interesting. "Volunteer" . . . it has an innocuous ring to it. It suggests that he doesn't really have to be there . . . almost like, "If they say I have to take my medicine I will, but I really don't need it."

Dr. Console: That's a good point. He doesn't say it but the implication is that "I volunteered" . . . which has a self-sacrificing meaning.

Dr. Vis: There's a quality of martyrdom.

Dr. Console: Offering himself. Yes.

> *Patient*: So . . . I volunteered. Because I feel that my problems are a lot stronger than my wife's.

Dr. Drucker: He recognizes some of his own pathology.

Dr. Console: Yes. The word *stronger* here means that he feels that he has made a *stronger* or a *greater* contribution to the child's difficulties. But no one has made mention of his use of the word *undergo* earlier.

Dr. Cohen: I think his choice of words is interesting and important. The word *undergo* makes me think of a passive position . . . a passively experienced situation.

Dr. Console: Yes. How do we ordinarily use the word *undergo*?

Dr. Cohen: To describe an operation.

Dr. Console: An operation! Yes . . . where you are rendered unconscious, insensate and immobile. So Dr. Cohen feels that the use of this word in such a context strongly suggests a quality of passivity in the man. Now what implications would you read into that, in terms of eventually treating him? What can you say about the nature of the work to be done? The nature of some of the difficulties that you can expect to encounter?

Dr. Drucker: I have an entirely different feeling about the word *undergo*. I think of it as undergoing an ordeal . . . a trial or situation of great tribulation. I think it implies that aspect rather than one of passivity. To answer your question more specifically, I would, in light of the *undergo*, get the feeling that he's going to be a tough patient. He's going to be resisting the therapy. If it *is* a trial and if he *is* a bit on the passive side, he's going to be resistant.

Dr. Console: What would be the difference in the manner in which he approached and dealt with treatment if it were as Dr. Cohen describes, primarily and overwhelmingly a matter of passivity, or if it is as Dr. Drucker describes, in the nature of a trial? What difference would you expect?

Dr. Redley: If he was passive in his orientation, he would expect you to be doing something for him or to him.

Dr. Console: In other words, he's just going to kind of sit there and wait for you ... and in the other circumstance, what might happen?

Dr. Redley: He would be more active.

Dr. Console: In what sense?

Dr. Redley: He would feel the need to explain himself or to defend himself.

Dr. Console: Yes ... I think he would be somewhat combative about it all.

Dr. Vis: He would have to provoke you.

Dr. Console: If it's a trial he would be in a much more actively defensive posture. So, I think that we'll have to try to resolve this dilemma in the course of the next few minutes ... and decide whether he's leaning in the direction that Dr. Cohen suggests or in the direction that Dr. Drucker suggests.

> *Patient*: ... I feel that my problems are a lot stronger than my wife's. They go back a lot deeper. My childhood has been anything but pleasant. My mother was ...

Dr. Marcus: He volunteers so quickly to tell you about his childhood. You didn't even have to ask him about it. It makes me think that he's a bit more on the passive side.

Dr. Console: Can you be more specific about your reasoning here? Keep in mind that he's seen Dr. Thomas.

Dr. Marcus: Well, I think that he knows what you want to hear, and he's being cooperative and trying to please you.

Dr. Vis: I get the feeling that this man is struggling with many guilt feelings and that there is going to be the quality of a confessional in the interview.

Dr. Console: So he has said that his childhood was anything but pleasant. He's volunteered this immediately. If we think about guilt, we might also think that he is attempting to explain and cover up the guilt. That these dreadful things were visited upon him as a child and it's not really his fault.

> *Patient*: ... My mother was very, very strict. I'll give you an example of that ... I was usually a good student as far as conduct goes. Average student as far as work. But one time I brought home a D in conduct. For what reason, I don't remember—possibly I had a friend sitting next to me who wanted to talk during class ...

Dr. Console: "Possibly I had a friend sitting next to me who wanted to talk during class" ... what are we observing here?

Dr. Drucker: It sounds somewhat defensive, defensive about himself. He tells you about this incident from childhood and of course we're assuming that his own child is emotionally disturbed. There may be guilt feelings about what he's done to his son or something like that. He seems to be making a connection between his son and his own actions.

Dr. Console: You're saying that at some level he is identifying with his son and I agree. But let me focus your attention on what he suggests in the incident of his having gotten this one bad conduct report. He says that there was a kid sitting next to him and there was some talking. In other words, there is a suggestion of a tendency, in his accounting of the incident, to avoid any responsibility for his own behavior.

> *Patient*: ... possibly I had a friend sitting next to me who wanted to talk during class. So she got very angry and she took pots and pans and threw them at me. I put up my hand and (*raises hands over his head*) I didn't get ... I wasn't injured. But this is an example of what went on. I can remember the traumatic experiences that I had. I can remember them very well but I don't remember any happy times as a child.

Dr. Console: Do you have any feeling about his description of this incident? That his mother took pots and pans and threw them at him.

Dr. Vis: I think he's trying to elicit sympathy from you ... especially when he says that he can't remember any happy incidents in his life.

Dr. Drucker: I may be jumping a bit too far but I can't help but think that his mother is psychotic.

Dr. Console: I think that is jumping a bit far. You see, if a patient comes to you and expresses a concern that the people living upstairs have an X-ray machine and they're sending down harmful rays specifically directed toward him, you can be reasonably certain that the man is paranoid. If this same man reports to you, however, that he goes to his mailbox and frequently, when he's expecting mail, there is none, and that he has a feeling that his next-door neighbor, with whom he has had some disagreements, is responsible for this ... your task is a much more complicated one. You cannot come to the same conclusion that you did in the first circumstance, unless and until you know that indeed the neighbor is not crazy or destroying his mail. So here ... we have no idea of what really happened. "She took pots and pans" ... it could be a gross exaggeration on his part. It's premature to make the assumption that she's that impulse-ridden. Now, suppose I tell you that when we first looked at this tape and we reached this point, Dr. Adams, who had seen him the day before, pointed out something that was very curious and interesting. The man had described this incident in precisely the same fashion and with the same mannerisms to Dr. Adams the day before.

Dr. Iglesias: It sounds as though he's built a nicely structured story to serve his own defensive purposes and it's going to be difficult to get him to give up those defenses.

Dr. Farber: It could reflect his attitude toward treatment and toward psychiatrists in general. They are the ones who are throwing questions at him and he has to defend himself from this assault. It could be the tone for the entire interview. This is the first memory that he's produced in the interview. I think it's symbolically important.

Dr. Vis: I think that his ability to describe it so vividly in the same manner would point to its having really happened, which might be the reason he can describe it so well and repeat it exactly.

Dr. Console: All right . . . you've called this a vivid description. Maybe this is what we should consider.

Dr. Iglesias: I think he's enjoying telling this story.

Dr. Console: Yes, I think there is some gratification in this for him. I would suggest that there also is an infantile or childish quality about it, a childish quality in that when coming home from school, the child often tells his mother about an incident that occurred that day. The child's ego is such that he is much more prone to literally act out what happened . . . with his body and arms and so on . . . whereas the adult with a more mature ego, uses his capacity to describe a situation with words and doesn't have to gesture. Now, I don't mean that one never uses gestures but here I am struck by the specificity of this piece of behavior . . . that he went through precisely the same gestures with Dr. Adams.

Dr. Cohen: The idea of his having used the same words and the same gestures in the beginning of each interview . . . I've noticed this a number of times in different patients. I think the most striking thing about it is how little really gets communicated to other people. I get the impression that they've told something many, many times before and that it doesn't matter to whom they're talking.

Dr. Console: Yes . . . it would seem that the primary purpose for someone like that is to relive the experience. The purpose is not so much to inform you but to reexperience the event by the description of it.

Dr. McDermott: I also get the feeling that he's trying to tell you that he's suffered "the slings and arrows of outrageous fortune" . . . as well as pots and pans. That he's really a nice guy and that whatever he does may not turn out well.

Dr. Console: We would want to check this out as we go along. He does convey the feeling of helplessness. After all, if it's true, what can a kid do in such a circumstance? You can extrapolate from this incident and read it into his adult behavior but in fact, as a child, the avenues open to him for retaliation, or even defense, were very, very few.

Patient: . . . but I don't remember any happy times as a child. I cannot remember them. Another method of her discipline was I'd lie . . . I mean, I'd have to lie in the middle of the floor and she'd kick me. . . .

Dr. Console: What has he said?

Dr. Iglesias: "I'd lie on the floor and she would kick me."

Dr. Bond: He said, "I'd *have* to lie on the floor . . ."

Dr. Console: He says . . . "I'd lie . . . I mean, I'd have to lie on the floor." . . . What about that? Isn't this in the nature of a slip?

Dr. Kent: The slip indicates to me that he wanted to lie on the floor. That it was a voluntary act on his part and then he tried to correct it in the interview and describe it as his *having* to lie on the floor.

Dr. Console: OK. He suggests very strongly in the slip that he would lie on the floor and his mother would kick him. But, having said "I'd lie,," he then said, "I'd *have to* lie" and Dr. Kent's comment is a valid one. It suggests, at the very least, compliance, and beyond that, some kind of wish.

Patient: I'd have to lie in the middle of the floor and she'd kick me and step on me. I wouldn't really get hurt. I don't think she did it hard enough. But, these have always stuck with me . . . these experiences.

Dr. Console: What confirmation is there in the remainder of his description of these events?

Dr. Vis: He said that he didn't get hurt because she didn't do it hard enough.

Dr. Console: He denotes the fact that there was no real pain inflicted on him. So perhaps in these experiences, instead of pain there was pleasure.

Dr. Cohen: I'm just wondering if we can assume that, implicit in his comment that she didn't kick hard enough, is the statement, "It would have been better if she had kicked me harder."

Dr. Marcus: He seems to have quite an investment in describing himself as having been the recipient of all these bad things.

Perhaps he's really describing his mother's having played with him
... rolling him on the floor in an affectionate kind of way.

Dr. Console: Well ... there are many possibilities here. We would
want to understand what, if any, was the pleasure that he derived
from this kind of activity. So let me make a conjecture. There was a
time when little girls were admonished not to come to school
wearing patent-leather Mary Janes. Do you all know what Mary
Janes are?

Dr. Bond: I think they're the shoes with the strap across the
front. The front part is rounded and quite shiny.

Dr. Console: And what does the front part ... the shiny part do?

Dr. Clarke: It acts as a mirror.

Dr. Console: Yes. It becomes a reflector ... a mirror. And it would
poison the minds of little boys who looked at this and saw what
was underneath the dress. Now when he says, "I'd lie ... I mean, I
would have to lie in the middle of the floor and my mother would
kick me and step on me" ... it may be in the same ball park. The
"kick me and step on me" may be his own idiosyncratic addition ...
This is an old game that little boys play. They lie on the floor
because of their sexual curiosity. It's not easy to lift dresses and get
away with it ... but they can lie on the floor and look up.

> *Patient:* These are the things that come to mind. Little bits of
> my childhood that I can bring out. These are the things I
> remember rather than an overall picture of happy times. I
> was always very shy ... quite withdrawn, didn't have many
> friends. I didn't participate in any sports. I was afraid of any
> kind of competition. Later in life I think this might have
> changed a little. I'm not as shy now as I was then. I'm
> interested in music. At one time I used to play in bands up at
> hotels and this exposure helped me to overcome a lot of my
> shyness.
>
> *Dr. Console:* You've told me that when Dr. Thomas
> suggested that one of you go ...
>
> *Patient:* Yes.
>
> *Dr. Console:* ... you volunteered to do so. You say that
> you're doing it on the basis of your own unhappy childhood.
> What do you know about your wife's childhood?

Patient: Not too much. A couple of the problems that she has told me about, seem to be similar to my own.

Dr. Meyer: I wonder if this is an indication as to how he relates to his wife. He doesn't really think about her as a specific individual with significant past events that are different from his. I wonder if it could indicate a relationship based on identification with his wife. Perhaps she is even a transference figure ... based on identification with his mother from the past.

Dr. Console: It's a very valid thought. Let's keep it in mind and see what he tells us.

Patient: A couple of the problems that she has told me about seem to be similar to my own. One example might be that if either of us had done well in something, we would never be complimented. I don't remember being complimented by either of my parents. And she has said that she'd never be complimented by her father. He'd always say ... "Do better next time." You'd bring home a ninety on a report card ... "Now, let's try for a ninety-five or one-hundred." It would never be, "I'm proud of you ... you're doing well now." It would always be, "Aspire to something higher."

Dr. Console: In his elaboration of his wife's childhood, he ends up showing us how similar they were. His description of her childhood makes it interchangeable with his own. So, Dr. Meyer's suggestion of a strong identification with the wife may be quite accurate.

Patient: This has always been the case.
Dr. Console: So, insofar as this factor ...
Patient: This factor, right ...
Dr. Console: ... is concerned, then the two of you may have made an equal contribution to what has been happening to your child.
Patient: Absolutely ... right. ...
Dr. Console: So, why should you volunteer?

Dr. Console: Now, what about his two responses here? As I start talking to him, he's almost repeating my words and then ends up saying, "Absolutely . . . right." What feeling do you get from that?

Dr. Kent: I get a feeling of great compliance here. Whatever you say is fine with him . . . it's right and has to be so. He's not even going to try to support his initial statement that his problems are worse than those of his wife.

Dr. Meyer: Maybe he's very compliant in his saying "right, right" . . . but he was interrupting you while you were talking. In a sense, he wasn't even listening. I thought there was more resistance here than compliance. He doesn't want to listen.

Dr. Cohen: I agree. I felt that when he was saying "right," he wasn't really listening to you. It wasn't really penetrating. He was resisting any attempts on your part to really touch him.

Dr. Vis: I see his saying "yes, yes" before you even complete your sentence, as his being extremely anxious to comply with you. There's a tremendous compliance in this man.

Dr. Rubinstein: We can try to integrate the two views by seeing the compliance as being a defense . . . an attempt to disarm the questioner. The compliance is his way of resisting a comment or confrontation made to him.

Dr. Console: Yes. What I am trying to underscore is that there is a lack of vigor in this man's defense. His resistance, his not allowing me to penetrate and so forth, is done with *no* vigor at all. It's done in the compliant and anxious-to-please fashion that Dr. Vis describes.

Dr. Console: So, why should you volunteer?

Patient: Well, uh—I . . . I don't know. I suppose that—I've always thought about undergoing therapy for a long time now. It never assumed the importance it does until now.

Dr. Console: It's really more likely that rather than its having become important now, the opportunity or avenue has been given him. In the seeming service of his child's treatment, he could be coming because of an awareness of problems that he has himself. This is very common.

Patient: So when Dr. Thomas had seen both of us separately and I told him approximatley what I'm telling you now . . . afterwards I felt an emotional upheaval and I went home that afternoon and I started to cry. I was by myself. There was no one home. It was the first time that all of these thoughts had come out. I admitted them all at one time. But then I tried to repress them. And when they came out I felt an extreme emotional upheaval. I wouldn't ask the doctor to try to find me someone I could talk to, but when he did suggest it, I just suddenly felt this great need. It was very important to me. I couldn't help my son without helping myself first. I've seen many of the fears that I had as a child . . . he seems to have them now. And this is something that I did not realize at the start of his therapy. I still don't understand how he could acquire through some sort of osmosis (*laughs*) these same things that I had as a child. I see them happening. I can't possibly hope that he can be helped without myself doing something.

Dr. Console: So when Dr. Thomas made the suggestion, what did your wife say?

Patient: She was silent at first and then . . . she was very . . . how should I put it . . . the first words out of her mouth were, "This is gonna be expensive." She still says that now. Between both my son and myself in treatment. I don't know about her true feelings. The fact that she keeps harping on that . . . she had always thought all along that I should have some help.

Dr. Console: What made her think that?

Patient: Well, we have a very poor . . . a lack of communication. We don't really talk things out. For a while, when my son was undergoing therapy, we had something in common to talk about. But it didn't last too long because my son was talking about his experiences in therapy, but he doesn't talk about it too much anymore.

Dr. Console: So the boy, for a while, was talking about his experiences in treatment, but he stopped doing that after a time.

Then, the communication between the parents, this man and his wife, dropped off. What does this suggest to you?

Dr. Meyer: Perhaps they can mobilize whatever relationship they have specifically around the son's problems. That could be one of the causative factors in the son's illness.

Dr. Console: In general then, what feeling do you have about these two people's means of communicating with each other? What about the state of things?

Dr. Marcus: There's a chronic lack of communication.

Dr. Console: Yes. It suggests very strongly that they really do not talk very much to each other. As Dr. Meyer suggests, when there's a critical problem, there's some talk. But when the child stops talking, they're back to par. They simply do not talk to each other.

Patient: But there is this great need welling up inside to talk to each other. There's such a great need and it never seems to come about.

Dr. Console: Now while it is true that he is our patient and he's the person to whom I'm talking, so far he's made it pretty clear that it's a two-way street. His wife participates or does not participate to the same degree. So, whatever problems or conflicts he has, seem to be shared by his wife. While I'm not a family therapist, I am suggesting that there's a great deal going on in this family and we're getting some picture of what the family is like . . . at least the relationship between the mother and father.

Patient: I come home at night, for instance . . . and my wife is sleeping at the kitchen table.

Dr. Console: What time might this be?

Patient: Ten . . . ten-thirty. Not every day. I work late some nights. So, from there on, she lifts her head up to say hello, something like that . . . and right away her head goes down and she's sleeping again. So, I immediately fall into a very melancholy mood.

Dr. Console: So, apparently on the nights that he works late, he comes home to find his wife asleep. She is aware of his coming into the house, says hello, and is then asleep again. And he falls into a very melancholy mood. What about that?

Dr. *Meyer*: He comes home after a day's work and this is the greeting he gets. He says he gets depressed but it sounds as though he becomes enraged at that point.

Dr. *Console*: If he's angry at her, what does he do?

Dr. *Vis*: I think that in addition to the anger, he realizes that he's helpless and he can't do anything about it.

Dr. *Rubin*: Why doesn't he try to wake her up and talk to her?

Dr. *Console*: Yes. Why doesn't he do that? Dr. Vis suggests that his passivity is so great that he is overwhelmed by the situation and reacts with a sense of helplessness. We don't know yet what he does in the face of her sleeping but we have to try to understand his statement that he falls into a melancholy mood.

> *Patient*: So, I immediately fall into a very melancholy mood. I'm not that way at work. I'm a completely different person when I'm working. I get along well with other people at work and uh—my opinions are respected, so to speak. . . .

Dr. *Console*: What has he just told us? In elaborating that he's a completely different person at work, that his opinions are respected and so on, he's told us that this is *not* the way things are at home. He's made a clear, bald statement . . . by indirection to be sure. By citing the difference between what happens at home and what happens at work, he gives us the specificity of, "My opinions are respected at work," but, "My wife does not respect my opinion."

> *Patient*: . . . my opinions are respected, so to speak. I feel as an equal many times.

Dr. *Console*: So he compounds it by saying that at work he feels as though he's an equal. And you can rest assured that he is going to make it clear that he doesn't feel equal to his wife. Now, people don't have to spell these things out. But you, in your thinking, can complete the sentence for yourself.

Patient: . . . my opinions are respected, so to speak. I feel as an equal many times. But not at home. I don't feel as an equal there. Very rarely . . . when she can't help herself . . . she very rarely asks my opinion on matters.

Dr. Console: Are you saying that you regularly work until ten o'clock at night?

Patient: No. I don't.

Dr. Console: What about on those days when you come home earlier? She's not sleeping then, is she?

Patient: No, that's true. We have dinner with the children and after dinner the children go to sleep about eight, eight-thirty, and we either watch television or we read. But there's still no communication. And uh—it's only a matter of an hour or an hour and a half before she's off in slumberland again. She doesn't usually go to bed before three A.M. in the morning.

Dr. Console: I wanted to establish that he was describing a regular pattern. He makes it clear that on the occasions that he comes home early, they have dinner, the kids are off to bed, and then what happens?

Dr. Marcus: "Slumberland."

Dr. Console: Where?

Dr. Marcus: At the kitchen table.

Dr. Console: So it doesn't make a great difference . . . it has little to do with the time of day. And here, perhaps you can feel a little more of the hostility by his use of the phrase "slumberland." This gets him angry. But his major response is one of withdrawal. She doesn't usually go to bed until three A.M. in the morning. What does that suggest if she's already asleep at the kitchen table?

Dr. Zimmer: She doesn't come to bed.

Dr. Console: Probably . . . and where is he all this time?

Dr. Zimmer: Probably in bed.

Patient: She doesn't usually go to bed before three A.M. in the morning. Then she'll come upstairs to go to sleep. And I'm already asleep by then. And uh—many times I hear her, so I wake up and I take a look at the time. The other night it was five A.M.

Dr. Console: What is she doing all that time?

Patient: She's sleeping at the kitchen table. Nods her head down and just falls asleep.

Dr. Console: And then you go up to bed without disturbing her? You go to bed yourself?

Patient: Right. And this has become increasingly disturbing.

Dr. Console: How has it become increasingly disturbing?

Patient: Well, naturally the lack of communication. We have extreme sexual problems. We haven't had intercourse since my younger son was born and he's five years old now.

Dr. Console: "We haven't had intercourse since my younger son was born and he's five years old now." What about that?

Dr. Marcus: That's a long time (*group laughter*).

Dr. Waldemar: To go for five years with no intercourse points out that it couldn't be that disturbing to him.

Dr. Console: Yes. This is not so disturbing to him. He has suggested that both of them make a contribution to the situation. He says that it's been five years. If the younger son is exactly five years old at the time of this interview, how long has it been since they've had intercourse?

Dr. Marcus: Five years and nine months.

Dr. Console: Five years and nine months! Now, do we want to say anything more about this? Here is a man who is in his thirties, a young adult, who has not had intercourse for five or more years. Can you conceive of the magnitude of the inhibitory forces at work here?

Patient: Part of it is my problem. I'm not very aggressive and my wife is extremely passive at any advances that I might make.

Dr. Console: So how does this relate to the business of her sleeping at the kitchen table?

Patient: Uh—I don't know how it might but I feel that all this has contributed to my not making any advances. . . .

Dr. Console: I asked him, "What has all this to do with your wife's sleeping at the kitchen table?" What am I trying to point out?

Dr. Zimmer: I think part of what you're trying to point out is that he plays a part in his wife's sleeping at the kitchen table.

Dr. Console: All right. What else is there here?

> *Patient*: Uh—I don't know how it might, but I feel that all this has contributed to my not making any advances. . . .
>
> *Dr. Console*: Well, if she's asleep at the kitchen table and you're asleep upstairs in bed . . . there's very little chance of making advances.
>
> *Patient*: Absolutely! Right!

Dr. Waldemar: This man has a tendency not to assume responsibility for what occurs. I think you tried to point out that there's a reasonable connection between his not making any advances and her sleeping at the kitchen table.

Dr. Console: And what about his response? What have I conveyed to him in making my somewhat abrasive and confronting statement?

Dr. Zimmer: I think you were trying to point out that there isn't a chance in the world that anything sexual is going to happen with him upstairs in bed, and her downstairs in the kitchen.

Dr. Console: Yes. It's very hard to make advances when the two of them are on two different floors of the house. And he says, "Absolutely! Right!" So what have I conveyed to him?

Dr. Cohen: I think you made very little impact on him.

Dr. Console: I agree.

> *Dr. Console*: Well, if she's asleep at the kitchen table and you're upstairs in bed . . . there's very little chance of making advances . . .
>
> *Patient*: Absolutely! Right!
>
> *Dr. Console*: So, what do you think the relation is between the fact that you go to bed without saying anything to her . . . you don't shove her and say, "Come on. Get up. Let's go to bed."
>
> *Patient*: Yeah . . . uhm . . . I think I've given up on that point. I

don't feel that it's worth trying anymore. To even wake her
up. I feel also that the more she does it the more I feel that
there's something wrong with myself. Uh . . . I can't, I can't
. . . I know that she doesn't want to go to bed with me
anymore. But I don't understand why and I feel that it's
hurting me very much. Maybe there's something wrong with
me. Uh—I'm possibly not a good sex partner, and so forth.
  Dr. *Console*: You said "the children."
  Patient: Yes—two boys, eight and five.

Dr. *Console*: Now this seems to be a real shift. He's been talking
about his marital life and the sexual difficulties, and I bring him to
his children. The reason is that I want to get as much history as
possible and for the time being, I've gotten enough information
about his sexual functioning without having him give me a
calendar of when, how and so forth. There's ample time for that.
My purpose in an initial interview is to get as broad as well as
precise a picture as possible. We have an indication of the nature of
his relationship with his wife. Let's find out how he feels about the
children.

  Dr. *Console*: And you've been married how long?
  Patient: About eleven years.
  Dr. *Console*: And you're how old?
  Patient: Thirty-five.
  Dr. *Console*: And your wife?
  Patient: She's also thirty-five.
  Dr. *Console*: Can you kind of give me a brief chronology of
your life. Growing up.
  Patient: That's part of my problem. I can't relate my entire
life's experiences . . . only the traumatic points. I was a very
shy child, as I said. My interests weren't very many except in
music. I could express myself . . . I played the trumpet by the
way. I used to practice five hours a day.
  Dr. *Console*: A good deal has taken place before you started
practicing on the trumpet.
  Patient: Yes. Right.
  Dr. *Console*: Tell me about your parents and brothers or
sisters. About how you grew up.

Patient: Uhm—Well, I have a sister. When she was younger, let's say about anywhere from five years old to ten years old or so we got along very well together. Many times my parents would leave me with her because I was old enough to take care of her.

Dr. Console: How much older are you than she?

Patient: I'm about five or six years . . . six years older. And when they'd leave me with her, I would be a very good brother. We got along very well. After a while though, it changed. There was very little outward sibling rivalry. My parents would also say that. I say outward because my inner feelings were different.

Dr. Console: You said, "My parents would also say that."

Patient: They told my wife many times, how well . . . you know, when they see my two sons fighting with each other, they can't understand it. They told my wife how well I got along with my sister.

Dr. Console: But isn't that kind of a self-serving observation? Aren't they saying, "See what good parents we were"?

Patient: I suppose so.

Dr. Console: I'm just curious about the way in which you said this. You said that they would say this. Of course they would say you didn't fight. It's in their interest.

Patient: Right, right. But on the other hand, my wife would never say that about my children. She admits that every once in a while there would be sibling rivalry.

Dr. Console: It would be difficult for her to say that there is no rivalry when they're scratching each other's eyes out.

Patient: That's true . . . yeah.

Dr. Console: You see, I've made a series of somewhat abrasive remarks here. His responses to all these confrontations are quite similar. You're going to see this very commonly. You say something that may be critical and the patient says, "Right, right, I never thought of that."

Dr. Chassen: It seems that he's compliant in the service of not hearing what you're saying.

Dr. Console: His compliance is overwhelming. It's almost as though he would agree with anything I say to him, even the most critical statement.

> *Patient*: But uh . . . I did get along with my sister very well. My inner feelings were a bit different. Every once in a while I would feel that I had to uh—uh—hurt her. I would . . . when I would take care of her I would . . . especially when she was younger . . . I would bend her finger and make her cry. It wasn't anything that kept going on. It was just occasionally that I felt that way. I had to see her cry once in a while.
> *Dr. Console*: Just once in a while you let her know who was boss?
> *Patient*: Yes. That's right.

Dr. Console: Now that's a mistake. That's a gratuitous comment of mine, and I cannot explain why I made it. It's a lousy intervention and it's of no use whatsoever. As I have said on other occasions, with an intervention like that and fifty cents, you can get yourself a subway ride (*group laughter*). The only justification for such a remark would be if he was becoming so anxious that I wanted to reassure him. I didn't have the feeling that that was the case. I made the comment and it's a mistake. I want you to understand that whenever you find yourself interjecting a gratuitous comment, you are making an error. Because it is not calculated to bring out further material. Actualy it tends to close off further material.

Dr. McDermott: I sometimes have trouble knowing which of my comments will be helpful and which will only block the patient from producing more material. Could you explore this a little further?

Dr. Console: First, let me say this. If a patient has finished talking and a thought comes to you and you're unsure if it is going to be helpful, don't say anything. Sit tight. Now, I had commented earlier to him about his parents having made self-serving remarks. I did not feel at the time that it was a criticism, but perhaps it was. And now I am smearing some ointment on the wound. It was not

conscious on my part but even so it is out of place. What I managed
to do was shut off the faucet. What I've said to him in effect is, "I
know that you didn't want to kill your sister. You just wanted to
show her who's boss." That's a mistake, because indeed he really
did want to kill his sister and I deflected that idea.

Dr. Meyer: I was thinking in terms of sadism and masochism
while he was describing this situation with his sister. When he was
younger he used to bend the sister's finger, but I wonder what
happened when they got older?

Dr. Console: Interestingly, we've talked a little about this man's
masochistic trends and he's now describing a sadistic piece of
behavior. The two trends always go together. All masochistic
behavior has sadistic elements and sadism always includes a
masochistic component. That's the reason for the saying, "If a
married pair comes to you because of sadomasochistic difficulties,
you really have four patients to treat."

> *Patient*: When we were older though, my sister sort of
> became very independent. She was always very strong-
> minded, more strong-minded than I was . . . always more in
> command than I was. Just as my younger son is to my older
> son.

Dr. Console: What identification has he made very clear?
Dr. Cohen: He compares himself to his older son.
Dr. Console: Yes. He is identifying with the older boy who is in
treatment . . . who has some difficulty. The younger boy is
independent and headstrong and the older boy is the same as he.

> *Patient*: My younger son is independent and strong-minded.
> He does everything for himself and refuses almost any help
> besides his basic needs. My sister was the same way. Exactly
> the same way. Whereas I always needed help with every-
> thing. I would follow my mother around by her apron strings.
> She would go shopping. I'd follow her. My sister never did
> that. She was always playing with her friends. Many times
> she would get herself in trouble because my parents didn't

bother finding out who she was hanging around with after a while. You know, and she'd never do anything by herself . . . it was the kids she was with. They did a lot of things that got her in trouble.

Dr. Console: What does that remind you of? His sister was not a bad girl but was with bad company and hence would do bad things. What did he say that was similar at the beginning of the tape?

Dr. Meyer: The incident at school when he brought home a bad grade for conduct. There had been someone sitting next to him who was the cause of the trouble.

Dr. Console: Yes. So here is the externalization again, the putting of the responsibility on the circumstances and not upon the person. He has not read Shakespeare and has not remembered the remark that Cassius made to Brutus, "The fault is not in our stars but in ourselves." In fact, there is very little of human wisdom that was not expressed at one time or another by Shakespeare—and he was never analyzed! Now, there's a very interesting aspect to the remark he makes in describing his younger son's independence. "He refuses any help besides his basic needs." What can he be referring to when he talks about *basic needs*?

Dr. Rubin: Food and clothing no doubt, for somebody that young.

Dr. Console: This really illustrates the point I try to make so frequently, that everything a patient says has an enormous amount of meaning. You could not possibly, sitting with a patient for the first time, be able to understand all the implications of what he is saying. I stopped the tape at this point to highlight his reference to basic needs and the distinction he makes between his two sons. The meaning of this, will, I think, become apparent later. But again it underscores a major issue . . . that human behavior is not random. We operate under the fundamental principle of psychic determinism. In the psyche of humans there is a well-ordered and lawful set of rules and regulations, just as there are laws and rules governing the movement of the planets. The task, of course, is, to understand which unconscious concerns determine psychically the patient's statements at any given moment.

Dr. Console: Tell me a little more about your parents.

Patient: Well, my parents were Jewish immigrants from Germany. They were very strict and old-fashioned. And, as I said, my mother had the idea . . . her way of discipline was to make me feel very guilty about anything that I did. When I was really good . . . the best . . . the happiest moments of my days were when I ate.

Dr. Console: So after a brief description of his mother, he then mentions feeling guilty. Then he makes the statement, "The happiest moments of my days were when I ate." Dr. Drucker, you're shaking your head. What does that mean?

Dr. Drucker: I have a feeling about people with eating problems. It seems that they eat when they feel badly about themselves. He switches from feelings of guilt to a statement about the happiest times being when he ate. The oral incorporation is a way of covering over things.

Dr. Console: Well, we can be a little simpler than that, I think. Let's just examine the content of this concept . . . "the happiest times were when I ate."

Dr. Farber: It seems that he would feel less guilty if he ate . . . that eating must have been subtly encouraged.

Dr. Console: But what do you think of a person who, groping for an expression of pleasure, of feeling good, of satisfaction, relates that the only time such a feeling is available is when he eats?

Dr. Waldemar: He's telling us how miserable his life really was.

Dr. Console: Yes. Let's take a kid. We don't know the exact age he's talking about, but, with the exception of the first six months or so of life, a kid growing up has many pleasures. *His* only pleasure was eating. What about the nature of that developing ego? What about the paucity of outlets . . . the paucity of areas of pleasure, of satisfaction, of gratification? "Only when I ate." It's a very significant statement. What kind of situation could that have been? That a person can look back to his childhood and say that the only satisfaction or contentment was eating. It's pretty grim.

Dr. Zimmer: I was just thinking about how this connects to his statement that his younger son only requires that his basic needs be met. I was thinking that he may feel this to be so because it's all he knows how to give. Since this was his only pleasurable experience, it may be the only thing he can imagine himself giving to a child—food.

Dr. *Console*: Well, as I've suggested, we'll see the extension of that a little later in the interview.

> *Patient*: I am really a true compulsive eater. I've been on thousands of diets in my lifetime. I recently lost seventy pounds. About three years ago . . . through Weight Watchers. And I've gained fifty of them back now and I'm working into the same problem. Food is my greatest enjoyment. I think of it constantly. The happiest part of my days was when I was eating. My mother . . . she would always make me finish everything on the plate. One time, I remember . . . this is another traumatic experience . . . she would . . . I couldn't finish a hamburger on the plate and she stuffed it down my throat. I remember choking on it and I was crying for a long time. She made me finish it. And for a long time I remembered this. And I still remember it today. Well, my father on the other hand . . . his method of discipline was to take off his belt and whip me. He wouldn't talk very much. He would just stand there and whip me.

Dr. *Console*: What is he describing? The father's method of punishment was to take off his belt and whip him. He wouldn't talk to him . . . "He would just stand there and whip me." What does this imply? What's the quality of this experience?

Dr. *Zimmer*: I feel that this may have been a very sexualized experience for him. The father's not talking to him while this was going on, almost removes the punishment aspect of it. It's not, "I'm doing this because you've been bad" . . . rather it's, "I'm taking off my belt," which might be a sexual thing and that's it . . . no words, no explanation.

Dr. *McDermott*: The result of such a practice could be that the child is never sure of what he's being punished for. He might expand it beyond the reasons for the punishment . . . to many other things. Perhaps the father wasn't even sure of the reasons.

Dr. *Console*: He denotes that the father whipped him and didn't talk to him. So the whipping might just as well be done how . . .?

Dr. *Farber*: By a machine.

Dr. Console: By a machine! Without affection, without concern, without anger, without any sort of feelings at all. I think that this is the important aspect . . . the whipping might just as well have been done by a robot. When I was a kid, we had this fantasy that in the principal's office they had a spanking machine. My own fantasy was that it was kind of like a converted sewing machine with a treadle and paddles that revolved and your tail was put there and it was repeatedly hit. A machine! (*group laughter*).

Patient: Usually it would be on the behind. Sometimes he'd get overanxious and it would be on the arms. I never really had a rapport with my parents. Like we never . . .

Dr. Farber: If the punishment was given in a nonverbal and impersonal manner, could this lead to his masochism?
Dr. Console: It could very well be a source of masochism, in that if the parents did not talk to him and if the punishment was mechanical and impersonal, he would have to convert the punishment into something acceptable and pleasurable. The derivative of that could very well be a fundamentally masochistic posture in his relations to the rest of the world. He would unwittingly repeat situations in which he would be punished, humiliated and embarrassed because this was the only currency of interchange with his father.
Dr. Farber: Also, he seems to have expressed disapproval when the punishment was given somewhere other than on the behind. This could imply a sexualization of the punishment. A submission to a higher, masculine authority. I suppose this could also predispose him to a homosexual orientation.
Dr. Console: Yes. It possibly could.

Patient: Like we never talked.
Dr. Console: What was your father's work?
Patient: He had his own store. He was a baker.
Dr. Console: Did you live in the same place as the store?
Patient: No, the store was in Manhattan. We lived in the Bronx.

Dr. Console: So he would have to leave early in the morning?

Patient: He would leave early in the morning and for a long time . . . especially when I was very young, he would come home very, very late at night.

Dr. Console: You didn't see very much of him.

Patient: I didn't see much of him at all . . . until later on. Then his hours started getting a lot earlier. He would alternate with his brother who was his partner. He would come home early one week and his brother would come home early the next week and so forth. So I got to see a lot more of him.

Dr. Console: So his father had his own bakery. Since this man is thirty-five years old, we've going back thirty or more years before the time of the supermarket, to the individual baker. The small bakery store meant long hours . . . arriving early in the morning to make fresh bread . . . and staying open late at night. So, for a while he didn't see much of his father. What else can we say about this? His father worked late hours. What has he already told us?

Dr. Zimmer: That's what he's doing himself. He comes home late at night also.

Dr. Console: Yes. He is repeating this in his life and with his family. There are nights when he comes home late also.

Patient: Now, my mother would say to me, "I'm going to tell your father what you did." So I would run downstairs and see him coming about halfway down the block and tell him the whole story before she got to him. I felt that my father had a little more understanding and that I could talk to him about things like that . . . about how my mother hit me or the things she did to me. I guess that he was too tired to really get excited about it . . . unless it happened while he was there. So, by the time she'd tell him again, I had already told him and it wasn't a great shock. I wasn't reprimanded as hard. This would constantly go on.

Dr. Console: What were your experiences in grade school?

Patient: Well, I was an average student. I was always very quiet in class. I didn't contribute too much. I did my work diligently. I couldn't get too much help from my parents. My

mother couldn't read. My father would try to help me with
my homework but he was impatient about it. So it would end
up as a crying session. Every day. It got to be quite an
experience. I never liked school very much. I had a teacher . . .
I don't recall what grade it was . . . probably third or fourth
grade . . . who was very, very strict. She used to make the
children run up and down two flights of stairs about five
times or more, 'till they'd get out of breath. It wasn't so
terrible but the idea was that she scared everyone so much
and I happened to be more sensitive to it than the rest of the
kids in the class. And I remember I could not control . . .
almost every day, I could not control my bowel movements.
Before school ended . . . about a half hour before school ended
I would go in my pants and I would have to walk home from
school. It would be pretty messy by the time I got home. And
this went on . . . I don't remember if it went on after that term
or if it was just because of this teacher. I remember that it
happened around that time. Another thing, she used to lock
children in the closet and a couple of times I got locked in the
closet. I wasn't bad in conduct . . . just once in a while I would
talk to somebody. Unfortunately I got caught. So, a couple of
times I was locked in the closet but that didn't last too long.

Dr. Console: So he describes that at the age of about eight or nine
years, he had daily encopresis in school.
Dr. Farber: It's certainly an aggressive act toward the mother.
Dr. Console: I'm thinking about his remark concerning the
difference between his two sons and his reference to basic needs. I
wonder if we would include the matter of the toilet as a basic need?
Let's keep this in mind as we inquire further about the kind of
problems the older son has.

Patient: I remember being quite afraid of closets for many
years. I wouldn't open a closet for a long time. And the bowel
movements happened only on weekdays when I went to
school. Never on Saturdays or Sundays or holidays . . . only
on school days. I understand that my toilet training was
normal.

Dr. Console: Tell me about high school.

Patient: Well, it was about the same thing there. I never enjoyed high school. I never participated in any sports. I had one teacher that I do remember, that I liked very much. It happened to be the one time where my grades were above average, without even trying any harder than I had before. I got a certificate in Spanish. I related to this teacher very well. Each student was an individual to her and I felt very good about it. I got through with the term and I was told that I was eligible for honors if my grades kept up for one more term. But they didn't because I had a gym teacher who would stand there with a ruler and whip the kids. So, that was it. I just was completely turned off by that.

Dr. Console: Because the gym teacher is whipping the kids you're turned off from everything?

Patient: Well, I was just turned off by him. My learning process seems to have been affected that way. I didn't feel happy about school at all.

Dr. Console: I've indicated my incredulousness here. He was doing well, headed for honors and then a harsh gym teacher caused everything to go to pot. It's a bit unrealistic. In high school most kids aren't that concerned or intimidated by the gym class or the teacher there. What does that have to do with the process of learning in other areas? A gym teacher who is not the most pleasant person in the world causes the whole curriculum to go down the drain for this boy? It's a little strange.

Patient: I remember feeling nervous about walking into school every day. You'd think that after a couple of months I wouldn't be nervous any more but I always was. So I couldn't learn anything very well because I couldn't relate very well to the teachers. After that my college experiences were better. I enjoyed it a lot more. I had more of a mature feeling about school. Then I got a job in a small store. There was only myself and the boss. Most of the time I would be left alone in the store after I'd gained enough experience and I enjoyed it. I was able to actually talk to a lot of people. It was a good feeling because it was something that I'd never had a chance to do before. I overcame much of my shyness. I was the all-important man there; I was in charge of a couple of other people that worked there also. The store recently went out of business and I got a job now in a very large store where I'm working with a lot of other people. Things are working out all right there. But I get the feeling that I'm trying to run away from something.

This past summer I checked into jobs in Arizona. I told everyone ... I told my wife that it was for retirement purposes. I'd be able to work there if we ever went there to retire ... but I have to admit to myself that it wasn't that at all. I really want to move out there. And it isn't because of any better position or anything like that because certainly the benefits I get through the union here are a lot better than they are out there ... but ... somehow I have this great need to move ... and ... I have a couple of friends living out there. They've been trying to talk us into going out. I couldn't say no. This sort of triggered something that made me happy. I harped on it for a long time. It created a feeling in me of hating my neighborhood, despising almost all the people in it.

Dr. Console: What common fantasy is this man giving expression to?

Dr. Farber: That the grass is always greener on the other side.

Dr. Console: "The grass is always greener on the other side." As psychiatrists, I think we have to inquire into the universality of this saying and elaborate what the most likely fantasy is. Here is an expression which has endured for years and years. People are all familiar with it and if something endures in this way, it contains a universal truth which relates to a common fantasy ... a fantasy that is present

Dr. Meyer: It's something in the order of thinking that if the *world* were different, then *I* would be different.

Dr. Console: OK. The common fantasy of people who are troubled ... and those are the people we see ... is that if they could change this thing, this situation or dilemma, then everything's going to be all right afterwards. If he could just move to Arizona, it would take care of every problem he has. If he could just make that one change. So it has the quality of the child's conception of the world and the child's belief in the use of magic to solve life's problems. A change will make a magical difference. This is a fantasy. I think that many patients bring such fantasies to treatment. I've often had to tell patients, "If you don't know how to play the violin before you start treatment, you're not going to be able to do so afterwards. The treatment doesn't remake you into a person other than who you are . . . with certain assets and certain liabilities and limitations. You do not become a superperson. You will still be confronted with anxieties." What we hope to do is to enable the person to deal more realistically with the facts of his life rather than to be governed, as he is now, by the fantasies in his life. So we try to replace fantasies with the realities of life. Now this is a very clear-cut fantasy on the part of his man . . . that if he could only move to Arizona, there wouldn't be any more troubles for him. Everything would be just lovely and, of course, this is not so.

> *Patient*: I couldn't be friendly with anybody. I couldn't talk to any people on my block because of this. I had the great urge just to move out. I'd still like to. I think if my wife would say "all right" . . . I don't want to move without her saying it would be all-right, because if she's not happy there and I have to work all day, I don't think it's fair.
> *Dr. Console*: Tell me about meeting your wife . . . originally.

Dr. Console: Now again, we are in an initial interview and the function of such an interview is to learn as much as you can about who this person is and how he functions. It is my feeling at this point that I understand the fantasy of the magical move and there's no further pay dirt here. There's no reason to continue an elaboration of this and since he has mentioned his wife, I use the opportunity to get the history of himself and his wife. I'm going to try to get a chronological account of the meeting with his wife . . . the courtship, marriage and so on.

Dr. Meyer: When he talked about moving to Arizona, he said that one of the main things was a friend of his there who was trying to convince him to make the move. I would like to know more about his relationship with this male friend.

Dr. Console: That's important, but I personally would hold off until later. When you see the patient for the first time, you want to get some idea of how big the forest is, what its boundaries are and in general what it contains. We cannot do this if, having come across a certain tree, we now inquire about every branch and every leaf of that tree. The hour is going to be over and we won't know where the hell the forest ends. So while you may want to have this information, you can save it for a later time . . . tuck away the question and save it for a later date. By the way, I'm not even doing that in this instance, because I seriously doubt that there's much of a friendship there. Up until this point I am not convinced that the nature of his object relations would include any relationship with a friend who is important enough for him to seriously contemplate uprooting himself from where he was born and brought up, to go to Arizona. No, it's magic that is involved there. I feel confident that it's magic and nothing more.

Dr. Adams: I would have to disagree. It seems to me important to inquire about the quality of his relationships with various people. It has predictive value because of the kind of relationship he might make with a therapist in treatment.

Dr. Console: Thats' true. It's a very important clue as to how he's going to relate to you.

Dr. McDermott: We may find that whenever he has to leave someone or something, he has to hate that object . . . as a way of handling his separation anxiety.

Dr. Console: I think that's a very good observation.

> *Dr. Console:* Tell me about meeting your wife . . . originally.
>
> *Patient:* Yeah. We met through a blind date. My cousin arranged the date and we . . . I picked her up and because of the late hour we went to a drive-in. It was very pleasant. We talked well to each other, you know, I felt that we were relating very well to each other. Well, for some reason she had gotten a stomach virus at that time and she messed up my father's car (*laughs*). But . . . other than that it was a good time.
>
> *Dr. Console:* She vomited?
>
> *Patient:* Yes, she did. She was worried about it. I was very

understanding. In a way, I was able to ... Well, I wasn't unhappy about the situation because I was able to show my understanding.

Dr. Console: Now, on the first date with his wife there was this unfortunate incident. She was ill and vomited all over his father's car. And he was not too unhappy about this situation. She was embarrassed but he could show his understanding.

Dr. Drucker: He seems to like the idea of being in this position relative to her ... the position of being above her. She's below him and owes him something.

Dr. Kent: It also puts her in the position of having messed up his father's car. It could be an angry thing on her part.

Dr. Cohen: We've talked about his tendency to see things as happening to him . . . . as fate ganging up and punishing him, and his reaction to that. I think that her illness is a familiar situation for him ... one that he can relate to.

Dr. Console: A familiar situation in what sense?

Dr. Cohen: The pain is familiar for him. She's suffering from the virus and I think he relates well to that. He can be either a victim or a punisher ... interchangeably. In this case ... there was somebody else experiencing the pain.

Dr. Console: Well, put yourself in his position. You have a date with a girl for the first time and she has a stomach virus and vomits. Now, you can feel compassion; you might go so far as to feel her pain and distress. But what about the quality that he suggests when he says that he was not unhappy about this? What about the quality of the girl's having established herself as having the potential to be sick? To return to Dr. Drucker's comment about one being above or below the other ... there's some greater specificity here. Above in the sense that here is a woman who expresses some kind of weakness or deficit, some capacity to be sick. And he is not unhappy about this. Could it be that he is not unhappy about this *because* she has indicated deficiency? All he is worthy or capable of is a relationship with someone who is deficient. Here was an opportunity for him to indicate that he did not find this disgusting. He did not find this threatening or annoying. I would like you to focus on his finding this a somewhat

welcome occurrence ... an unusual one to say the least, and for
him, a welcome one.

Dr. Adams: Not only would he perhaps choose someone who is
vulnerable, but there's the question of his identification. You can
safely assume that he does identify with this woman's illness. In a
sense he gets an identity for himself this way. In a sense also, he
identifies with the aggressor. He has shifting kinds of identifica-
tions which enable this to happen.

Dr. Console: If you're going to say that, you have to take it one
step further, to the nature of the identification with his mother. In
the face of this girl's vomiting, he cleaned it up. He has already told
us that he had this unfortunate difficulty in school with encopresis
and that his mother would have to clean him up. Now he's cleaning
up the contents of her gastro-intestinal tract ... the other end to
be sure, but the meaning is the same.

> *Patient*: We got married about three years after we met. She
> was a secretary.
> *Dr. Console*: She was working at the time?
> *Patient*: Yeah, that's right. When we met she was just
> finishing college. She wasn't working yet. Afterwards she
> started working and while I was going to school I wasn't
> working at all. She was supporting me.
> *Dr. Console*: So that when she started working you were still
> in school.
> *Patient*: That's right. Yes.
> *Dr. Console*: And when you got married had you finished
> school or were you still in school?
> *Patient*: I was still in school when we were married.
> *Dr. Console*: So that for a while she was supporting you?
> *Patient*: Yes. She was.

Dr. Console: So for a while here, there was the reversal of the
usual roles. She was the breadwinner and he was being supported
by his wife.

> *Dr. Console*: During that period ... you mentioned that it
> was a three-year courtship ... what were your sexual
> experiences?

Patient: Premaritally? None at all. Uhm ... I did make advances but not very strong ones. And my wife ... uh ... turned them down. It was all very polite ... and uh ...

Dr. Console: Let's focus for a moment on the premarital experience.

Dr. Drucker: He used the word *polite*.

Dr. Console: It's an interesting word, isn't it?

Dr. Zimmer: You asked him about sexual experiences and he interpreted your question in a very narrow sense. There are sexual experiences that people have premaritally, other than actual intercourse. When he said that he had none, I think he was focusing only on intercourse.

Dr. Console: Yes, I'm interested in the general nature of the premarital relationship. Now, we already have the information about the first date, in which the girl whom he eventually married threw up and where he wasn't disturbed about this.

Dr. McDermott: He said that he had made some minor advances and that they were not very strong. My impression is that he made an advance because he felt that he was expected to and that he was probably hoping that something would intervene ... such as her vomiting.

Dr. Console: Well, this man has told us that he wasn't very aggressive. Now, in this context, what does the word *polite* mean?

Dr. Waldemar: That he was very passive. I think he tries to convey the impression that he was active and that she rebuffed him, but that doesn't seem to be the case.

Dr. Console: Yes. What might he think is the opposite of polite? His concept of being impolite includes what idea?

Dr. Vis: Being forceful.

Dr. Console: Yes. For him, being impolite means pressing the point ... if you'll excuse the expression (*group laughter*). This is what he is telling us. He believes that it would be impolite, boorish and insulting if he pursued what ordinary people pursue with a certain ardor and vigor.

Patient: It was all very polite ... and ... uh, when we got married, we did have many sexual acts. ...

Dr. Console: "When we got married, we did have many sexual acts." What has he told us?

Dr. McDermott: I think he's being a little defensive here, almost as though he's beginning to worry that you may think that he's had sex only once in his life. . . .

Dr. Console: Twice . . . because the children weren't twins (*group laughter*). I would bet that he could almost count the times, even give you the dates—there were really so few. The chances are that intercourse occurred very infrequently. There were long intervals between sexual acts.

> *Patient:* . . . we did have many sexual acts . . . but I had trouble myself during the act . . . not initiating it necessarily, but in keeping an erection. Uh—almost losing interest after a few minutes. Sometimes—occasionally, I felt a fear of having sex. . . .

Dr. Console: What is he describing to us? Difficulty in maintaining an erection, then almost losing interest and sometimes experiencing fear.

Dr. Farber: Premature ejaculation?

Dr. Marcus: Partial impotence?

Dr. Console: Yes, but why? What is he describing?

Dr. Kent: Castration anxiety.

Dr. Console: Yes. He's describing the inhibitions he feels consequent to castration anxiety. He is giving a clear-cut description of castration anxiety that is overwhelming and that inhibits his functioning. He is afraid that something will happen to his penis and he's going to protect it as best he can. He puts it in there . . . it gets soft and it falls out. He doesn't pull it out . . . it falls out. This is a classical description of castration anxiety.

> *Patient:* . . . Sometimes—occasionally, I felt a fear of having sex.
>
> *Dr. Console:* What do you mean . . . a *fear?*
>
> *Patient:* Uhm . . . I honestly don't know. I've been trying to think about it a lot myself. I don't know what the fear was.

Possibly it was because I wouldn't reach an orgasm. It would take a long time. And many times I would give up before reaching an orgasm.

Dr. Console: So, Dr. Farber, he responds and makes clearer the point you raised about premature ejaculation. As in many aspects of human functioning, we have two extremes which may be derivatives of the same fundamental conflict. One person will deal with his castration anxiety. by ejaculating prematurely, while others will be unable to ejaculate. It denotes some differences as well. In a general way, we can surmise that the ejaculation has many profound meanings for him and that he must avoid it at all costs. The paradox in all of this is that these people tend to have no difficulty at all in what . . .?

Dr. McDermott: Masturbation.

Dr. Console: Yes! In masturbation they are always able to maintain an erection and they enjoy full control over the timing of the ejaculation, and this is because in masturbation they do not have to deal with their fear of being inside the vagina.

Patient: And many times I was afraid that my wife would say something about it to me . . . that I would be put down.

Dr. Console: Did you have any sexual experiences prior to your wife?

Dr. Drucker: I have something on my mind and I'm afraid that I may almost sound heretical here.

Dr. Console: Good for you! Go ahead!

Dr. Drucker: This castration anxiety. I have a feeling that . . . well we see here that he's anxious. He's afraid that it would be the greatest put-down if he failed . . . if he didn't satisfy his wife. I'm not sure that this can best be explained as castration anxiety. Can't we see this as a problem with manliness and self-esteem? He has fears of not being able to perform adequately. Do we have to use the psychoanalytic concept that all this is a function of castration anxiety? I have problems accepting this.

Dr. Console: Again I say, good for you! Let's see if the patient can give us an answer to your question.

Dr. Console: Did you have any sexual experiences prior to your wife?

Patient: Just a couple.

Dr. Console: When were they?

Patient: When I was younger. I went out with a group of fellas and we had a five-dollar prostitution experience. That wasn't very successful. The same thing happened. And uh— actual intercourse didn't come about until I was married. Petting and so on happened. I could take care of that.

Dr. Zimmer: I think that he feels quite castrated with this line of questioning and with the way the interview has evolved, and that he's trying to salvage a little bit of his self-esteem by stating that there were no problems with petting.

Dr. Console: Let's assume for a moment that this comes from his heart, rather than from the pressures of the interview. Let's assume that he's pretty accurate in this description and that long before he ever saw me, he was perfectly able to handle necking and petting, and that he did not have intercourse until he was married. What about all of this?

Dr. Drucker: I'm thinking of a bad pun . . . that petting isn't, for him, where the knife meets the butter. It's not where the crunch occurs.

Dr. Console: "Where the crunch occurs." "Where the knife meets the butter." Dr. Drucker, you're the one who questioned the concept of castration anxiety. That was a very rapid conversion! (*group laughter*).

Dr. Drucker (*smiling*): Well, I certainly accept the idea of the penis being representative of the manly weapon . . . the source of manliness. That's "where you've got it or you don't." It's just that I have trouble seeing this more specific idea of castration anxiety.

Dr. Console: Well, let me say that you'll hear many men say to you that they handle the sexual situation very well . . . perfectly well, so long as they have their pants on! (*group laughter*). As long as the penis is kept well covered and protected everything is fine. These people have absolutely no difficulty in rubbing against a woman to the point of orgasm but it's through the clothes, and usually both the man's and woman's genitals are covered. But with exposure, the threat becomes overwhelmingly real for them. In men the threat takes on the specificity of castration. For women the danger is more in the area of some kind of genital mutilation as a result of penetration. And keep in mind that in both sexes, underlying these dangers at the oedipal level, are much earlier and more primitive fears of losing the object, or losing the object's love—both of which can be subsumed within the overall concept of separation anxiety. And in the psychotic patient the most primitive fear of all emerges—the fear of annihilation and total body disintegration.

> *Patient*: I could handle that very well. I had no fear along those lines.
> *Dr. Console*: You were able to maintain an erection?
> *Patient*: Oh yes. No difficulty at all.

Dr. Console: So, he elaborates that there is no difficulty at all. The difficulty in maintaining an erection is present only when there is a possibility of intercourse. It's almost a precondition that there be no likelihood of intercourse for him to be able to function well. This is a form of protection. The man knows that he's not going to be called upon to perform.

> *Patient*: I always felt . . . I still feel today, that I'm not very proficient in that way. My wife somehow feels the same way. Not about me necessarily—but about herself. She doesn't— she would prefer not to have intercourse.

Dr. Console: So, the two of them share their inhibitions. In response to Dr. McDermott's observation of a while ago, about the patient hoping that she would rebuff him or that something would intervene and prevent intercourse . . . he wasn't hoping at all—he *knew*. Again, marriages *areee* in heaven. By that I mean that there is nothing accidental or happenstance about the choice of a partner in marriage. The two of them *knew* that intercourse was not going to be a problem for them. It wasn't going to be a problem because there wasn't going to be any intercourse.

Dr. Console: So that you're able to gratify each other by touching . . . petting?

Patient: Well, it's a one-sided affair. She doesn't do very much. She'll be lying there like a rock. Just not be moving at all. This has been going on for some time.

Dr. Console: This is currently happening?

Patient: No . . . currently there's nothing. Nothing has been happening. Once, once this past year there was some sex. I guess she just got tired of sleeping at the table that night. But other than that, nothing has happened at all in the last year.

Dr. Console: Is anything ever said about it?

Patient: No . . . I was just going to say . . . nothing at all. I always want to bring it up but I can't bring myself to discuss it. It again points to the lack of communication that we have.

Dr. Console: He anticipated my question and wanted to mention that he and his wife never speak about this state of affairs. How can we interpret this in terms of wishes, needs or desires for intercourse?

Dr. Kent: There just don't seem to be any wishes in that direction.

Dr. Console: The two of them have entered into collusion to avoid sexual intercourse and we have to conclude that neither of them has very much interest or desire.

Patient: We spoke to the doctor about it; afterwards, we talked a blue streak about it between ourselves but it didn't last too long. We felt that our problems were aired out. It was a good feeling to be able to just discuss it. That's as far as it goes. A slight discussion and that's it (*pauses*).

Dr. Console: What was it that brought your son to the clinic?

Patient: First of all, bed-wetting. We let it alone for a while because we felt that there was the possibility that he might grow out of it. He was too young and we thought that if he was given a chance he'd grow out of it. The doctor had given him Tofranil and that didn't work. He had taken another antispasmodic and that didn't work either. He had all the tests and they were normal.

Dr. *Console*: This was the pediatrician?

Patient: The pediatrician and a urinary specialist.

Dr. *Console*: I must say that this is one of those unfortunate things that parents unwittingly visit upon their children. It's also one in which the medical profession plays a significant supporting role. We've heard enough about this man and this woman to reasonably speculate that their relationship is lacking in many areas. There is a great sexual inhibition and a great lack of communication. There is the peculiar behavior of the wife's sleeping at the kitchen table and when he comes home, nothing is said and he just goes to bed without her. And then the little boy becomes enuretic and it is to our shame and regret that some pediatricians and family doctors will refer these children to a urologist, who will then cystoscope them, perform an IVP, subject them to God knows what, all without even considering the nature of the emotional difficulties in the household. The frequency of an organic reason for enuresis in a little boy is next to nothing; the overwhelming majority are caused by psychogenic factors. The regrettable thing is that these investigations and manipulations tend to fix the idea of organicity and make subsequent psychotherapy much more difficult.

Patient: After a while his work habits in school began to be very poor. He's a very bright boy. He has much better capabilities than he shows. His teachers, both his kindergarten teacher and his first-grade teacher, have commented that he tends to sit and look out the window all the time. The same thing happens at home when he gets dressed in the morning. He procrastinates . . . daydreams quite a bit. We let it go a while because he was still growing up and possibly this would stop. But after this term . . . after the second-grade teacher mentioned it, we decided that something had to be done.

Dr. *Console*: So what was happening to this boy? The teachers describe him as always dawdling and daydreaming and this is also

happening when he's supposed to get dressed in the morning.
What's happening to this boy? I think he's responding to what he
probably senses ... the stress and the lack of harmony in the
household. The boy is not seeing a loving father and mother,
either toward himself or toward each other. I think he is now
overwhelmed by fantasy and daydreaming and this is as much an
attempt to solve his dilemma as to escape from it.

> *Patient*: In other words we didn't really want to put it off for
> too long but we wanted to see if he'd grow out of it. But all
> these factors considered, we decided that there was really a
> problem. We were determined to seek help (*pause*).
> *Dr. Console*: Do you dream very much?
> *Patient*: No. I don't at all.
> *Dr. Console*: Not any dreams?
> *Patient*: I used to. But lately I don't recall any dreams at all.

Dr. Console: I just want to make a point about my having asked
him if he dreams very much. This is not necessarily a question that
you should routinely ask a patient in therapy. I am doing it on tape
because I want to demonstrate that we can anticipate a
characteristic dream in this man. First there is the customary
resistance about dreams ... he feels that he doesn't dream very
much. Well, I'm a bit persistent here and when I do this I
frequently get a dream. Hooowever, you should not go about
eliciting dream material in this fashion because many patients will
be quite compliant and flood you with dreams ... not only in the
session where you ask for one but in many sessions thereafter ...
and the dreams become the major resistance. If the patient
spontaneously brings up a dream, well then, of course you pay
attention to it. Now, as I mentioned, I want to anticipate the kind
of dreams this man has. Can anyone do this?
Dr. Clarke: I think that his dreams will be ones where he's being
attacked or threatened.
Dr. Vis: I agree. The content of his dreams will be very
frightening to him. The theme of punishment will be prevalent.
Dr. Waldemar: I would like to address myself to the wish aspect of

it. I think he would dream about being cared for and fed ... nourished.

Dr. Farber: I think that he may have perceived your question about dreams as an attack ... When you asked him, "Not any dreams?" he then covered himself over with his sweater.

Dr. Console: Well, *attack* is a strong word but I think there's something to that if we consider it from the point of view of my making an inquiry ... my kind of getting into him, as though he has some awareness that dreams are from the unconscious, as though I would be peering into him. In that sense I think the word *attack* may apply.

Dr. Kent: We've seen him as a very passive man in most of his relationships with men and women. I wonder if his dreams might entail the very opposite of what goes on in his life. He may beat women or be very aggressive in his dreams. There might be a complete reversal ... something opposite of what he ordinarily does.

Dr. Console: All right. Let's see what he tells us.

> *Patient*: But lately I don't recall any dreams at all.
> *Dr. Console*: But before that, there were dreams that you can recall? Any dream?
> *Patient*: Yes. Mostly they were sexual dreams.

Dr. Console: Are you surprised? Nobody mentioned sexual dreams. Now, having established that they were mostly sexual, what is their content going to be? Is he going to dream that he happened to meet Raquel Welsh and that she was enchanted with him, and that in short order they tore off their clothes and jumped into the sack and had themselves a lovely time? Will his dreams be like this?

Dr. Clarke: I still stick with what I said before ... about an attack. Even in a sexual dream, he'll probably dream that the woman is the one who makes the approach.

Dr. Console: All right. He's going to be approached and what's going to happen?

Dr. Clarke: He'll be the one who says no ... there will be some sort of inhibition on his part.

Dr. Console: Let's be more specific. What's he going to tell us about sexual intercourse in his dreams?

Dr. Drucker: That he has great potency? That he can satisfy a woman and that he's a great lover?

Dr. Console: Here's a man who's told us that insofar as making advances toward his wife is concerned, he gave up. Here's a man who has not had intercourse for six years. He's thirty-five years old. I think that many of you are trying to straighten him out . . . you know? If he's not doing it in real life, he should at least be doing it in his dreams (*group laughter*).

Dr. Marcus: I think his saying that he *used to* have dreams and that he doesn't have them any more, is an indication that the dreams will proceed in the direction of frustration and inhibition.

> *Patient*: Mostly they were sexual dreams (*pause*). Not with my wife but with other women. They were very short dreams . . . they had no . . . (*pause*).
>
> *Dr. Console*: What happens?
>
> *Patient*: Mostly they would just involve petting—uh—no intercourse would ever be involved in my dreams at all. I would be with a group of friends and . . . it would be during my teen-age years . . . even though it might be when I was in my twenties, I would still think that I was a teen-ager at the time. And uh—(*pause*) that's about all. The rest of it would be—the rest of the dream would involve the act of petting. And uh—no story behind the entire thing and nothing afterwards. I don't have any nightmares.

Dr. Console: Now, first of all, Dr. Drucker, what has he gone back to? That they're sexual dreams but there's no intercourse . . . only petting.

Dr. Drucker: As if his anxiety . . .

Dr. Console: What anxiety?

Dr. Drucker: Castration anxiety? (*group laughter*). It's able to inhibit his functioning . . . even in his dreams.

Dr. Console: All right! Now in his elaboration he says, there's only the petting . . . there's no story before and there's nothing afterwards. "I don't have any nightmares." What has he said to us in so many words?

Dr. Zimmer: That dreaming about sexual intercourse would be a nightmare.

Dr. Console: Yes! That if the dreams progressed to intercourse, it would be a nightmare. Isn't he really saying that the whole idea of intercourse and of exposing his penis and putting it in this dangerous place is a nightmare?

> *Patient*: . . . I don't have any nightmares.
> *Dr. Console*: With these dreams would there be an ejaculation?
> *Patient*: None at all.
> *Dr. Console*: No.
> *Patient*: And . . . I don't know if there would even be an erection. No . . . there would be no ejaculation at all.

Dr. Drucker: Is there a general rule about dreams? Do they follow anxieties in the same way that the anxieties manifest themselves in conscious life . . . inhibiting the dream also? Or is there more of a wish-fulfillment quality to them? Or is it that you just can't be sure and you have to go by what a particular patient is like and what his conflicts are?

Dr. Console: Well, why break it up into categories? Why can't a dream accomplish all these things? His anxiety is there and so is his wish fulfillment. What is his wish here?

Dr. Zimmer: To be taken care of and not to have to get sexually involved with someone.

Dr. Console: His wish is to be cuddled, to be stroked, to be held. That's his wish. Keep in mind that in a fantasy or in a dream, you can arrange to meet a better class of people. You can arrange to meet the hottest thing on two legs (*group laughter*). The whole world is yours because you can arrange whatever you want. There is a story of a woman who is asleep and she is dreaming. The dream is that she's lying in bed alone, and suddenly she thinks that she hears something at her bedroom door. She is scared stiff. She stares intently at the doorknob and lo and behold, it is so . . . the

door knob is turning slowly. The door opens ... slowly. A huge
man walks into the room and slowly approaches the foot of the bed
and stops and looks at her. She is paralyzed with fear. She says,
"What ... what are you going to do?" He says, "Madam, this is *your*
dream. What would you have me do?" (*group laughter*).

> *Dr. Console*: Is masturbation something you do?
> *Patient*: Yes ... I ... there has to be some way I have of
> relieving myself of these sexual tensions, and I occasionally
> do resort to that.

Dr. Console: What do you think about his language here? "I
occasionally do resort to that."
Dr. McDermott: He feels very guilty about giving in to this
impulse.
Dr. Console: Yes. He reports it as something he has to *resort* to.

> *Dr. Console*: When you do, what do you think of?
> *Patient*: Someone ... some girl I've seen lately, that I've
> taken more than a second look at. Possibly someone I met at
> work. Someone who takes my interest. By the way—I never
> cheated on my wife. I'm not saying that I wouldn't if I had the
> opportunity but I wouldn't go out and look for someone.
> *Dr. Console*: You say, "If you had the opportunity."

Dr. Console: I was looking for a masturbatory fantasy and then he
made this statement about not having the opportunity to get
involved sexually with another woman. To me this was a
remarkable thing to say, and I abandoned my question concerning
masturbation and turned my attention to this statement. Since he
works in a retail store, what can I say to confront him with the idea
of there indeed being an opportunity?
Dr. McDermott: He must meet a hundred attractive women each
week when they're buying underwear (*group laughter*).
Dr. Console: Of course!

> *Dr. Console*: You mean the opportunity never comes into the
> store?

Patient: Uh—I don't advance toward opportunity. It might be there ... not openly ... it might be there. I'll put it this way ... to satisfy my male ego I would try to make advances, probably even more than most, but only in a sort of kidding-around manner ... But if the girl would ever say yes, I think I'd be awfully frightened and I'd start backing off. But naturally I have to make these advances.

Dr. Console: So what is he telling us?

Dr. Adams: He seems to be saying that he has appetites but that his castration anxiety is so overwhelming that he has to quickly abandon any attempt to fulfill them.

Dr. Console: Why does he have to make these advances?

Dr. Farber: I think it's an attempt to deny his tremendous castration anxiety by a pseudo-attempt at seduction ... at demonstrating his masculinity.

Dr. Console: Yes. This has to do with the conflict between giving the appearance of being a "full-blooded man" and the dangers attached thereto. So he makes the advance in a kidding fashion but beats a hasty retreat if there's a positive response. His statement about having a male ego is basically correct. He has to satisfy a certain image of himself. But it is a fantasy. He has to make himself believe that he is as virile as anybody else, by going through this little charade with a customer.

Dr. McDermott: I would think that he would somewhat enjoy a positive response on the part of the girl. His act is succeeding.

Dr. Console: Yes. But remember that it's a double-edged sword. The positive response causes his retreat. I think that the woman's response is not important to him. More crucial is his playing out his pseudo-aggressivity ...he plays it out for *himself*.

Patient: But naturally I have to make these advances. I guess it's to show everybody around me.

Dr. Console: You know, people used to kid about the back room of a retail store. Half the time is spent in filling inventories and the other half engaging in more arduous activities. That is, if the girls would make themselves available.

Patient: In this case there are seven other people who are with me at work.

Dr. Console: There was a time when you said you worked alone.

Patient: There were no women in the store working with me for a long time.

Dr. Console: You can see how obtuse he becomes ... an obtuseness which is one hundred percent defensive. He long since established that he used to work alone in the store when his boss was out ... before this job. So he then thinks that I'm referring exclusively to the other workers. I'm not concerned with the workers. I'm concerned with the customers. This is the population of people where occasionally someone will take a shine to the salesman and make herself available. Or to the dentist or the doctor or the lawyer or the plumber or to anybody else.

Patient: When I was alone ... oh, I see what you mean. When I was alone at the store I never made any advances toward any woman that came in the store.

Dr. Console: So, when the potential for some kind of getting together existed, he wouldn't make the advances, not even in a kidding fashion. He didn't need the masculine image then because the potential with the two of them alone in the store was too great. Something might happen and this would be too threatening to him.

Patient: If I did, it was so slyly that I would be absolutely certain that they would never take it as an advance. Just as sort of a compliment.

Dr. Console: You never had a feeling that maybe a customer, a woman, took an interest in you?

Patient: I think that happened once or twice but I became very frightened at that time. I never admitted it before this, but it's the truth. I have experienced that and it's been very frightening. I would not pursue it. My boss where I work ... he occasionally, well, I don't know if it ever happened—he would pursue a kind of person like that and I was turned off by it. I didn't want to hear about it. At times to be polite I would listen but . . . sort of with disinterest.

Dr. Console: Tell me, yesterday, how did you feel? You were seen by Dr. Adams and he asked you if you would mind being interviewed by one of the members of the staff. How did you feel?

Patient: I immediately, without any reservations, said that I had no objections. Because I have . . . I can see this great need that I hadn't felt before. But now, I can see the importance of it . . . to get help for myself.

Dr. Console: Did you feel that you needed help from two people?

Patient: Well, the way he explained, it was that this would be just a sort of consultation and it would be a teaching situation. So I was glad to help out. I don't know . . . maybe I feel that there's a need for this exposure and the fact that a lot of people will be listening. . . .

Dr. Console: This is the most common, really almost the standard fantasy of virtually everybody I've taped. That many people will be watching this. They entertain the fantasy that the universe will be watching them. Their exhibitionism rears its head—and their need for help. The ease with which many people will assent to being taped is astounding and those of us who can learn so much from these tapes must be grateful for that.

Dr. Drucker: I'm puzzled by the exhibitionism. Does anyone want to show off all his troubles . . . his sexual difficulties and inhibitions?

Dr. Console: Well, it depends on your conception of exhibitionism. It's simply the desire to show oneself. And the showing of oneself definitely includes the blemishes. Some people will be more defensive about the blemishes, while others will revel in describing every detail specifically. But remember, we have already imputed to this man a certain need. It was manifested in his vignette of his mother who would kick him while he lay on the floor.

Dr. Zimmer: His masochism.

Dr. Console: Exactly, his masochistic needs.

Dr. Adams: It's interesting. He described how he would have to run and tell his father what he had done, before his mother could get to his father. I think he really wants someone to listen to him . . . especially to listen to his shortcomings.

> *Patient*: . . . and the fact that a lot of people will be listening.
> *Dr. Consolee*; It's not such a lot of people.
> *Patient*: Well, I don't know. I remember walking into Dr. Adams' office and I don't remember even saying hello to him. I just immediately blurted out why I thought I was here and why I thought I needed help (*laughs*).

Dr. Console: Why do you think that he has reminded himself that when he saw Dr. Adams, he didn't even say hello? What might it represent?

Dr. McDermott: Probably a hope that Dr. Adams will watch this tape and he wants to make an apology now.

Dr. Console: So you have a feeling that he senses this as a rude oversight on his part. Anything else?

Dr. Zimmerj; I think he's describing how desperate he was when he first walked into Dr. Adams' office.

Dr. Console: Yes. I think he is telling us how terribly anxious he was.

> *Dr. Console*: So how much time did you spend with him yesterday?
> *Patient*: Forty-five minutes.
> *Dr. Console*: Forty-five minutes.
> *Patient*; And uh . . . (*pauses*).
> *Dr. Console*: Have you noted any similarities or differences in the two interviews?
> *Patient*: Uh—just about the same. The only thing, I did feel yesterday that I hadn't apologized to him. My thoughts were so jumbled . . . he also wanted to know about my childhood, my parents and so forth . . . and I could not give him an overall picture. Just those traumatic experiences were the only thing.
> *Dr. Console*: So you feel that this was an easier experience?

Patient: Yes.

Dr. Console: So there were some things you have told me that you didn't tell him then?

Patient: Uh, yes, especially about my sexual experiences. I don't know whether it was an oversight on my part or not . . . before I saw him I kept thinking about what I was going to say so that by the time I got down to it everything just blurted out (*laughs*). My thoughts were so jumbled that afterwards I wasn't sure I had made myself understood.

Dr. Console: Are there any questions you want to ask me?

Patient: Well, on the basis of what you've heard today . . . I think my problem is extremely serious, although I didn't before. But every time I tell you or someone about it, it becomes more serious to me.

Dr. Console: Serious in what sense?

Patient: Well, that it's affecting my life. It's affecting the people close to me. Although I can function properly I feel that I have a great neurosis which probably will not become better but will become worse. I just wonder . . . I see a lot of elderly people who cannot handle themselves—cannot handle the fact that they're getting older, and if I have this feeling complicated by my neurosis, what will this do to me in later life? I have this great anxiety about that. So, I'd like to know whether or not you feel that my problem is minor, major, or if it really would complicate my life.

Dr. Console: Well, you say that it's complicated your life up until now.

Patient: Yes, definitely. That's true . . . so I can answer my own question (*pause*). Especially with these sexual experiences. I keep thinking to myself . . . I'm getting older. How much more time do I have to enjoy myself sexually. I guess that's a very important part of everybody's life. And I don't want to miss out on these things.

Dr. Console: Focusing again for a moment on the question that many patients raise in this situation, namely, "Am I crazy?" or some variant of it, the situation will be a bit different in private practice. When you see a patient in these circumstances, the question at the end of the initial interview will often be, "Do you think I need treatment?" It is my practice in that circumstance to turn the question back to the person in much the same way that I did here. Simply by reviewing with the patient his symptoms, his description of the distress, his confusion and problems, he is often able to answer his own question. So, you don't have to be a salesman and try to convince the patient that treatment is indicated. You only have to ask him what *he* thinks in light of the symptoms.

> *Patient*: I said to my wife one time ... I said, "Look, it's important that I go through this because when our kids are not home any more, all we will have is the two of us to worry about ... no one else. And we've got to live together and it's very important that we think of ourselves." As a matter of fact, I didn't actually think about coming for therapy for myself ... or for either of us individually. We thought of going to a marriage counselor.

Dr. Console: I would like to look for a moment at his last statement. He makes a projection ... not in a psychiatric sense ... but a temporal projection when he takes a look toward the future and realizes that the children will grow up. That eventually he and his wife will be alone and they really don't talk much now and there is no sexual life. What is going to happen? There is a real sadness here in the matter of his anticipation that life in the future will be bleak indeed. Now the children take up a lot of effort, energy and interest on his part, but he anticipates the emptiness of their future together once the children are gone.

> *Patient*: We thought of going to a marriage counselor. I thought that would solve the problem but I think I need something deeper than that.
> *Dr. Console*: When Dr. Adams spoke to you, he said that he would meet with you on this coming Thursday. He was not aware that this would be on Thanksgiving. ...
> *Patient*: Thanksgiving. I thought about that too but I thought that he might be here.

Dr. Console: Dr. Adams had been unaware that the Thursday in question was Thanksgiving. He says, "I thought of that too." But he didn't say anything. There is nothing in the direction of a realistic, aggressive posture where he might politely decline the appointment because of the holiday. Now, I mention a realistic and aggressive posture that this man did not adopt. Unfortunately, the term *aggression*, over the years, has taken on a pejorative connotation. I believe this is unfortunate because not all aggression is unhealthy or dangerously obtrusive or in violation of other people's sensibilities. There is such a thing as well-modulated and healthy aggression ... or perhaps, aggressivity. That is, the ability and the willingness to demand what is one's rightful due in the way of consideration and respect, which does not connote stepping on another's toes. To politely decline an appointment because it conflicts with prior plans or because it falls on a holiday and you would rather spend that time with your family, does not constitute an aggressive or hostile act. It is healthy and realistic and reflects a reasonable level of good sense and self-esteem.

> *Dr. Console*: You thought about it but you didn't say anything ... ask about it?
> *Patient*: I thought about it afterwards.
> *Dr. Console*: I see *(pause)*. If you call the clinic and ask for Dr. Adams, he'll arrange for another appointment for you.
> *Patient*: OK. Fine.
> *Dr. Console*: All right. Thank you very much.
> *Patient*: Thank you. *The Interview Ends*

Dr. Console: OK. Now, we've gone over this tape in great detail and in light of this, I would not be surprised if you don't remember everything that we've tried to dissect and understand. Nonetheless, I'm going to ask you to give me your impression of the totality of this interview. Your impressions in these terms: This man is now your patient. You're going to see him in therapy. How do you feel about it? What do you think? What's going to happen?
Dr. Drucker: I think that he has some motivation. He wants to

improve his life. I think there's a lot of fertile ground here for change and improvement. Despite his immense anxiety, there are many positive features. He seems intelligent. He seems to have a certain amount of insight, or maybe I should say that he's inclined toward having some insight. I don't think that, in his present state, he has very much but he seems to be directed in that way.

Dr. Vis: One thing is for sure: if he entered treatment he would come to every session. He would always be on time.

Dr. Console: Of that you can be sure.

Dr. McDermott: He impresses me as an extremely passive man. Hard to get hold of. He isn't at all self-assertive. But, I think he could probably be helped after a long initial period of waiting and frustration.

Dr. Kent: I think it would take a long time for this man to make any progress in treatment. I have some reservations about his willingness to change and really make an effort to do so. I think it would be a lot easier to treat someone who has a little more bite to his bark than he has. I wonder if his passivity is not so great as to make him almost untreatable. I don't know if I could answer that question at this point.

Dr. Waldemar: Well, we've seen how compliant he is. We have to look at the total picture. He's severely neurotic and might be the kind of person who would sit passively and wait for instructions from the therapist . . . advice from the doctor. He uses denial and intellectualization a great deal and I would think that his therapy would proceed very slowly. Perhaps we should have goals in mind that are more in line with his difficulties rather than trying to get him to the point of having a very active sex life and all of that. Perhaps more modified goals such as getting along better with his wife, establishing more of a dialogue with her, and at least beginning to have some sexual relationship with her.

Dr. Rubin: I think that he's the kind of patient who would let the therapist's interpretations roll like water off a duck's back. It would be difficult to treat him and I think it would be a very frustrating experience. I think he would be extremely compliant . . . the way he was in this interview. You just wouldn't be able to get through to him and that could lead to trouble in tolerating your own frustration. I think you could end up interpreting away with him, and finding it had accomplished nothing.

Dr. Kent: I'm thinking back to the very beginning of this tape when he mentioned his *undergoing* therapy. I think that word reflects on his ability to handle insight. He would let the doctor do all the work and in the name of compliance he would say anything that the therapist wanted to hear ... or that he thought the therapist wanted to hear. I think we also have to consider that he's continued in his present life style for many many years now and never sought help until this point.

Dr. Console: Yes, and I would suggest that the quality of this man's willingness to talk about his troubles has a distinctly masochistic tone. It is in the nature of a self-deprecating confession. Now, we really don't have to wonder too much about the answers to the questions that you've raised, because since approximately Thanksgiving of 1973 ... right after this interview with me ... he has been in treatment with Dr. Adams. He was presented at a continuous-case seminar last year and is still in treatment with Dr. Adams. So I suggest that you direct your questions to Dr. Adams. What do you want to know about this man? He's been in treatment all this time—for over a year and a half.

Dr. Vis: Would you like to continue with him for another year? (*group laughter*).

Dr. Farber: Has he missed any sessions?

Dr. Adams: I gather from the consensus that the group mainly expects that he didn't miss any sessions. You're correct. He's hardly ever missed a session.

Dr. Farber: What were his responses to interpretations?

Dr. Adams: Let me make things a little easier for everybody by saying that in the main, your comments about this patient, his defenses, his disposition toward treatment, in particular your comments about setting more realistic goals in his treatment ... have all been borne out. They've all been borne out remarkably, and I'm impressed by the accuracy of your predictions based on the material that emerged in an initial interview. To spare you the effort of many questions concerning relatively minor issues, let me say that most of your comments have been right on target. The things that you've been saying have been confirmed in my treatment of this man. I wanted to say that first so that if there are any more specific questions that you would like me to elaborate on, I'll be happy to try.

Dr. Kent: I'd like to know if he's any different now than he was when he first started treatment. Has he been able to make any changes over the time he's been with you?

Dr. Adams: Would you think that there's been a big change in him?

Dr. Vis: No. I would guess that there's been very little.

Dr. Adams: That's right. There have not been many changes, at least not changes of the kind that we hope to see in a patient that involve his defenses and basic character structure. This is not to say that there have been no changes at all ... specifically along the lines that Dr. Waldemar brought up. In terms of more limited goals and more limited expectations, there have been some changes.

Dr. Kent: Has he had intercourse since this tape was made?

Dr. Adams: He has not had intercourse. He has avoided it like the plague. I would like to preface some of what I'm going to say about this, however. I think it came out on the tape that Dr. Console had interviewed this man the day after I had done so. In this session, every expression and anecdote that he related was virtually a verbatim recital of what he had told me the preceding day. Over the last year and a half or so, there have been recurring vignettes and stories told in the same intellectual way ... without any attempt to get beyond or beneath the semantic content.

In the treatment, we've talked about this. We've talked about his immense fear that something terrible might happen to him, and also the other fear ... that he might inadvertently do something terrible to his wife ... destroy her or hurt her. He unconsciously views the sexual act as something aggressive, violent and destructive ... fraught with danger. However, over the last month or two, he's been able to begin making some sexual overtures to his wife. They've opened a dialogue about some of their difficulties. Although it sounded as though they had had sort of a dialogue and had talked about marriage counseling and their problems before, don't buy that. There was very little communication. The routine in this man's home was one in which he would go to his neutral corner and his wife would go to hers, with little or no talk. It was absolutely forbidden that they talk about anything that might lead to any closeness or intimacy, or that might force them to face their feelings . . . whether that might imply intercourse or anything else. Again, in the last month or so, he has spoken with his wife about his distress over their asexual marriage. She, quite correctly perceiving something about the nature of the treatment, said something like, "Those doctors, that's all they're interested in." So, you can see, it's a long time off before they'll have intercourse.

But intercourse is only one aspect of the problem. It's almost like a phobia at this point, in that the avoidance is spreading. Lately he's been reluctant to talk about anything that might remind him that intercourse may be at the end of the road. But I'm not sure that that's the main difficulty. There was an acute problem in the home . . . namely the trouble with his boy. This was the child who was in treatment.

Dr. Console: He did not mention in the interview that in addition to the enuresis the boy also had the same trouble that he had had as a child . . . encopresis. Tell them about how this was handled.

Dr. Adams: Well, part of this certainly came out in the tape. There is a tremendous identification with the son. It's almost more than an identification. In a sense, he may have more difficulties than just neurotic symptoms or a neurotic character structure. There really are times when he's not quite sure who he is. In the service of his wish to gratify his own need to be taken care of, especially his own anal concerns, he has become vigorously involved in taking care of his son. There's a special bond or arrangement that they have. In addition to bed-wetting, the boy also soils himself. And whenever the son is encopretic, he is "unable" to clean himself up. This is a boy who is now nine or ten years old. When the encopresis occurs, the father runs up to the bathroom and washes the boy off. He plays with the boy and with the feces and is intimately involved in a wish of his own . . . one that goes back to his own childhood. If you remember, he discussed his own experiences as a child in school. He would rush home and have a bowel movement on the way. In a sense this is a man who has the capacity to split objects. Thus, the teacher in school was the horrible mother who would beat him up or lock him in a closet, and he could come home to the wonderful, good mother who would do what he does for *his* son . . . bathe him and cleanse him. In this context, perhaps you won't be surprised to learn that his own mother was wiping his rectum after he had his bowel movements until he was about twelve or thirteen years old!

Dr. Console: Tell them about the Mallomars.

Dr. Adams: Well, he talked about his urge to eat constantly and how this was one of his greatest pleasures in life. He almost sees himself as a little boy of two years of age, whose main interests are eating and defecating. Sex is something that he recognizes as existing, but he's retreated from that into a different world. In this connection he mentioned a good friend of his at Weight Watchers. This friend would take his Mallomars and found that they fitted nicely into a roll of toilet paper . . . he would sequester them there. When he went to the toilet he could sit there and eat the chocolate Mallomars.

Dr. Rubinstein: Do you all know what Mallomars are? (*group laughter*).

Dr. Adams: They're chocolate-covered marshmallow cookies. If it's slightly warm or humid, the chocolate will melt and get all over your hands, which can lead to chocolate-covered hands (*group laughter*).

Dr. Console: Well, it's more than just over one's hands. They're put in with the toilet paper. You can imagine what a very real fascination this story had for him. As he cleans his son, as Dr. Adams mentions, he delights in handling and touching and playing with feces. Here an even more primitive urge is suggested—to eat the feces. A soft Mallomar on toilet paper is quite clearly representative of such a striving.

Now, let me elaborate a bit on the beginnings of this case. The doctor who was treating his son was aware that we were seeking someone for the continuous-case seminar, and he offered this man as a made-to-order patient for such a proceeding. I asked Dr. Adams to arrange for a taping and having sat with this man for maybe five minutes, I had the impression that he was not nearly so good a patient as he first appeared . . . particularly in terms of what

Dr. Waldemar described . . . the matter of reasonable goals and so forth. The goals here would have to be quite restricted. Now, unquestionably all of the psychopathology would be very interesting and the identification and fusion with the child would be instructive. But, in terms of the kind of patient in whom there would be significant changes and improvement over the course of a year, I felt with this man very little would happen. I must say I'm delighted to see how well all of you perceived that in the initial interview. This is not a case that's going to move very quickly.

Dr. Rubinstein: Dr. Adams, would you share with us some of your feelings about your experience with him? It's been a bit over a year and a half that you've been treating him . . . what has it been like for you?

Dr. Adams: It hasn't been a bad experience. I've enjoyed it. It's been a challenge and a chance to learn a great deal. I've had to be somewhat imaginative in trying to figure out ways to help him. I couldn't just sit back and adopt a passive or "analytic" role; if I did he would become very anxious. I had to learn to be somewhat more flexible and different in my approach and that's been an education. I've made attempts to interpret his resistances . . . and it's been a fascinating process. If, however, my expectation had been that when I came up with a clever interpretation, the resistance would melt away and the treatment would progress rapidly, I would be miserable right now. I would have been sorely frustrated. I really don't expect that that's ever going to happen. I really think that some of what I say to him is as much for me as it is for him. I try to make an interpretation because I think it applies dynamically to his difficulties, but he hardly ever shows the capacity to use interpretations. His responses are, "Yes, you're right. I know what you mean", and so forth. He doesn't use interpretations for growth, insight or any sort of consolidation.

There has been a change though. We've talked about his difficulty in standing up like a man. He realizes that his father was not someone with whom he could identify strongly. This ties in with some of his rage, because he's afraid that if he expresses rage he will either kill or be killed. He's begun to channel some of these angry feelings in a more appropriate way. What used to happen was that his boss at work, whom he used to call "the animal," would say something to him and the patient would not say a word and just stew in his juice. He would say to me, "I showed him how angry I was by not saying anything," and no one would know that he was angry. He would go about his business in the most compliant way but would feel enraged inside. In the course of the last eight months or so, he's been able to respond more appropriately in an angry way. On one occasion when he did this, he said to me in a session soon afterwards, "You know, when I did that, I didn't spend the rest of the day hating this man. When I came home, I didn't think about killing my wife." What happened prior to this was that he felt that he couldn't get angry at his boss at work. He would come home full of anger and would want his wife to understand him . . . almost by reading his mind . . . which she couldn't possibly do. He would then feel that she didn't care for him and he would want to kill her. His defensive response to this would be to go to his room and hide and then she would respond by falling asleep at the kitchen table. He's been able to stick his neck out a little and has begun to find out that nothing terrible happens when he gets angry.

This past year, he was asked to be the regional representative for his union. He would represent the entire borough of Manhattan. It scared him to do this but it's a measure of the fact that somehow he's now able to give people the idea that he is competent and capable. He's been able to arbitrate disputes at work and to handle some of his feelings of anger in various areas of his life. There's been an increase in his ability to look into his feelings. This applies particularly to feelings about being destroyed or hurt. He's been able to test the water a little bit and find that it's not quite as dangerous as he had imagined it to be. In view of this, his self-esteem has increased meaningfully. I think that what is involved here is the fantasy that I'm behind him, reinforcing him and giving him power in some kind of loving, paternal way. I'm the good father enabling him to do things that he could never do before. The effect of this, again, has been a measurable increase in his self-esteem, which has been helpful to him in dealing with his family, particularly with his wife. He's been able to go to his wife and say, "Look, I think we should be able to talk about such and such." He's had relapses when he's blown up and almost lost control, but the quality of these outbursts has changed. Many of the self-destructive, world-destructive ideas have begun to be replaced by questions about how he could behave more appropriately. How should he act with his wife? Is he doing the correct thing with his son?

Along this line, a vignette is worth mentioning. He was sitting at the table and had buttered his younger son's bread (now seven years old). His ten-year-old son wanted him to do the same for him and instead of feeling that it was a good thing for a child to grow and become more independent, he felt badly that he had to "deprive" the son of having his bread buttered. He has a terribly inverted idea of what it means to grow up. He sees it as a deprivation rather than as an expression of mastery and independence. He felt badly for his older son in the context of his own identification with him because he himself is afraid to grow up. He now recognizes the very strong urge that he has to infantilize his children and keep them small. In this first interview, he gave evidence of this concern ... what will happen when he loses the children? They are a tremendous source of gratification for him and in a sense he lives through them.

Just one other vignette, this one in response to Dr. Drucker's earlier question about castration anxiety. It is indeed quite specific and quite overwhelming in this man. We had been working for a long period of time on the fact that his relationship to me in the treatment is very much an attempt to reenact his earlier relationship with his mother. He would bring in all kinds of "crap" to every session and he would want me to clean it up and send him off feeling that he had been tidied up and cared for. In addition, his whole concept of his sex life is a degraded one. The vernacular and vocabulary of his sexual experiences is the vocabulary of the toilet. "I want to sit there ... I want to do it ... I don't want to have to produce ... I don't want to give what I'm supposed to give" ... and so on. What emerged eventually was an immense phobia linking his castration anxiety to the toilet. To this day he has a phobia of toilets, but it is no longer restricting his activities to the degree that it once was. While he was an adolescent, he would have one foot out of the door before he flushed the toilet and when he did flush it, he would run for his life. This fear is still there for him.

He's terrified of being overwhelmed and drowned, and of losing parts of his body in the toilet, specifically his genitals. So an understanding of castration anxiety, and the way in which it can bring about a regression to earlier and more primitive fears and anxieties, is absolutely essential if one is going to be of help to this man in psychotherapy.

CHAPTER SEVEN

A Suicidal Young Woman

Dr. Console was asked to interview a female patient who was on the treatment ward of the psychiatric hospital. He taped the interview and in the following session the tape is reviewed with the ward staff. Both Dr. Simons and Dr. Rubinstein were present at this meeting.

Dr. Console: Why don't we begin with Dr. Bond's giving us some of the history pertinent to this patient's case.

Dr. Bond: The patient is a twenty-year-old, white English woman who was transferred to the psychiatric ward in March, after having been evaluated on several other services at Kings County Hospital where she has been hospitalized for four months. She was initially admitted with a chief complaint of hematuria and severe abdominal pain. During the time that she was being evaluated for these complaints, she developed fever and spiked temperatures of 102 and 103 degrees. She was then thoroughly worked up for the additional problem of the fever but no causative condition was found. Since coming to the hospital in November, she has undergone laparoscopy, cystoscopy four times, exploratory laparotomy, culdoscopy, two renal biopsies, two liver biopsies, and has received almost every conceivable laboratory study.

She has been presented at two Grand Rounds meetings on Internal Medicine and Surgery and has been the subject of three interdisciplinary conferences among the Departments of Internal Medicine, Obstetrics and Gynecology, Surgery and Urology.

She has never refused any procedure that her doctors have proposed for her and has not been known to complain of any discomfort or pain resulting from such procedures, whether it be an unsuccessful venipuncture where she would be pricked at five or more different sites before a necessary blood specimen was obtained, or whether it be a surgical exploratory procedure. She has stated that she would deliberately try to confuse her doctors and tell them whatever she thought they wanted to hear. Before undergoing the exploratory laparotomy she told the surgeon that it would be all right if she died because she didn't deserve to live anyway. Furthermore, the patient had been receiving fifty milligrams of Demerol, six times daily for a number of weeks and was noted to be suffering from a mild withdrawal syndrome when it was discontinued.

At various times her abdominal pain has been relieved by placebos. She's complained of dark, tarry stools but has never been able to show these to the staff. For four months prior to admission, she complained of night sweats but no such phenomenon was observed while she was in the hospital. At one point she was placed on Elavil but she complained that the medication was causing her to feel nauseated and to vomit, at which time it was discontinued. At various times throughout her stay she has been treated with Streptomycin, Isoniazid and Penicillin, and had developed an apparent serum sickness from the Penicillin.

One month prior to coming into the hospital, the patient relates that she broke off a relationship that she had been having with a thirty-two-year-old, married, and very sadistic cousin, of whom the patient said, "He's too much like my brother and anyway . . . he's too close to the family." Also during this time, the patient had been seeing a man who is a medical resident at another hospital.

She had been employed at a prestigious store as a secretary and had a good work record. She had also been taking a number of courses in child psychology at a local college.

The patient has also begun suffering from insomnia, because when she fell asleep she would have a repetitive dream in which she would be having pleasurable sexual intercourse with a youthful and handsome man, only to have him suddenly change into a huge, dark, horrendous monster.

She has been hospitalized twice in the past for psychiatric illness, once at age sixteen when she was treated for fainting spells and the second time when she was treated for depression and a suicide attempt. She has attempted suicide at six different times in the past, not to mention other gestures. After slashing her wrist on Easter Day of last year, she denied any memory of what had occurred. For the past three years the patient has attempted suicide on or around Easter time.

She underwent an appendectomy at age sixteen, and at age fourteen was hospitalized for two months because of fever of undetermined origin. At age seventeen she deliberately splashed a caustic solution into her face because she was having severe headaches. On one occasion last year she suffered total body paralysis which lasted for about twelve hours. There have been a number of other hospitalizations for the same presenting symptoms that brought about this hospitalization. Also, at age eighteen she developed bladder stones while following a restricted-calorie diet. Last year she was treated by means of hypnosis for her recurrent fainting spells. After being transferred to the psychiatric ward, the patient began requesting injections of tranquilizers.

Dr. Console: Why was she transferred to the psychiatric ward? How did this come about?

Dr. Bond: Basically because no explanation for her chief complaint could be found by the other services involved in her stay at the hospital. It was then discovered that she had a psychiatric history. At this point she threatened to commit suicide if she was discharged and sent home. One of the first things that she said when she came to the ward was that it was a good thing that she hadn't been sent home because she felt at the time that she would have killed herself.

Dr. Harvey: I think there's another element. I think that after all this trouble, the medical people started to get annoyed with her because there were some comments made that implied that her symptoms were all fictitious. I would expect that it was really more than a discharge . . . something more in the nature of throwing the patient out. At that point she indicated that "If you do that, I'm going to harm myself."

Dr. Console: Yes. It's customary that if anyone presents these myriad symptoms and is the subject of an obviously intensive study . . . Grand Rounds and Interdisciplinary Seminars and so on

... and they don't come up with a satisfactory answer, the physicians get frustrated. Then if there is talk about suicide or anything of that nature, this is their way out. They present her to the Department of Psychiatry. When it has gotten to the point where the patient starts climbing out the window, then the psychiatrist is called in as a consultant. I think that a consultation is indicated long before that. It is indicated whenever a patient is evaluated over and over again and nothing organic is found. I think it's going to take a long time to get this across. I've spent almost thirty years of my life trying to teach medical students in this regard. I've tried to help them to think in terms of potential psychiatric difficulty early in the course of someone's complaining, rather than waiting until the patient is climbing the walls or threatening to sign out of the hospital or to kill himself. By that time the psychiatric consultation may be too late.

Dr. Bond: After being transferred to the psychiatric service, she began requesting injections to "calm her nerves," as she would put it. She would either refuse to take oral medications or would take them and then return to the nursing station about twenty minutes later and state that she had become nauseated and had vomited and would again ask for intramuscular medication. The patient continued demanding injections in order to sleep. The medication for sleep would often be obtained from the night resident on call, until the entire staff was requested not to provide her with intramuscularly administered medication. In the early weeks of her stay on the ward the patient complained of nightmares and frightening hypnogogic phenomena, with subsequent insomnia, despite which she continued to refuse oral medicines, hoping to be given intramuscular medication. Further, she frequently refused to eat but was observed later to be secretly eating in her room or in the utility room or with visiting relatives.

Her relationships with people on the ward have been turbulent. Initially she alienated most of the other patients, particularly other women, while relating seductively to many of the male patients. One in particular is a gregarious, married man. She would also spend a great deal of time moping in her room or lying in bed crying.

In psychotherapy, the patient relates in a negativistic and noncommunicative manner. At least she did for about the first three weeks of her hospitalization. Throughout this time she has remained aloof from the therapeutic community and has been oblivious to peer-group pressure. Her individual psychotherapy sessions are dominated by silences, demands for medication and complaints of physical illness. One Friday afternoon at 4:30, immediately following a therapy session, she was observed by another patient to be attempting self-strangulation, saying that she could not go on living. She continued threatening to kill herself unless she was given intramuscular medication. At that time she was transferred to a closed psychiatric ward for acute cases, where she stayed for six days.

Since returning to the therapeutic community ward she has been continually agitated or depressed, but improves as the week draws to a close and she manages to obtain a weekend pass. She is frequently visited by medical doctors, including some of her former physicians here at the hospital. It has also been learned that the patient attempted to communicate information to her therapist through the other doctors, while at the same time stating that she had nothing to say during regular therapy sessions. Last Wednesday she was observed to be wrapped in a blanket, lying on the floor, trembling and crying for a period of two to three hours.

Dr. Console: Was that Wednesday evening?

Dr. Bond: Yes, it was.

Dr. Console: The interview on tape was done Wednesday morning.

Dr. Bond: Yes, that's right. At that time she said only that she was nervous and depressed and wished to be left alone. More recently, over the past three days, she has been participating more in community activities but continues to insist that she's a worthless creature who doesn't deserve help or even kindness. At the same time she relates to most people in a cold and haughty manner.

Dr. Console: It may well be that in seeing this girl I had an advantage in having heard virtually none of this history or information. If I remember correctly, Dr. Harvey did suggest that this was indeed a very interesting patient with some interesting problems, but I think that all I knew was that she had been admitted to the hospital because of hematuria and fever. I didn't realize that there had been a four-month period on the other services, but I think that Dr. Harvey did tell me that she had had all kinds of tests and that they could find no basis for the bleeding.

You have heard this very fine description that Dr. Bond has given us and I want you to think about the characterization of this girl in terms of her negativism, her noncooperation and her histrionic and hysterical behavior ... her demanding, her tyrannizing, her statements, "I'll kill myself unless you give me this or that," and so on. Now, let's turn on the tape and look at the interview.

Dr. Evans: Before we begin, Dr. Console, I would like to mention that we presented this patient at another case conference on the ward about six weeks ago. It was very early in the course of her hospitalization. I think that we had raised several questions about her and I hope that we can touch on them today. One of the questions was and still is that of the diagnosis. Some people are concerned that she may be schizophrenic. She may be sicker than she initially presents. The second question has to do with problems during her hospitalization. We certainly realized that she was an atypical patient for our ward ... that she would place great demands upon us and upon her therapist, and the question is how and if we can meet those demands. The third question involves a concern as to what would be the best approach with her in individual therapy. I would appreciate it if we could keep these questions in mind and perhaps at the end of the tape we can discuss them.

Dr. Console: All right. Now, I'm going to show you this interview, which unfortunately is not my customary one-hour interview. We sandwiched it in between the start of the day at 9:00 in the morning and my commitment to give a 10:00 lecture to the medical students. So it was a somewhat hurried interview. But I would ask one thing ... that you be very careful about how you use the information that we derive from this tape because it is my intention to see this girl again, maybe two or three times more. I think she will be willing to be taped again, so we can have a follow-up.

(The videotape machine is turned on. The patient and Dr. Console are seen sitting in their respective seats, facing each other. The patient is a young, attractive, white woman, in her early twenties, casually dressed in slacks and a blouse.)

Dr. Console: Tell me, you've been in the hospital for some time now. Why are you in the hospital?

Patient: I came in at first because of hematuria, fever and pain.

Dr. Console: Hematuria, fever and pain. And you've had this for how long?

Patient: Before I came in?

Dr. Console: Yes.

Patient: I've had this hematuria for about two years. And the fever since I came into the hospital.

Dr. Console: Hematuria for two years?

Patient: On and off.

Dr. Console: And what were you told about this? What was causing this hematuria?

Patient: They couldn't find out.

Dr. Console: They couldn't find out. What do you think was causing it? Do you have some idea?

Patient: No, not really. I was thinking that maybe it was my kidneys.

Dr. Console: Maybe it's your kidneys.

Patient: But I couldn't know for sure.

Dr. Console: Would you watch for this? Whenever you urinated you would look to see whether there was blood in the urine?

Patient: Yes . . .

Dr. Console: You would. As though you expected something to be there.

Patient: Yes. I would say so.

Dr. Console: I see. What about the first time? You said two years ago. How did you discover it originally?

Patient: I discovered it after I had a pain in my back.

Dr. Console: A pain in your back?

Patient: Yes. And I went to the doctor and he tested my urine and told me that there was blood there. At that time it was microscopic.

Dr. Console: So, point number one. She had pain in her back and she went to a doctor. He tested her urine and he told her there was blood in the urine. And it wasn't visible. She was *told* that there was blood in her urine.

Dr. Console: How old are you?
Patient: Twenty.
Dr. Console: Twenty. Tell me about yourself—in general. Where you're from.
Patient: Well, originally I'm from England.
Dr. Console: You're from England.
Patient: Yes.
Dr. Console: And how long have you been here?
Patient: Ten months.
Dr. Console: Ten months. Can you tell me about your family? What it was like being a little girl?
Patient: I had a pretty happy childhood but when I turned thirteen I became . . . I don't know . . . I became withdrawn. I stayed by myself.
Dr. Console: When was this, you say?
Patient: Around thirteen.
Dr. Console: Around thirteen. You became withdrawn and stayed by yourself.
Patient: Yes. I would stay by myself.
Dr. Console: Why was that?
Patient: I liked to be alone.
Dr. Console: You liked to be alone. What did other people say about this? What did your family say?
Patient: My mother didn't like it. She would get mad.
Dr. Console: Can you tell me about your father and mother?
Patient: My father is quieter than my mother. He wouldn't yell at the kids. He was understanding. When I was withdrawn he would come into my room and talk to me. My mother was the opposite.

Dr. Console: So your mother would kind of try to chase you out of the room into some activity. . . .

Patient: Yes. . . .

Dr. Console: Whereas your father came and talked to you in your room. Just the two of you?

Patient: Yes.

Dr. Console: . . . and then he left without making any demands.

Patient: He would just say "You should get out" but he wouldn't push and push.

Dr. Console: So, let's establish some of this girl's family orientation. She makes the distinction immediately between the strictness of the mother who urged her to get out, and the attitude of the father. We can extrapolate from this the frustration that the mother must have felt. She must have repeatedly challenged the girl with "Why don't you go out? Why are you staying in your room?" Perhaps she would even become a bit annoyed. The father on the other hand was soft. He came to her room and sat with her and talked with her and he was nice and did not make these demands. So she's made a very definite distinction in her attitude toward her father and mother.

Dr. Console: Tell me about your brothers and sisters.

Patient: I have four brothers and sisters. There are five of us. The oldest is my sister and then come two boys. Then me and then my younger brother.

Dr. Console: So there's a boy before you and a boy after you.

Patient: Yes.

Dr. Console: Do you think that has anything to do with the way you look at things? That you had a brother and then you came along and then you had another brother? So here you were kind of sandwiched in there.

Patient: Yes. I felt that there was a lot of protection of me by them.

Dr. Console: You felt a lot of protection.

Patient: Yes. And my father was there too. He would protect me in case my brothers got too rough with me.

Dr. Console: And what about school? As a youngster.

Patient: I started school at about four years old. It was a church school. And a year later . . . my teacher died. I saw her. I saw her when she died.

Dr. Console: You saw her when she died? Meaning . . .?

Patient: It was lunchtime. She had the school right at her house. When it was hot she would take a bath at lunchtime. I liked her a lot and I used to wait for her to come out. But that day she didn't come out so I went in to see her and there she was in the bath . . . dead.

Dr. Console: And you were then . . .

Patient: Five.

Dr. Console: Five years old.

Patient: I was so shocked. I wouldn't go back to that school . . . ever again. I was too scared ever to go back.

Dr. Console: Indeed . . . you must have been scared to come upon a teacher whom you liked . . . to find her dead in the bath.

Dr. Console: So here is trauma number one, and a trauma of considerable magnitude. That a teacher whom she liked was found dead by her in this fashion. Now, those of you who are familiar with my usual method of interviewing may be aware that I'm pushing along quite rapidly here. I'm really working by the clock because of the limited time available. I think the total interviewing time turned out to be only about thirty-five minutes. There are many areas that I would have liked to discuss more carefully, but you will observe me from time to time glancing at my watch. However, we can appreciate the magnitude of this incident in the light of what we already know of her feelings about her mother and father. We can postulate that here was the "good mother" . . . the teacher . . . in place of the "bad mother." This was someone whom she liked. At age five she discovered this woman dead in the bath. So perhaps her death wishes toward her mother had now been realized. So, there may be here one of the first important sources of her masochism . . . of her guilt. Her wish came true in that the mother or mother substitute died. It might have been fruitful to have explored what it was that she saw. How did the teacher die? As a general rule, of course, it's a good idea when hearing of an incident that may be so important in a patient's life, to obtain as many of the details of the situation as possible but I just did not have time.

> *Dr. Console*: So what happened after that? You say that you didn't want to go back to school . . . which is understandable.
> *Patient*: Yes. Well, my father was a dentist and he was moved to another borough and then I was able to go to another school.

Dr. Console: So again, if I had had more time, I would have inquired in more detail about this situation. I would have specifically inquired about the father who was a dentist. What I would want to know would be the nature of his professional arrangement. Namely, was his office in the house where the children could see or be aware of the patients who came and went? Just think of what it might mean to a child who is three, four, five or six . . . who sees people come, hears people scream and cry, who senses the anxiety of people going to a dentist and who sees them walking out, perhaps with a piece of gauze, bleeding and so on . . . all of which provides rich material for many fantasies concerning what the father does to people. So this is very important. In my experience, the children of dentists have a hard time in their lives if they have observed the father at his work.

Dr. Simons: Isn't there another dimension, too? Wherever the office might have been, she may very early have gotten the idea that the only way to get really close to her father would be to become a patient in one form or another. This may have great meaning in view of her life over these last few years and her involvement with a whole series of doctors. All of them may represent her father.

Dr. Console: Yes. This is characterized by the joke about the child who has a psychiatrist for a parent, or where both parents are psychiatrists and they have their practices in the house. Visitors come for a social event and someone asks the child, "What do you want to be when you grow up?" And the child answers, "I want to be a patient" (*group laughter*).

Dr. Simons: She may also have identified with her dentist father and be doing to herself what her father once did to his patients, especially if she was one of his patients. It may be that, in some way, she actively causes the hematuria by some sort of conscious or unconscious manipulation, or by the insertion of something into her urethra.

Dr. Console: Yes. I think this is a definite possibility and is something that I would ask the nurses to look for very carefully.

Dr. Console: You say that he was moved to a different borough. Did he ask to be moved to a different borough because you wouldn't go to the school? Do you remember that?

Patient: Yes. I think he wanted to move anyway and this just helped it all along. I did all right after that. In general I could say that I had a happy childhood.

Dr. Console: Well you say, "I had a happy childhood," but what changed at thirteen? Now your happy childhood becomes a solitary one.

Patient: It was really at age fourteen.

Dr. Console: At fourteen.

Patient: Well, I had a really bad experience *(pause)*. I got raped at a party.

Dr. Console: At a party?

Patient: Right.

Dr. Console: So this was another frightening experience.

Patient: Yes. And I became pregnant and I had an abortion. I didn't tell anybody but I had it taken care of.

Dr. Console: How was this taken care of . . . without telling anyone?

Patient: I went to the doctor and he swore not to tell anybody.

Dr. Console: I see. And your parents never knew about it?

Patient: No.

Dr. Console: Did you like this boy?

Patient: I didn't know him.

Dr. Console: You didn't know him. And he forcibly . . .

Patient: Yes.

Dr. Console: So it was after this that you became withdrawn? Started to stay by yourself?

Patient: Yes. I was very distressed, upset and unhappy.

Dr. Console: And there was no desire . . . no need to tell your parents about this awful thing that happened?

Patient: No.

Dr. Console: They must have asked why you were staying in your room and so on.

Patient: They tried to find out what was wrong but I wouldn't tell them.

Dr. Console: What other experiences did you have after that? What other things happened?

Patient: Well, two years ago my boyfriend died. In a crash. He died in a car crash.

Dr. Console: Were you in the car with him?

Patient: No. But I was supposed to go with him.

Dr. Console: You were supposed to go with him?

Patient: Yes. But I didn't want to go.

Dr. Console: Why not?

Patient: I had changed my mind. I was going to but I decided not to.

Dr. Console: Was he angry with you that you didn't want to go with him?

Patient: No. He wasn't. But if I had been with him he might have been more careful (*pause*).

Dr. Console: Now what about your general physical health? You've had this hematuria and cystitis which you've mentioned. You had this pain in your back. Have you had any other illnesses?

Patient: Well, I have migraine headaches.

Dr. Console: Migraine headaches. Starting when?

Patient: At about thirteen.

Dr. Console: At thirteen.

Patient: Yes. But they stopped at about seventeen.

Dr. Console: Any other things?

Patient: I had an operation here about two months ago.

Dr. Console: What was the operation?

Patient: An exploratory laparotomy.

Dr. Console: An exploratory laparotomy. Because of . . .?

Patient: Because of the pain and the fever of unknown origin.

Dr. Console: Because of the pain and the fever (*pause*). Do you know how much fever you had?

Patient: Sometimes it would go up to 103 degrees. Then it would go up and down. For a while the doctors thought it might be an infection in the tubes but they didn't find anything.

Dr. Console: Did you have any further sexual experience after the rape?

Patient: About two years after.

Dr. Console: About two years after. Can you tell me what happened? You knew another boy?

Patient: Yes.

Dr. Console: And . . . you liked him and he liked you?

Patient: Oh yes. It certainly wasn't a bad experience. I had a really good relationship with another boy about four years later.

Dr. Console: And up to that time you had had other boyfriends?

Patient: Oh Yes. Many.

Dr. Console: And there were intimacies with these boys?

Patient: Yes, with most of them.

Dr. Console: And how did you feel . . . in light of having been raped as a fourteen-year-old girl? Now you were having intercourse. Did you have any feelings about it?

Patient: Sometimes, while I would be having intercourse I would get very depressed. Several times afterwards, I would try to commit suicide. I would get very down on myself and then I would do silly things.

Dr. Console: Like what?

Patient: I would get so depressed that sometimes it would be like I didn't know what I was doing anymore. I would take pills. I tried it three times. I took overdoses.

Dr. Console: And this happened three times. The first time . . . what happened?

Patient: I took the pills. It was while I was at nursing school. But I was found by my roommate.

Dr. Console: And the second time?

Patient: I couldn't sleep at night and I kept taking pills and more pills to get to sleep. I just wanted to sleep forever. The next morning . . . I was on nursing duty . . . and was walking to the hospital and I passed out. It was about ten o'clock.

Dr. Console: About ten o' clock. And you say you were on nursing duty?

Patient: Yes, I was studying nursing. I studied it for a year but I didn't like it.

Dr. Console: So the second time, you passed out in the morning?

Patient: Yes . . . I ended up in the hospital.

Dr. Console: You said there was a third time as well.

Patient: Yes. At that time I was in the hospital.

Dr. Console: You were in the hospital already?

Dr. Simons: I'm not so sure that she really wants to kill herself. I have more the feeling that what she really wants is to go on living so that she can suffer.

Dr. Console: Well, let's look at these gestures. To begin with, she's a nursing student and she didn't show up at her post. So someone is sent to her room at the dorm and she's discovered. Secondly . . . she can't sleep and is taking many pills. So at ten o'clock in the morning, she continues to take pills and gets up and walks out in the street and apparently collapses. On the third occasion, she is in a hospital and manages to get hold of some pills. Now here is a one-time nursing student . . . an obviously intelligent girl who cannot manage to overdose sufficiently. So we can have great question as to what was taking place, but there should be no question as to whether this girl is really attempting suicide. She is not. This girl is going through dramatic suicidal gestures to bring the environment to its knees, and to get the people in the environment to look after her. As Dr. Simons says, she really has no intention of killing herself. Her nursing experience helps to explain the ease with which she mentions these various procedures such as exploratory laparotomy and so on.

Dr. Bond: I think, also, that her having been a nursing student may help explain why her symptoms may be as convincing as they are.

Dr. Console: Yes. They have a certain coherence to them . . . a credibility.

> *Dr. Console:* What was it that made you depressed at these times? Were you going with a boy at the time?
>
> *Patient:* Everything seemed to be going well at the time but I was just very, very depressed.
>
> *Dr. Console:* Well, isn't that a strange thing to say . . . "Everything was going well at the time" . . ?
>
> *Patient:* Yes . . . but I was still depressed. I didn't want to live.
>
> *Dr. Console:* Were you brought up as a religious person?
>
> *Patient:* Yes.
>
> *Dr. Console:* What religion?
>
> *Patient* Anglican.
>
> *Dr. Console:* Anglican (*pause*). Do you think that plays any part in your feelings about being depressed and feeling that you're bad?
>
> *Patient:* In a way I blame myself for having that abortion. Because that's a life . . .

Dr. Console: She blames herself for having had the abortion because "that's a life." So she feels she committed murder. She killed somebody.

> *Patient:* Because that's a life . . . I killed somebody. And . . . going out with different boys . . . I'm very unclear about that. I think that was wrong too. But to kill *yourself* is not wrong.
>
> *Dr. Console:* But tell me, in light of what has been happening for the past few years . . . that women believe that their bodies are theirs and they have the right to have an abortion if that's what they want. It's upheld by the Constitution of the United States.
>
> *Patient:* I know. I feel that way too. But subconsciously I don't know if that's the way I really feel.
>
> *Dr. Console:* So, consciously you agree that women have the right to have their own lives and control over their own

bodies and the lives inside them . . . but somewhere else, you don't feel that way (*pause*). What about psychiatric treatment?

Patient: What about it?

Dr. Console: Well, since this is a matter of your feeling guilty, how are we going to take this away? How are we going to help you with it?

Patient: I don't know. I just feel bad about everything. I just start to feel down and no good. It takes very little to get me upset and crying. I start thinking about killing myself.

Dr. Console: Now tell me. What do you think that all of this has to do with hematuria?

Patient: It's not connected.

Dr. Console: It's not connected. The hematuria is just something . . .

Patient: The doctor told me they just had another case like mine, where there was just blood from childhood on. It's not really my biggest problem . . . it doesn't really bother me now.

Dr. Console: You say the hematuria doesn't bother you?

Patient: I guess I've gotten used to it by now.

Dr. Console: Let's look back to when you were fourteen years old . . . when you were raped and unfortunately became pregnant. So you had an abortion. And you had an abortion under these clandestine circumstances. What happens immediately after? You went home . . . what did you do?

Patient: Yes . . . I went home.

Dr. Console: And then . . .

Patient: That's when I made up a story about headaches. For the next three days I had migraine headaches so I could stay home.

Dr. Console: But what did the doctor tell you was going to happen as a result of the abortion? What did he tell you to watch for?

Patient: He said I would have occasional bleeding.

Dr. Console: He said you would have occasional bleeding.

Patient: Yes (*pause*). I knew that doctor pretty well. I asked him not to tell my parents what had happened.

Dr. Console: And he was good enough not to betray you and tell what had happened. But again, he told you that you would have occasional bleeding. You would have some bleeding afterwards. So you had the headaches and were able to stay by yourself because you had that as an excuse.

Patient: Yes . . . that's right.

Dr. Console: You could go to the doctor whenever you felt the need, and no one would know that you were bleeding.

Patient: I figured that if there was any blood then I could make it look like I was just having my period.

Dr. Console: But you do tell me that your depression and your three suicide attempts are in some way connected with the abortion. Your feelings of guilt about the abortion.

Patient: I hate myself for it . . . for having been bad.

Dr. Console: For having been bad (*pause*). Normally when you're having your period and you go to the toilet, you look and see blood don't you? Some blood in the bowl?

Patient (nods): Yes . . .

Dr. Console: How do you know it's not hematuria?

Patient: Because it stops after a few days. The hematuria is always there. And, for the hematuria I don't have to wear anything.

Dr. Console: But every time that you urinate and there is some blood, does it remind you of anything?

Patient: No.

Dr. Console: No (*pause*). You don't think it might have anything to do with the bleeding that you did at fourteen?

Patient (smiling): I know what you're going to ask. . . .

Dr. Console (smiling): What makes you so smart . . . to know what I'm going to ask? (*group laughter*).

Patient: You think it's all psychological, when I bleed now . . . I remember the past.

Dr. Console: Not necessarily remember . . . no. But are you going to tell me that the rape and the abortion did not have a psychological effect on you?

Patient: It did. But not in *that* way.

Dr. Console: Not in that way.

Patient: No.

Dr. Console: And, you're a little annoyed that you knew I was going to ask that question.

Patient: Not annoyed . . . but I was waiting to hear it.

Dr. Console: Are you saying that you were waiting to hear it because you have been asked that same question many times before?

Patient: No, I haven't, but I knew that you would think that way.

Dr. Console: All right. You say that you knew that I would think that way. But you've talked to other doctors. Why didn't you know that they would think that way?

Patient: It's the way you get off the subject and come back to it later. Afterwards.

Dr. Console (smiling): You mean I'm pretty sneaky?

Patient (smiling): In a way . . . the way you ask certain leading questions. With something in mind

Dr. Console: Yes . . . very definitely. And I do want you to think about it (*pause*). Now, are you saying to me that no one else has suggested this linkage?

Patient: Nobody even knows about the abortion. I haven't even told my doctor here on the ward . . . so nobody even knows about it.

Dr. Console: Do you plan to stay in the hospital for a while?

Patient: Yes. But I feel badly about it. I'm wasting everybody's time.

Dr. Console: No. You're not wasting everybody's time. These things are not like operations, where we can go in and take the bad part out and throw it away in a wastepaper-basket and forget it. It takes time and it takes a deep understanding.

Patient: I know . . . but I get very nervous and they won't give me any medication. I'm not on any medication now and I get so nervous, I can't think. I get confused.

Dr. Console: The medication wouldn't help the confusion. It can slow things up in your mind so you could become more confused rather than less confused (*pause*). I think you'll be able to take care of this difficulty by developing a deeper understanding and a conviction as to how all this came about . . . what you are trying to accomplish in the unconscious . . . through the hematuria. And you'll learn better ways of

taking care of this, so that you don't really need to have
hematuria. You think about it and maybe we'll talk again. All
right?
   Patient: OK.
   Dr. Console: Thank you very much for coming.
   Patient: You're welcome. *The Interview Ends*

Dr. Console: All right. So again, this was an abbreviated interview
but I think that in a relatively short time some potentially
important dynamics were unfolded. This girl, who has been
cooperative, and who has that characteristic English accent, who is
a very attractive and intelligent girl, was disturbed to some degree
by the confrontation that I made, but at the same time she found
some pleasure in the situation. She's the focus of attention and is
aware that the interview is being recorded. Her exhibitionism is
being gratified to a degree and, strikingly, she suggests that she
has told no one else about the abortion ... including her own
therapist here at the hospital.

One of the very critical aspects of this girl's life history is the
abortion. And you can picture, as I did, a fourteen-year-old kid
whose father is a dentist, who goes to a doctor who is a friend and
is known to the family. The doctor knows something of the
general relationship of this girl to her parents and he enters into
collusion with her to protect her and not tell the parents. So the
parents don't know anything of what had happened. In that
circumstance, he's taking something of a risk. So he tells this girl to
watch for bleeding and so on and so forth. And lo and behold, she
watches for bleeding. Where does she watch for the bleeding? The
toilet bowl.

Now, she says that she has had the hematuria for two years. The
period of two years, at least temporally, coincides with the death of
her boyfriend. Two years ago he died in an accident. My asking her
if he had been angry with her because she didn't go with him on
that fatal trip, was an attempt to establish some of the sources of
her guilt. She says that he hadn't been angry but she nonetheless
feels that had she gone with him the accident might not have
happened and therefore in fantasy, she feels she killed this boy.

So, she killed the baby. She killed her mother-teacher. She killed this boy. And she has to pay for all of this. She has to suffer. What the specifics are in the matter of hematuria as one of the expressions through which she attempts to expiate her guilt, is something that I hope I will be able to unravel in further interviews with this girl. Now why don't we open things up for some further discussion.

Dr. Bond: I would like to add, before we go on . . . in connection with her father being a dentist. Many of the hypnogogic phenomena that she reported in the treatment were of a large, dark creature with claws . . . a creature that both approached her sexually and that was going to hurt her. Her father *did* work on her as well as on the other children.

As far as the oedipal material is concerned, I ought to mention that she left nursing after one year of study. She made that decision after an *elderly English lady* died in her arms. Also, she has on many occasions, entertained the fear that her father would shoot the mother when they argued. As a child, she remembered that he kept a loaded gun in the house and to curtail any arguments between her parents she would pretend to be sick so as to focus their attention on herself and away from the fighting.

Dr. Console: You can put that latter part a little more specifically. She was afraid that the father would shoot the mother and she had to prevent this because, at least in part, this was her wish.

Dr. Simons: Do you think that in light of what we know about this girl, it's likely that she invited the rape and perhaps even unconsciously sought it out? One reason that she might feel so guilty about the abortion is that she killed the baby that unconsciously she may very much have wanted.

Dr. Console: Again, by virtue of the brevity of this interview, there are many details missing. In the interview I asked her if she liked this boy and she informed me that she didn't know him. Well, it was at a party and I have serious questions about her not having known him. This probably was a party of young people . . . she's fourteen at the time. It may even have been chaperoned. I agree with Dr. Simons that there's a great likelihood that she had a greater involvement in this than she tells here in this interview, and it's something I would like to clarify in another talk with her.

Dr. Harvey: I would like to mention her capacity to pick out from the environment people who will gratify her masochistic wishes. She's had many encounters with other patients and with staff on the ward. Some of us have been talking about the almost persecutory posture that she adopts. I'm not sure whether it's persecutory or masochistic.

Dr. Simons: I think the two are very closely related. I suspect that rape fantasies are probably central in this girl's dynamics and have to do with what she imagined her violence-prone dentist-father was doing to his patients and to his wife. She is really reenacting these rape fantasies and also reenacting the abortion with all of the physicians and surgeons who have operated on her and probed her with instruments. There's a strong element of projection in any rape fantasy: "It's not me who wants this ... it's the man who's going to do it to me." Furthermore, with the failure of all of these tests and procedures and operations to find any cause for the hematuria, she has the opportunity to blame the physicians for not really having understood her. She does this on the tape. Nobody has yet understood her. So I think that the two themes ... the masochism and the persecutory, projective trend are very closely related.

Dr. Console: Absolutely. They have the same roots.

Dr. Rubinstein: Do you think that there's some real chance that she is in fact instrumenting herself or rather, that the hematuria is an unconscious symbolic and expiative conversion symptom?

Dr. Console: Both of these things are possible. My own feeling was that in response to my question about her temperature, she revealed some of what is truly going on. Here's a girl who has been a nursing student and must be familiar with many of the techniques by which patients can elevate their temperatures ... or at least make it appear that way on a thermometer. So I do indeed wonder about this girl's inserting something into her urethra or vagina. Now the story about her having had bladderstones because she was on a diet and so on ... I would have liked to ascertain the actual chemical composition of those bladder stones. This kind of person is capable of masturbating by inserting something into her urethra. I remember, as a medical student, we were shown an X-ray of a young man with bladder stones. The surgeons operated and removed the stones, and lo and behold, the "bladder stones" turned out to be a fine watch chain, encrusted in calcium and other chemicals. The urologist went on to say that this man had "gone fishing" in his bladder with the chain and he had lost the line. So, this is not a terribly uncommon thing. People will often masturbate by introducing some kind of filament or device into the urethra. And occasionally there is the chance that the object will slip and wind up in the bladder. This is easier in a girl, of course, because of the shorter urethra.

Dr. Bond: Last weekend, she had one of her tantrums for about three hours. She was sitting on the floor and had a blanket wrapped around her and was rocking back and forth. Do you think that she was masturbating then?

Dr. Console: I would certainly have to say that it was some sort of regressive acting out . . . a regressive phenomenon. It's hard to characterize it with the specificity of masturbation. I just don't know. It occurred after the interview that we've just watched. I had pointed out to her that she was a little annoyed with my confrontation, as indeed I sensed, and she admitted it. And one of the most striking things is her statement, "I knew you were going to say that." How in God's name did she know I was going to say that and how come she never knew that other doctors were going to say it? And this is a bright girl! She says in effect that I built up the story . . . "You were leading up to it." But she was with me every step of the way . . . leading up to it. So she shows absolutely no surprise at my confrontation that the hematuria represents a reenactment of the bleeding at the time of her abortion.

Dr. Alper: And moreover . . . if she is instrumenting herself, it's a reenactment of the entire procedure.

Dr. Console: Yes. She probably had a curettage.

Dr. Alper: Also, it struck me that in her relationship with you there was a reenactment of the circumstances of the abortion, insofar as the doctor knew about it while her parents—in this case her therapist—did not know. She's confided in you about the abortion and I wonder if in some way she wishes that the doctor had told her parents.

Dr. Console: It's a valid conjecture.

Dr. Rubinstein: Very valid. She chooses to "confide" in Dr. Console on television. She must know that her therapist will see this videotape.

Dr. Harvey: I would like to mention something else. Since we've stopped giving her any medication on the ward the complaints about having fever have completely stopped. More important, she had complained that the hematuria of two years duration had become worse over the last two months. We asked her to call the nurse to observe, when she noticed any bleeding into the toilet . . . that is, when she saw hematuria. When she did call the nurse, it was apparent to everyone that the patient was having her period at the time. Since then, the complaint of hematuria has not been repeated on our ward. We haven't heard anything more about it.

Dr. Evans: I have a question concerning her diagnosis. We have many people here today who have had one sort of contact or another with this young woman and many who have ventured a diagnosis.

Dr. Console: Well, this is one of those situations in which any one diagnosis is not going to be entirely satisfactory, but I am persuaded that her hematuria is either an hysterical conversion or that it is brought about by her deliberately through manipulation.

Dr. Evans: Well, there are some people who aren't sure as to whether or not she's psychotic.

Dr. Console: I don't think there's any doubt that she's a sick girl. But I think we ought to avoid falling into the trap of conceptualizing everyone who is very sick as schizophrenic. I don't think that this girl is psychotic. On the basis of my interview with her I don't consider her to be so. I do not recall any overt manifestations of psychosis during the interview. She related in a friendly, cooperative and appropriate fashion and there was no evidence of any failure to test reality. At least none that I could elicit.

Dr. Evans: There are some people who feel that the childish and even primitive quality of her acting out on the ward can be considered psychotic or perhaps borderline. That this is the kind of patient who appears to be more healthy than she really is and who functions on an extremely primitive level.

Dr. Console: Well, childishness and regressive potential need not be considered as borderline or psychotic functioning. There's no doubt whatsoever that this girl is histrionic, childlike, prone to regressive outbursts of angry behavior, and has a good many realistic difficulties in her ego functioning. But to consider her psychotic or schizophrenic on the basis of the clinical material that has emerged here, is, I think, erroneous.

What may occur, and what I think must be guarded against, is that this young woman will manage to convert those people with whom she interacts into angry and hostile antagonists. This is in keeping with her posture vis-a-vis the rest of the world, and is apparently the way she interacted with the people in the medical, surgical and obstetrical departments. As part of the sadistic hostility that she engenders, she will get the involved physicians to see her as being sicker than she really is. She provokes them into an overzealous therapeutic and diagnostic approach, which, when translated into action, results in her getting far more manipulations and procedures than the true pathology would call for. On the psychiatric ward, she virtually demands that she be stuck and punctured again and again, and that she be medicated as though she's sicker than she really is. And that's the way she might be seen by those around her. The willingness to see her as psychotic may be partly a function of this constellation of dynamics.

Dr. Simons: I would like to add to what Dr. Console has just said. We are reminded every day in our clinical work that sexual functioning and overall ego functioning in terms of diagnosis cannot be equated. We all know of schizophrenic patients who have excellent orgastic capacity. And we also know of very well organized, productive, well-integrated patients—with essentially characterological problems and with conflicts primarily at the phallic-oedipal level of development—who may be markedly inhibited .sexually, and who may suffer from all variations and degrees of potency and orgastic difficulties. I think we need to remind ourselves regularly that the same holds true in regard to prognosis and treatability, namely that we really cannot make an equation between a patient's diagnosis and his or her potential for therapeutic change. Our lives would be simpler if all these equations held up, and I think we sometimes twist our diagnoses around, and sometimes even resort to diagnoses like "borderline state," in order to try to make the equations work and say everything with one label—and then we end up saying nothing.

This girl is an example. I agree with Dr. Console. I do not see anything in the interview that indicates the presence of either a schizophrenic process or a psychotic depression. She is depressed—no doubt about that. But I believe this depression is a consequence of a profoundly masochistic character disturbance and not a psychotic or borderline state. However, I can think of many patients who are psychotic, and indeed more seriously disturbed than this young woman in terms of their diagnoses, who would be eminently more reachable in treatment. I think that her masochism and her guilt are of such an order that effective psychotherapy is going to be extraordinarily difficult, even for an experienced therapist, let alone a resident in training. So here is a situation where the patient is not psychotic, where indeed the patient is unusually bright and perceptive, and yet where the potential for therapeutic change is, at least in my opinion, very questionable. Because hand in hand with her masochism goes a great capacity to provoke angry and rejecting countertransference reactions in all those who will want to help her.

Dr. Harvey: I think that some of the events going on on the ward now substantiate this hypothesis. I think that there are many staff members who are very angry at her and are feeling frustrated, particularly in terms of how to deal with her. There seems to be a move afoot to discharge this patient. She wants to stay on the ward and, as Dr. Bond has already mentioned, for the past few days she has begun to interact in a more appropriate way. This may be because she now senses the frustration of the staff and is trying to guard against discharge . . . really trying to guard against expulsion.

Dr. Console: Which is what happened on the medical ward. She ended up being expelled and packed off to psychiatry. I would be extremely careful about discharging this girl at the present time. I don't think she means to kill herself, as I think she's never really intended to cause herself harm, but there's always the outside possibility that what starts out as a gesture may end up a genuine suicide. This patient is certainly burdened with enormous feelings of guilt and self-contempt, and a premature discharge at this point might tip the scales.

Dr. Bond: It seems to me that your interview technique with her was quite supportive. Do you feel that support plays an important part in her treatment at the present time?

Dr. Console: I certainly do. I think that she needs all the support and structure that the therapeutic ward can provide her . . . even if she elicits angry responses from the staff. That's part of her pathology. I think that the proper amount of support, combined with interpretations concerning her abortion and the guilt . . . really the dynamics that emerged in this interview . . . will bring about some initial relief of her depressive symptoms and will enable her to work further in treatment.

By the way, Dr. Bond mentioned that the patient seems to make a suicidal gesture or to feel like committing suicide on or around Easter time. I interviewed her on May tenth and she was admitted to the psychiatry ward on March twenty-seventh. I recall that Easter fell early this year . . . somewhere around the end of March. I would wonder if the anniversary of the abortion is around Easter time. Again, there's so much more that I would like to find out about this girl . . . much more than such a short initial interview would permit.

There's one other thing that I feel I have to mention at this point and that is the incredible number and variety of surgical and diagnostic procedures to which this girl was subjected. She's been probed and punctured, opened and closed, and evaluated for every conceivable thing on four separate services of the hospital, and has managed to confound and confuse a host of doctors.

It shouldn't surprise us that the doctors were confused by the myriad symptoms and complaints that this young woman presented to them. It shouldn't surprise us because we already know that an X-ray machine or a laparoscopy tube . . . or whatever instrument you want to pick . . . can only see something that organically protrudes or that is visibly abberrant in some way. These instruments cannot see an *idea*. And this is, unfortunately, what the other physicians were searching out, albeit with the wrong tools—an idea. *They were looking for a fantasy.* I think that some of the fundamental aspects of that fantasy are revealed in this interview. That on both a conscious and an unconscious level, there is a need to suffer and to place herself in the hands of doctors in the fashion she has been doing, and thus expiate some of the

guilt that has burdened her over the years. Even if some of her
behavior is determined consciously . . . that is, even if she has been
purposely instrumenting herself, the reasons are most certainly
beyond her. They are not consciously accessible to her, and the
physicians are employed as tools in the playing out of an
unconscious fantasy on the part of this young woman.

So again, the doctors have been using all their diagnostic skills
and instruments in a search for some organic pathology when
there is none. They have been unwittingly drawn into collusion
with the patient's guilt and have themselves been the instruments
of suffering and expiation—without ever having realized it. They
never thought of searching for the idea—the fantasy behind all
this behavior. This, I think, is the primary lesson that this young
woman has to teach us.

Now, I intend to see her a few more times in a brief
psychotherapy. I would like, if I can, to continue seeing her until
her discharge and to have a videotape record of our therapy
sessions. I hope that in a relatively short time, I can help her to see
some of what she has been doing—the masochistic and self-
destructive behavior and some of the roots of that behavior. I
would like to engage her in a brief therapeutic situation and see
what evolves. It might be both helpful to her and instructive to the
residents. I think residents rarely have the opportunity to see how
any of the senior staff people would actually conduct a therapy
session, or for that matter, an entire brief treatment. I would like
to have such a treatment on videotape.

Addendum

Dr. Console and the patient met for an additional six sessions
over the course of the next few weeks. She was in the process of
being discharged from the hospital despite having clearly stated
her wish to continue treatment on the ward. In addition, her first
ward therapist could no longer treat her and the patient was about
to be reassigned to another resident for outpatient psychotherapy.
This new therapist was about to leave for a vacation.

It was under these circumstances that Dr. Console began
meeting with the patient. It was fully understood that this would

be a temporary measure. In their last session together Dr. Console told the patient that he would be following her case closely (he had planned to supervise her new therapist in her treatment). Soon after the last session with Dr. Console, she began sessions with her new therapist.

He reported that the patient's initial phase of psychotherapy was characterized by frequent lateness and by many missed sessions. This may have reflected her rage at having been discharged from the hospital, as well as having been transferred to another therapist and not being able to continue with Dr. Console.

Some weeks later, Dr. Console suddenly died at the age of sixty-two. The patient was never told of his death and we do not know if she ever learned of it. There is a possibility that she may have, because she continued to see some of her former physicians at the medical center and she may have learned of Dr. Console's death through them. This possibility raises some intriguing questions. If she did learn of his death, it is reasonable to speculate that she may have felt partly responsible, because of her many feelings about Dr. Console and about her situation at the time. She had been discharged from the hospital against her wishes, had seen Dr. Console for a brief period of time during which they had formed a relationship, and she was then transferred to another therapist. Her treatment was therefore enormously complicated by these multiple transfers and discharges, and there can be little doubt that she felt frustrated and angry toward the hospital, toward the ward, toward her new therapist, and toward Dr. Console.

Because of this it is conceivable that she could have fantasized that she was partly responsible for Dr. Console's death. She was a survivor again . . . having survived the teacher, the unborn baby, the boyfriend, and she now survived Dr. Console. While we will never know her feelings or fantasies about all of these events, they might have been crucial, because shortly after Dr. Console's death, the patient impulsively terminated her therapy with her new therapist. She ended her treatment after only ten sessions, and left New York for another state, perhaps fleeing a situation that so frighteningly recreated her own past.

So, after having spent many months in the hospital and after having engaged many physicians in frustrating, sadomasochistic relationships, the patient left New York City to begin a new life in another state. She left behind a videotaped record of her seven sessions with Dr. Console. However, this was not the last we were to hear of this young woman, as shall become evident in the next chapter.

CHAPTER EIGHT

The Beginnings
Of A Psychotherapy

Several months later, the first-year residents who had been with Dr. Console for the preceding year, having now started their second year of residency, asked Dr. Simons and Dr. Rubinstein to conduct a seminar on the techniques of beginning a psychotherapy. We decided to study the initial interview that Dr. Console had conducted with the young woman in the previous chapter. This first session was viewed with few interruptions and most of the discussion took place at the conclusion of the tape. Present at the proceedings were Dr. Simons, Dr. Rubinstein, the residents, as well as Dr. Jorge Steinberg and Dr. Howard Welsh, who helped moderate the seminar. The discussion with the residents dealt primarily with the techniques of interviewing and of beginning a psychotherapy. We will now present this discussion, along with a few short excerpts from the first session, after which we will present the second therapy session without interruption.

THE INTERVIEW ENDS

Dr. Cohen: I was a little puzzled at the outset of this interview. Very early on, Dr. Console asked the patient what it was like being sandwiched between an older and a younger brother. I'm not really clear what he was trying to get at.

Dr. Simons: What were your impressions at that point in the interview? Your impressions either of her or of the interaction that was going on.

Dr. Kent: It struck me that when he pointed out that she was a girl between two brothers, and her chief complaint was blood coming from the genital area, he was looking for conflicts about not having a penis. He was looking for some concept of herself as a

THE FIRST ENCOUNTER

damaged person. Perhaps she views herself as injured or harmed in some way.

Dr. Drucker: There's a constricted and really depressed quality about this girl. She seems quite depressed. This was evident to me right at the beginning. She did not look at Dr. Console throughout the interview. There's a withdrawn quality about her, one that I suspect she's had for many years.

Dr. Simons: How is Dr. Console dealing with that?

Dr. Drucker: Having seen his other tapes of interviews with patients, I think he's relating to her in a more solicitous way. There's really a very fatherly quality that he adopts with this girl ... a more empathic quality than is generally visible in his interviews.

Dr. Marcus: Throughout the interview he's been repeating the last word or two that she uses.

Dr. Simons: Yes. Practically every interchange begins with his repeating something that she's just said. Do you get the feeling that this is an example of Rogerian technique?

Dr. Clarke: I don't really think that that's what he intended to do. I think he's trying to move very gingerly with this patient. She's the type who will screen everything that she says. At least that's the feeling I have about her.

Dr. Simons: Well, why don't we get back to Dr. Cohen's question. Where do you think Dr. Console is at this early point in the interview? What has he accomplished thus far, early in the interview?

Dr. Clarke: I think that he's moving in the direction of questioning her about penis envy, as was just mentioned. I think he's pursuing that line of inquiry.

Dr. Simons: Any other thoughts?

Dr. Zimmer: I was thinking that at this point in the interview, he has really engaged this person. I think most of us would find her a difficult patient to engage. She mentioned at the outset that she is a quiet and withdrawn person and she certainly appears to be that way. My feeling is that he's gotten her quite involved with him right at the outset. I think that she's interested in what he's got to say. She's spontaneously offering material that she might not offer with another interviewer.

Dr. Rubin: I'm impressed with the activity of Dr. Console in this interview. He's much more active than he had been in the other interviews that we've seen.

Dr. Simons: Are you surprised by that?

Dr. Rubin: Not really. She is a withdrawn girl and I think he's actively getting her more involved.

Dr. Marcus: Along with this solicitous quality, I think he's being protective of her. It strikes me that he's acting in a way similar to her father, who would go into the bedroom and talk with her . . . in contrast to the mother.

Dr. Vis: It seems to me that Dr. Console is coming across in a very empathic way with this girl. Empathic without being overprotective. I have a feeling that he is doing this by following the Rogerian technique. His repeating her last few words shows that he feels empathy for her.

Dr. Simons: Dr. Console, as you may know, was quite contemptuous of Rogerian technique. I'm not sure that he communicated that to you but he certainly was. He was contemptuous of it because, to him, it indicated that if a therapist is sitting there and doesn't know *what in the world* is going on with the patient, the easiest thing to do is merely to repeat the patient's last words without ever clarifying or interpreting or pulling anything together. I don't think that that's what he's been doing with this girl. I think that, as some of you have pointed out, he really is empathizing with her fear, her withdrawal, her shyness and her depression. I think he's trying with this technique to make her feel more comfortable and to draw her out.

To respond to Dr. Cohen's question . . . of course, in every interview you're going to be thinking of everything that the patient tells you, but what's so striking to me, what's so remarkable, is the amount of information that Dr. Console has obtained from this girl in just the first few minutes of the first interview. In about eight minutes he's gotten the presenting symptom. He knows something about her cystitis and something about a flock of medical examinations and admissions. He knows where she comes from. He knows something about her father . . . something about her mother . . . something about the father's work . . . something about the personalities of the parents . . .

something about her place in the family, who the other siblings were and where she fits in the family. He's found out about a very traumatic death that occurred when she was age five. He's found out about a rape at age fourteen. All of this in a space of seven or eight minutes.

I think *that* is what is so instructive about where Dr. Console was heading at the very beginning of this first interview. He's trying very actively to establish a relationship with the patient and not get caught up in some stereotype of how a psychiatric interview should be conducted. Some rule that says that you should be this way or that way. No. You should be the way the situation requires you to be in order to establish an alliance with the patient. And, in the context of the empathy that he is conveying, he is finding out a great deal about this young woman.

Dr. Welsh: I think it's also important to note how Dr. Console went about getting all this information in such a short space of time. He didn't linger over the chief complaint and try to get her to elaborate on it in detail. He established for himself, fairly quickly, that no organic cause was found for the hematuria and he pushed right ahead to the past history, and when he did that, her first association was that at age fourteen she became withdrawn. She was really saying, "My hematuria today has something to do with an event at age fourteen".

Dr. Meyer: She mentioned that after the rape she had become withdrawn. Dr. Console must have intuitively realized that if he became too intrusive and aggressive, she would withdraw and not give anything. I think this speaks to a very difficult point in the technique of conducting an initial interview, where you have both to get a history and establish a therapeutic relationship. You have to be forceful but you don't want to be experienced by the patient as aggressive and intrusive.

Dr. Alper: Yes. She had mentioned that her mother's efforts at drawing her out had made her withdrawn.

Dr. Cohen: Another facet of his technique that I found interesting was his comment, "Hematuria. Would you watch for this?" With this question he has made it a psychological interview as opposed to a medical interview. That was one of his very first comments to her. I think that it set the tone for the rest of the interview and perhaps it made her more willing to look at things in a psychological way.

Dr. Simons: I would like to go back to Dr. Kent's comment that, at the very beginning of the interview, he thought that penis envy might be the central conflict for this girl. However, within a very few minutes it became clear that her major struggle has to do with guilt. She feels guilty over the teacher's death, guilty about the abortion, and guilty about the death of the boyfriend. With just a few questions Dr. Console has arrived at something that is far more important in terms of a brief psychotherapy than anything that might exist on a deeper level, whether it be penis envy or anything else. Not that other conflicts may not be there, but it's easy to get entangled in the depths and miss something that's right on the surface, something that could be the major motivating fantasy or conflict. She survived the teacher at age five, the baby at age fourteen, and two years ago she survived the boyfriend.

Dr. Welsh: I think that Dr. Console made an important omission in the first interview. He didn't ask about how the teacher had died. He didn't inquire if she knew how that happened. I think that that was very important.

Dr. Clarke: Yes. Particularly since this patient's presenting complaint is one of bleeding. We don't know if the teacher might have hit her head or something like that and if the patient had seen blood.

Dr. Welsh: My fantasy is that the teacher committed suicide and that she was lying in the bathtub, dead, with blood coming from her wrists and that the patient saw the body and the bloody water in the bathtub.

Dr. Simons: It's an interesting speculation. Whatever may have been the case with the teacher, what can we assume about the death of the boyfriend? Even if she hadn't actually *seen* the accident, she certainly saw it in her mind. What would she have seen?

Dr. Welsh: Blood.

Dr. Simons: Plenty of blood. And at the time of the abortion?

Dr. Marcus: Blood. And possibly at the time of the rape also.

Dr. Simons: Yes. At the rape too. This demonstrates how important it would be in the treatment of this woman, really in the treatment of any patient, for us to see the ego conflict that we're going to try to work with? Can you see what a difference it makes if we conceptualize this young woman's most immediate concerns in terms of anxiety and guilt, rather than as more direct expressions of the drives, such as penis envy or incestuous wishes or whatever? Can you see how different our approach, our interventions and our interpretations would be? Everything would be different.

Dr. Bond: Just about everyone here knows about the many difficulties that this patient presented to the staff on the ward. All the battles for intramuscular injections, all the acting out on the ward and everything. Frankly, I was shocked at seeing the way she related to Dr. Console. I must say that I had never seen her so well organized as she appears in this interview. I had never seen her relate to anyone in such a positive manner.

Dr. Simons: How do you explain the way she related to Dr. Console in this interview?

Dr. Bond: Well, considering how close she had felt to her father, I guess I shouldn't have been too surprised.

Dr. Simons: Would you say that she was one of the most difficult patients you have ever observed on the ward?

Dr. Bond: Yes. For many reasons. One of them was the extraordinary number of people who got involved with her. Medical students, nursing students, residents—everyone who had any contact with her at all managed to become involved with her.

Dr. Alper: There were so many people caught up in her treatment that it was incredible.

Dr. Simons: It was chaos. But the chaos had a center—the patient. She created the chaos. Not consciously or intentionally of course, but as a part of what?

Dr. Alper: It was part of her medical experience all over again, where many different physicians on many different services were involved. Here she managed to get at least three attending psychiatrists and two residents involved in her treatment. It was a mess. It was almost as though these people were competing with each other in order to become involved with her. It was chaos.

Dr. Simons: Of course. But the chaos was ultimately in the service of what? Can we answer this question on the basis of what has emerged in just this one interview?

Dr. Zimmer: It was really a massive resistance that prevented anyone from treating her.

Dr. Simons: Can you be more specific?

Dr. Vis: It could be the result of her having been provocative.

Dr. Simons: In the service of what?

Dr. Vis: She could have been engaging other people in sadomasochistic relationships.

Dr. Simons: Yes! In the service of her masochism! It's so easy when we see a patient like this, to respond to the aggression and the sadism, and not appreciate that this behavior is in the service of something else. It's in the service of maintaining the illness. It's in the service of masochism. It's my impression that we frequently fail to recognize masochistic behavior because we're so often caught up in our anger toward the patient. We don't appreciate the fact that we're angry for a reason. The patient has provoked it!

Dr. Steinberg: I would like to comment on the fact that she had two somatic complaints involving pain, migraine headaches and abdominal pain. When a patient presents with a chief complaint of pain, especially migraine headaches, often underlying the physical symptom is a feeling of very great rage. She has difficulty expressing this rage directly and manages to turn it masochistically back on herself in the form of painful symptoms.

Dr. Simons: Yes. And the somatic symptom both expresses the rage and at the same time has a self-punitive aspect to it.

Dr. Cohena; I would like to get back to looking at the technique again. I was struck by an intervention that Dr. Console made about the abortion. I thought it was uncharacteristic of him. Could we replay that section of the tape?

> *Patient*: Because that's a life ... I killed somebody. And ... going out with different boys ... I'm very unclear about that. I think that was wrong too. But to kill *yourself* is not wrong.
>
> *Dr. Console*: But tell me, in light of what has been happening for the past few years ... that women believe that their bodies are theirs and they have the right to have an abortion if that's what they want. It's upheld by the Constitution of the United States.
>
> *Patient*: I know. I feel that way too. But subconsciously I don't know if that's the way I really feel.

Dr. Simons: How is that interchange uncharacteristic?

Dr. Cohen: I'm not sure that that was a remark I would expect to hear from a psychiatrist. I would really expect to hear that from a medical practitioner rather than from a psychiatrist. I felt that his intervention here was in the service of reassuring her . . . which is what medical people tend to do.

Dr. Meyer: I don't feel that he was merely trying to be supportive about the abortion. I think he was trying to clarify her earlier contradictory statement that she was feeling good but also wanted to kill herself.

Dr. Kent: I agree with Dr. Cohen. Dr. Console never tried to sell things like that. Compared to the way we have seen him conduct other interviews, he's talking a great deal. We're not used to seeing him this way.

Dr. Zimmer: He's behaving in an extremely supportive way.

Dr. Kent: Yes. It doesn't seem like him at all.

Dr. Simons: So you see a discrepancy between the way in which he's acting here and the way you feel he should behave as a psychotherapist?

Dr. McDermott: He's acting very much like the father she wants him to be. He's being extremely nurturing and parental.

Dr. Vis: I think that the patient's response indicates that Dr. Console's comment was a good one. He explained to her about the Constitution and the right that she has to make a decision about her own body, and in so doing he presented himself in a nonpunitive manner. As a result, his comment elicits from her the response that, while she intellectually knows it's all right to have an abortion, she's aware that there's another part deep within her that disapproves of it and makes her feel guilty. He has diminished her anxiety about the abortion and helped her to take a look at what might be going on underneath the surface.

Dr. Simons: So you feel then that his statement was not so much a value judgement but more in the nature of presenting a reality to her that made clearer the discrepancy between her own conscious attitude and her unconscious feelings about the abortion?

Dr. Vis: Yes, and it serves the function of opening things up further.

329 The Beginnings in Psychotherapy

Dr. Rubinstein: Yes. It initiates a reflective process on her part. It encourages her to make a comparison between conscious and unconscious.

Dr. Kent: I'm surprised at his comment because I can see Dr. Console already beginning a psychotherapy with this woman. In other interviews he was relatively neutral. We have never seen him this way. I think that's the main reason we wanted to see these tapes. We wanted to see someone *do psychotherapy* as opposed to just doing an initial interview.

Dr. Rubinstein: I think we're struck by this *apparent* difference, a difference that is really a function of our own misconceptions. I doubt that this woman would have responded at all to a neutral interviewer, one who was relatively inactive. I think that Dr. Console would have taken an active approach with her even if he had no intention of seeing her in a brief psychotherapy. In other words, I think that he was responding to her withdrawn and depressed state, and related to her in a way that he hoped would draw her out. All the other patients whom we've viewed on tape were much more verbal and spontaneous than this patient.

Dr. Steinberg: I want to comment on the reaction that the residents are having. There's absolutely nothing wrong with being therapeutic in the first interview. Psychotherapy begins in the first interview. Now, why Dr. Console seemed so very different in this interview than in other interviews is a question about which we can only speculate. I think that this woman was able to elicit from people a wish to rescue her, and perhaps this is what happened with Dr. Console.

Dr. Meyer: I spoke with Dr. Console about this after seeing this tape on my own a few months ago. I mentioned to him that in these sessions, he seemed different than I had ever seen him. I asked him why this was so. He said that he wasn't aware of being that different with her. He said that this was always the way he was with any patient he was treating.

Dr. Steinberg: Well, I think that brings up an important issue. Dr. Console seemed to feel at the outset that he was treating her. His answer to Dr. Meyer's question was that he identified this as a treatment situation.

Dr. Rubinstein: He felt that his role was to be that of a transitional object for this girl . . . an interim therapist. There was an imminent crisis ahead. She was going to be discharged from the ward against her will. She wanted to stay on the ward and it was his feeling at the time that she might inadvertently kill herself by making another suicide attempt or gesture. Also, her newly assigned outpatient therapist was about to leave for a vacation and I think that Dr. Console decided to intervene in what he felt was a crisis situation.

Dr. Welsh: Our entire discussion seems to be about whether Dr. Console is really being Dr. Console or not (*group laughter*). We began with this comment to her about the Constitution and we went on from there to wonder about the appropriateness of his activity. But Dr. Console always made a point of not differentiating between a diagnostic and a therapeutic session. As Dr. Rubinstein said a few minutes ago, if Dr. Console had been any less active in his interview with this patient, there wouldn't have been an interview. He *had* to be different with different patients. She was not a productive or communicative woman. He had to be more active. And the interview followed a very definite flow. He first established the severity of this woman's self-punitive behavior. He went through each suicide attempt and what had happened in each instance. After establishing how this woman had repeatedly punished herself, he then made it clear that her guilt was coming from inside her and that her reaction to the abortion was the result of conflict. I think he really had a very definite plan in mind.

Dr. Vis: I was just wondering. Could we go over the last few minutes of the interview again? I was struck by the interpretation that Dr. Console made about the hematuria (*the tape is replayed*).

> *Patient*: I figured that if there was any blood then I could make it look like I was just having my period.
> *Dr. Console*: But you do tell me that your depression and your three suicidal attempts are in some way connected with the abortion. Your feelings of guilt about the abortion.
> *Patient*: I hate myself for it . . . for having been bad.

Dr. Console: For having been bad (*pause*). Normally when you're having your period and you go to the toilet, you look and see blood don't you? Some blood in the bowl?

Patient (*nods*): Yes . . .

Dr. Console: How do you know it's not hematuria?

Patient: Because it stops after a few days. The hematuria is always there. And, for the hematuria I don't have to wear anything.

Dr. Console: But every time that you urinate and there is some blood, does it remind you of anything?

Patient: No.

Dr. Console: No (*pause*). You don't think it might have anything to do with the bleeding that you did at fourteen?

Patient (*smiling*): I know what you're going to ask . . .

Dr. Console (*smiling*): What makes you so smart . . . to know what I'm going to ask?

Patient: You think it's all psychological, when I bleed now . . . I remember the past.

Dr. Console: Not necessarily remember . . . no. But are you going to tell me that the rape and the abortion did not have a psychological effect on you?

Patient: It did. But not in *that* way.

Dr. Console: Not in that way.

Patient: No.

Dr. Console: And, you're a little annoyed that you knew I was going to ask that question.

Patient: Not annoyed . . . but I was waiting to hear it.

Dr. Console: Are you saying that you were waiting to hear it because you have been asked that same question many times before?

Patient: No, I haven't, but I knew that you would think that way.

Dr. Console: All right. You say that you knew that I would think that way. But you've talked to other doctors. Why didn't you know that they would think that way?

Patient: It's the way you get off the subject and come back to it later. Afterwards.

Dr. Console (smiling): You mean I'm pretty sneaky?
Patient (smiling): In a way . . . the way you ask certain leading
questions. With something in mind.

Dr. Vis: I found this section of the interview fascinating,
especially the patient's anticipation of Dr. Console's next
statement. It reminds me of Freud's case of Dora. Freud would
make an interpretation and Dora would say, "I knew you would say
that." Freud's response was something to the effect that, "It was
already in your mind." He considered this kind of a response to be
confirmatory of an interpretation. But I also want to make another
point. When Dr. Console asked these questions in the way that he
did, I knew what he was aiming at. I wonder if he might also have
implanted an idea in the patient's mind that he had already linked
these two events together and expected her to do the same. It
leaves us wondering what was really in her mind. What is the
reality?
Dr. Simons: Well, that's a question that will always be with us in
our work. Of course, there are different realities, aren't there? Dr.
Vis is raising a question as to whether this interchange confirms
some links that actually existed, or did Dr. Console put something
in this young woman's mind.
Dr. Farber: Well, I couldn't help but notice that she spontaneously
denied much of what Dr. Console had brought up. She denied it
even before he suggested it. I'm always suspicious of spontaneous
denials.
Dr. Simons: Why?
Dr. Farber: The denial suggests that she was indeed thinking
about the connection. That there is a connection.
Dr. Simons: That's a good working assumption. It doesn't
necessarily mean that it's always true, but it's a pretty good
assumption.
Dr. Vis: Dr. Console had asked her, "Every time that you urinate
and there is blood, does it remind you of anything?" The patient
said "no." To my mind, this would indicate that it did remind her of
something and that she was denying it. Otherwise she might have
thought about it for a moment or two and maybe not have recalled
anything or else have seen a similarity. The fact that her response

was a strong and immediate no, suggests that she had some memory or association with the blood in the toilet. But I don't know how much of it was a result of her having picked up from Dr. Console an idea of where he was heading. To what extent was he leading her?

Dr. Simons: Well, what about her affect during this interchange? Did any of you have any thoughts about that? Does that give any clue to the question that Dr. Vis has raised?

Dr. Vis: She was obviously amused during all this, in spite of her depression.

Dr. Simons: Yes. Why would she smile? She's depressed and supposedly suicidal. Why did she smile during this interchange?

Dr. Kent: I think she's smiling because she's having a good time giving Dr. Console a hard time.

Dr. Simons: Yes ... but she's been doing that throughout the interview. Why at that moment would she smile?

Dr. Kent: She had caught him at that moment.

Dr. Simons: Did she catch him? Is that why she smiled?

Dr. Kent: I think that she's openly playing a hostile game with him. She's been doing it throughout the interview. It's almost a game ... a sparring match.

Dr. Meyer: Dr. Console was also smiling at that point. I can't say for sure what's going on, but it does seem as though there's a game going on between the two of them.

Dr. Simons: Well, of course, we can't know for sure. We can't read their minds, but this is really the first moment that she is smiling in this way during the entire interview.

Dr. Steinberg: To me this is the most crucial moment in the interview. I don't know what will happen in future sessions, but I suspect that this is the moment when the future difficulties begin. If this interchange is a game, as Dr. Kent suggests, then this is the moment when both players are putting their cards on the table. Both of them are smiling, I believe, because this is the moment when both of them know exactly what the struggle is going to be, and therefore I would suspect that this is the moment when Dr. Console's difficulties in relating to this patient are going to begin. Because her resistances are going to become greater. It's going to be very hard from now on to get her to be willing to see these connections.

Dr. Welsh: Well, we can see the confirmation of that when he made the connection clearer to her. She seemed obviously annoyed and upset. Dr. Console even pointed this out to her. What we were talking about a moment ago was the problem of determining whether or not an interpretation is correct. Dr. Console made a very specific interpretation that linked her current hematuria to her abortion when she was fourteen years old. How do we know whether this or any interpretation is correct? The patient may agree enthusiastically with the interpretation and say that we're brilliant, and the interpretation may be completely wrong. Or, the patient may deny it, as in this case, and it may be quite correct.

The only way that we can find out about the validity of an interpretation is to listen to the patient's own associations and responses after the interpretation is made. This patient said something very specific in response to it. For me, this response clearly confirmed the validity of what Dr. Console said. She told him that she had not told any other doctor about the abortion. She was saying in effect, "Yes, I do have to defend myself. I *know* there is an essential connection between my abortion then and my hematuria now. I've been in the hospital for many weeks having all kinds of tests and have seen many doctors, including psychiatrists, but I have never told anybody about the abortion."

Dr. Bond: I just want to add something. The ward received a call the other day that this patient is back in a hospital for a cholecystectomy. This is a small hospital in another state where she's living now.

Dr. Simons: This is fascinating! How did you hear about this?

Dr. Bond: The doctor from the other hospital called. I had to go to the ward to see a patient and the nurses told me that a surgeon had called to find out about her.

Dr. Simons: What do all of you think about this?

Dr. Iglesias: That it is typical of the way she behaves. I've had the feeling all along that she was in control of the interview, not Dr. Console. She's a great chess player. Her king and queen are well protected by the other pieces, and by moving one pawn she gets Dr. Console to move his knights and bishops all over the place. I think that the entire treatment of this girl became an intellectual challenge to him . . . right from the outset.

Dr. Kent: I think that may have been one of the reasons why she was smiling. She had Dr. Console quite provoked. He said, "What makes you so smart to know what I'm thinking?" That's a pretty sarcastic confrontation to make to a patient.

Dr. Rubinstein: But they were both smiling at that point.

Dr. Kent: But the words themselves were hostile.

Dr. Rubinstein: I don't agree. I think that his tone was very friendly. In a way, I found this moment one of the most intimate and moving in the entire interview.

Dr. Simons: I think this discussion is a very important one. We are really talking about a patient's resistances. We all tend to have an idea that resistances are something bad. They should melt away and everything should be open and straightforward. But resistances and defenses are quite related. What are resistances, after all? They are simply the operation of the patient's defenses in the therapeutic situation. That's all. "Resistances" have a pejorative quality in our minds, probably because they require so much work on our part. But they are the stuff of which therapy is constituted. So I would encourage you to give up this way of thinking, namely that when we see certain resistances operating, it's like a chess game or a struggle to the death. Indeed it is a struggle in the sense that the patient's defenses are a part of the patient's symptoms, and patients are not going to give them up without a struggle and a great deal of work. And with a masochistic patient, the specific resistance operating is the attempt to provoke the interviewer or therapist. That is the essence of masochism. That is why working with a masochistic patient is so very difficult. And this is what we see here in this initial interview, in the very beginning of this girl's therapy. This is her pathology.

Dr. Iglesias: I think Dr. Console responded to her pathology. Everybody has been asking why he changed his technique with her. I think he did so because he was responding to her masochism.

Dr. Simons: That may be. I think we'll have a better chance to evaluate that as we get into the second session. But I want to get back to why she's smiling, because I think there is a dimension here that we haven't really talked about. I don't think she's smiling because she's trapped Dr. Console. I think she's smiling at this point because she feels that Dr. Console understands precisely what is going on in her symptomatology and in her masochism. He is the one person of all the people whom she has met thus far, on all the medical and the psychiatric services, who fully appreciates the depth and the dimensions of her masochism—masochism of such an extraordinary strength that she is willing to submit herself to countless operations, and here, right now before our eyes, is submitting herself to a cholecystectomy.

Dr. Iglesias: I disagree. I had a chance to observe her on the ward. She knew what her pathology was all about. It had been brought up many times. Her smiling here is, I think, her recognition that the two of them are involved in a highly intellectual struggle and that they are squaring off for the battle to come.

Dr. Simons: It's possible. All I can say is that if we feel that way about a particular patient, it's going to be difficult for us to work with that patient. If we see someone's conflicts only in terms of the aggression or sadism that is operating, then its going to be almost impossible for us to develop the empathy that will be necessary to work effectively with that patient in psychotherapy, especially a masochistic patient such as this woman. That view of the patient already reflects a feeling of anger, a feeling that the patient is an opponent rather than an ally. I think she's smiling at this point because she feels that Dr. Console does understand her and that he is strong enough and tough enough to be able to cope with her illness, and that he's not going to be frightened by her. I think that's what's going on. You know, we talk about so many different needs and wishes and impulses in psychotherapy. I think the need we hardly ever mention is probably the most fundamental human need of all and that's the need to be understood.

But I want to return to what I think is the essential point that this interview illustrates. To me, it graphically illustrates what is necessary in order for us to engage and work successfully with a masochistic patient. You cannot sit back. You cannot be passive. You cannot allow the patient's masochism and aggression to take over the interview. You must be appropriately active and know what you're doing, and you must make connections for the patient right from the beginning. I think *that* is what this interview can teach us. I also think that Dr. Steinberg's point is very important. This is the moment at which she clearly knows that here is someone who can help her and that knowledge brings with it all of her anxieties, all of her guilt and all of her need to sabotage the treatment.

Dr. Rubinstein: I think we should spend more time discussing the phone call to the ward. I think it's an amazing message from this woman.

Dr. Simons: Yes. Why should we be notified here that this patient is in another hospital in another state? The only way that this could have occurred is if she told someone to call our ward.

Dr. Steinberg: Her message to us is, "Pay attention because I'm going to do something to myself and *I want you to know about it*".

Dr. Simons: Absolutely! Now we can respond in one of two ways. We can say, "Dammit ... there she is again, playing her silly games. She's giving an indirect message to us. She's got herself in the hands of the surgeons again and she's doing the same damned thing. She's provoking us and she's provoking the surgeons and she's splitting the transference and ... she's not behaving properly" (*group laughter*). Believe me, that's the way many of us feel about masochistic patients. Their aim is to get the environment to hate them and to punish them and to drive them away so they won't feel guilty. And they need to do this over and over again. That is why it's such an extraordinarily difficult task for us to intervene properly as therapists and to maintain the therapeutic alliance. Their illness drives them to sabotage the treatment and there is no other patient for whom this is true in precisely the same way. It's not true with the schizophrenic patient. It's not true with the obsessional or hysterical patient. It's not even true with the profoundly depressed patient. But with the truly masochistic personality or the person with a masochistic perversion, this is one of the most difficult kinds of situation that we can encounter, because they are the patients toward whom our countertransferences immediately come into play. That is why this woman and this interview are so instructive. That is why this telephone call from her is so important.

If I had been her therapist, I think I would want to talk directly with the nurse who got this phone call. I would want to get the name of the hospital and the name of the surgeon, and find out what's going on. This girl should not have an operation unless there has been some extraordinary medical emergency that has intervened between the time she was a patient here five months ago and the present time. She's putting herself under the knife and the surgeon who's going to operate on her needs to know from us what he is dealing with here. I think he will be grateful for that information. I also think that *she* would be grateful for that communication. I believe that this call is a test to see whether we still care about her and whether we are willing to make the effort to still be of help to her.

Dr. Steinberg: It may also be her way of asking us how well we understand her.

Dr. Simons: Yes. She may have already had the surgery but we shouldn't be provoked by that. Unless she can be treated, she will have operations all of her life. I hope that someone on the ward did talk with the surgeon. It would be understandable if they didn't, but if not, it would be as a result of anger because of the difficulty that this patient caused everyone. No patient who has been on the ward in recent years caused the trouble or evoked the anger that this girl did. But that's part of her illness. And if we don't deal with it, who is going to deal with it? The surgeons aren't going to deal with it. They're going to cut her open. The internists aren't going to deal with it. They're going to give her medication. The gynecologists and urologists aren't going to deal with it. They're going to probe her. If we don't deal with it, no one is going to deal with it. That's what we're here for, and that's why we're psychiatrists.

Dr. Steinberg: If she has had the surgery, it would be very interesting to get a pathology report about this patient's gallbladder.

Dr. Simons: Yes. I would bet that they would be embarrassed to provide us with such a report because I think it would read, "normal gallbladder" (*group laughter*).

Dr. Kent: I may be reacting to her masochism, but one of the things that Dr. Console taught us was that it is not our mission in life to go out in the world and drive people sane! It seems to me that she clearly did not want to be in treatment any longer. She had stopped going to her sessions and she moved out of town. I think that if we contact her now, we will be trying to rescue her.

Dr. Simons: That's an important point. But can you see a difference between her therapist trying to cajole her back into therapy with letters and phone calls and all of that, and his responding to an inquiry that she arranged to be made? There is a difference. She's asking us to intervene. She may be asking in a confused and masochistic way, but she is asking. That makes all the difference in the world. It's not chasing after the patient. That would be wrong. Because then you would be entrapped in her masochism and there would be no hope of really helping her. This is different. This is a call for help.

Dr. Cohen: I'm remembering something from Dr. Console's tapes and it's becoming much clearer to me why he saw this woman so many times. I'm reminded of the polysurgery woman ... the one with a million operations, no teeth, and so on. There was a great deal of regret in Dr. Console's voice when he said that if someone had understood this woman earlier and had done something about it, perhaps her life would have been different. I think that here he was, faced with a young woman whom he saw going down the same path, and he felt that perhaps he could do something about it.

Dr. Simons: Yes. It is the polysurgery woman ... twenty years earlier. And if you could have seen the polysurgery woman's medical chart, you would have been amazed. It was a foot thick! It documented years and years of medical and surgical interventions. And there was not one word about the history of her twin sister's death when she was two years old and her mother's comment, "You will have to suffer for two." I think Dr. Cohen is absolutely right.

Dr. Alper: I am bothered by something else about this case. While this patient was on the ward, she had two different therapists as well as a supervisor who was also involved in the case. It seems to me that Dr. Console's having seen her for those seven sessions was one of the worst things that could have happened. She had therapists all over the place. She was playing the two therapists on the ward against one another, and then Dr. Console got involved. She knew that the treatment with Dr. Console would be brief. In fact, I wonder if the reason she related to him as well as she did was because she knew it would not be a long-term relationship. I really question why he got involved in a therapeutic relationship the way he did. I remember at the time, I was taken aback and after all these months I still feel the same way.

Dr. Simons: Dr. Alper, what do you think Dr. Console's reaction would have been if you had told him about your feelings in this regard?

Dr. Alper: I must say that I certainly wouldn't have wanted to be around to find out (*group laughter*).

Dr. Simons: I ask because I think that your criticism is quite justified, and it holds true whenever there's the kind of splitting of the transference that occurred with this patient. I can't tell you why Dr. Console got involved with her. I don't know. I can only guess. I do know that he didn't seek this patient out. The people on the ward sought *him* out. They asked him to see her in consultation because she was driving everybody crazy and he took it from there.

Dr. Alper: I think that's only partly true. The supervisor asked Dr. Console to see her because he thought that she was a very interesting patient. As a matter of fact, once Dr. Console began seeing her, the troubles on the ward intensified. Wouldn't it have been more appropriate for him to have talked with the patient's therapist rather than treating her himself?

Dr. Simons: If Dr. Console's therapy with her was not coordinated with her milieu treatment on the ward, that was a mistake . . . no matter who was conducting the therapy.

Dr. Kent: Look at how this woman has gotten us all stirred up this morning. We're excited, argumentative, maybe even angry. I think it's important to remember that her getting all of these people involved with her is a function of her pathology.

Dr. Simons: Absolutely. It's important for us to see that this is her masochism in operation.

Dr. Vis: As we said earlier, she has the capacity to evoke rescue fantasies in many of us. The very fact that Dr. Console saw her seven times meant that she was something special for him. And now, we have a call from another hospital. I am feeling a sense of urgency right now. We have to rush and get the surgeons to stop before they cut her open. She is a very attractive and seductive young woman with many hysterical features and we may be responding to her seductiveness.

Dr. Simons: Yes. She evokes these feelings in us and we have to be prepared to face them if we are going to work with such a patient. But she's not calling because an internist wants to give her some Librium capsules. She's calling because someone is going to cut her open and take something out of her body, and she isn't going to get it back once it's taken out. There's a big difference in the order of the masochism that's operating here. Her masochism can kill her and may kill her eventually, unless someone intervenes.

I would also like to comment on the observation that Dr. Vis made about her seductiveness. I don't think there's any question that one of the major ways in which this young woman tries to deal with her anxiety is through sexualizing her relationships. We can see that in her history, and we have some rather strong evidence to suggest that rape fantasies are an impelling, motivating force in her behavior. When we view the second interview with Dr. Console, you will also observe that she is dressed much more attractively than in the first interview. So I think that Dr. Vis is quite right in what he says. But a few minutes ago I urged you not to become preoccupied with the aggressive components of a patient's behavior, to the exclusion of his or her anxiety and guilt, and the various unconscious defenses mobilized to deal with that anxiety and guilt. I would now say the same thing about a patient's sexual drives and wishes. One kind of error is to deny their existence. A very different kind of error is to become overly concerned and preoccupied with them, again to the exclusion of the patient's ego. It's been my experience that this is especially common in a male therapist-female patient relationship. The homosexual transference that develops when the therapist and the patient are of the same sex is probably the most frightening of all to both therapist and patient. But the heterosexual transference is frightening enough. I think that male therapists too often try to deal with this by diagnosing any attractive woman who stirs them up as "hysterical" or "seductive," when in point of fact that may not be an accurate diagnostic or dynamic explanation of what is going on at all. The woman may be struggling with conflicts that are quite different. How rarely have I heard a male therapist describe an older female patient as "hysterical," and how even more rarely have I heard a male therapist describe a male patient as "hysterical" or "seductive." And yet there are just as many hysterical men as there are hysterical women.

Dr. Rubinstein: It's also important to recognize that there are many preoedipal determinants in what may seem on the surface to be "hysterical" and therefore oedipal. For many of these patients, their sexuality has very little to do with genitality but really reflects much earlier concerns.

Dr. Welsh: I think we can see the confirmation of that in this woman's pervasive and chronic depression. She said very dramatically in the interview that she's made several attempts at suicide and she doesn't know why she's alive. Perhaps she doesn't feel that she deserves to be alive, and maybe doesn't even deserve to be helped in treatment.

Dr. Simons: Dr. Welsh has made a very pessimistic observation, but I think a very accurate one. It's something we don't ever like to face as psychiatrists, the fact that there are some patients whom we may not be able to help. It confronts us with our limitations and our fallibility, just as the dying patient did when we were medical students and interns. And it may be that we can't really help this woman. But that doesn't mean we shouldn't try. You are going to encounter people where the drive to destroy themselves is of such intensity that no matter what efforts you make, they will find a way to wreck their lives and possibly even kill themselves. In my own experience, however, even the person who is determined to kill himself or herself will, in most instances, try to arrange for some way to be rescued. They will still make some desperate last minute attempt to get help.

Dr. Rubinstein: I think that what is amazing is that this patient may get *someone else* to kill her rather than doing it by her own hand. She seems determined to get someone to instrument her and kill her the way her unborn child was killed.

Dr. Simons: Yes. And you have to interpret that wish and that guilt and not be afraid to deal with it in treatment.

Dr. Rubinstein: I am also struck by what we learned here today about her impending surgery in another hospital. Here we are watching a videotape that Dr. Console made five months ago, and the very woman whom we're watching called the ward only a few days ago . . . or had someone call for her.

Dr. Vis: It could be that the reason she is calling us after five months reflects her feeling that the people here understood her and were trying to help her. I'm thinking about Dr. Simons' comment of a while ago . . . about being understood. Dr. Console made the statement to her that she was annoyed, but they were both smiling. I definitely had the feeling that they were in tune with each other. I think that they were sharing a piece of insight together. There was a feeling of concordance.

Dr. Simons: Dr. Cohen is shaking his head. He doesn't agree with you.

Dr. Cohen: That's right. I don't. I think there was *dis*cordance there and Dr. Console picked it up. Because if she was really in touch, *she* would have made the interpretation. He gave her plenty of opportunity to do that and I think the fact that *he* ended up making the interpretation is indicative of that discordance.

Dr. Simons: I dislike a moderator who tries to make everybody feel good by blurring disagreements, but I must say that I think there's something to what each of you are observing. I agree very much with Dr. Vis that there was an empathic relationship there at that moment. They were sharing something with each other. But as many of you have mentioned, there was also a great struggle going on. I think both things were happening at one and the same time. That's why it's such an instructive tape. Now let's go ahead and view the second session that Dr. Console had with this patient, and see what more we can learn about the beginning of this psychotherapy.

Session Two

(The patient and Dr. Console are seen sitting in their chairs. She is neatly dressed, in a short skirt and a blouse.)

Dr. Console: How are you?

Patient: I'm OK.

Dr. Console: Tell me, it's almost two weeks since we talked the first time. Did you have any thoughts about our talk?

Patient: I thought about it. It's not connected. I don't think it's connected.

Dr. Console: What's not connected?

Patient: Well, about the blood in the urine, right? And my being sick right now, right?

Dr. Console: Yes . . .

Patient: It has no connection. Because I wasn't thinking about it at the time.

Dr. Console: So the thinking you did about it is that it has no connection.

Patient: Yes.

Dr. Console (smiling): That's pretty quick.

Patient (smiling): Well, I didn't have to think much about it.

Dr. Console: Any other thoughts that you had after our interview?

Patient (pause): Not really.

Dr. Console: Well, tell me how you've been the past two weeks.

Patient: Well, I've been depressed now and again. Just severe depression. Without any cause. I don't know what brought it on. I just got very depressed. On Thursday, I got very depressed.

Dr. Console: Do you really believe that these things can happen without any cause?

Patient: No. I think there's something deep down in my subconscious . . .

Dr. Console: Yes . . .?

Patient: You know, that I don't really know about.

Dr. Console: But only a minute ago you said that there was no connection between the hematuria and the event at age fourteen because you weren't *thinking* about it. Now you tell me that deep down in your subconscious there are reasons for your behavior.

Patient: Well, I'm not *able* to think about it.

Dr. Console: Well let's see if I can help you to think about it. I'd like to go back over your life as you remember things, and let's start with the unfortunate event about your schoolteacher *(pause)*.

Now, give me a little more detail about what happened. You said that at lunchtime she would take a bath?

Patient: Yes. She'd go to her house, have lunch and then she'd take a bath. And then come back.

Dr. Console: And on more than one occasion you had gone over there?

Patient: Yes. I used to have lunch with her.

Dr. Console: All right. Now, on this occasion, you went as you had done in the past to have lunch with her. . . .

Patient: Yes. . . .

Dr. Console: . . . and now, exactly what happened?

Patient: Well, she used to leave me to have lunch alone. We used to have lunch together at times but not all the time. She used to be busy around the house. And then she would take a bath after her lunch, but when I was finished eating, I didn't hear her around. Usually she would take her bath and come back and get me, but she didn't come back. So I checked in the bathroom.

Dr. Console: And what did you see in the bathroom?

Patient: I saw her lying in the bath. Dead. It seemed as if she was dead. Her eyes were closed. She was under the water.

Dr. Console: How old a woman was she? Do you recall?

Patient: She was elderly.

Dr. Console: And afterwards, what did you learn as to what possibly had happened to her on that day?

Patient: I think she had a heart attack or something.

Dr. Console: And she actually drowned in her bath?

Patient: Yes.

Dr. Console: Do you recall what you did immediately afterwards?

Patient: I ran. I *really* ran out. And I told all the other children and some of them were frightened. They didn't want to go and see. And then, other teachers were around so they went and checked and they called the ambulance.

Dr. Console: Did you go back with any of the teachers to check and see?

Patient: No.

Dr. Console: You did not (*pause*). And it was after this that you said your father moved to another borough.

Patient: Yes.

Dr. Console: And you continued in a different school.

Patient: Yes.

Dr. Console: Now, what about these parties that you went to.

Patient: You mean later on?

Dr. Console: Yes, around thirteen or fourteen.

Patient: They were school parties, birthday parties. That sort of thing.

Dr. Console: And the party at which the *other* unfortunate event took place. What do you recall about that party?

Patient: That was a friend's birthday party.

Dr. Console: And there were how many kids there as you remember?

Patient: About thirty.

Dr. Console: And you didn't know all of them.

Patient: No, I didn't.

Dr. Console: Was this a big community?

Patient: Yes.

Dr. Console: I see. Again, if you will—just what took place? How did this happen?

Patient: Well, we were all downstairs dancing and there was this fellow. He kept looking at me, you know? He wanted to dance with me but I didn't want to dance with him.

Dr. Console: Why not with him?

Patient: I just didn't feel like dancing with him. And, well, it so happened that I went upstairs to the bedroom. I don't know what I went up there for. I guess, maybe . . . I don't know what I went for. But I went in the room without knowing that he was following me. Because there was a lot of noise going on. And, he . . . I went in the room and he followed me. He closed the door behind me. I asked him what he wanted. He said, "I wanted you all evening and I just couldn't get you and this is the only way I can get you." And I started to get out of the room and he threatened me. He said, "Don't make a move or a sound." And I was just shocked. I couldn't even move or anything. And it happened like that. He just pushed me on the bed and turned off the light.

Dr. Console: And then, how did you know that you had become pregnant?

Patient: Well, I thought I became pregnant. That's why I went to the doctor.

Dr. Console: The next day?

Patient: No. Not the next day. About . . . a few days after. I started having some bleeding. Unusual . . . a lot of bleeding. So I went to the doctor. And he did a test. He said I was pregnant. He did a urine test first. And an internal test. I had to wait a few weeks after it before the abortion could be done.

Dr. Console: I see. And when the abortion was done, did he give you an anesthetic?

Patient: Yes.

Dr. Console: He did. Then you must have stayed there for a while after you came to.

Patient: I managed to stay there without my parents knowing it. I stayed there for a while.

Dr. Console: Was it in the afternoon or something like that?

Patient: Yes. I told my mother I was spending the day with a friend. This friend, she came over and picked me up. Took me over to her house. I spent the night there.

Dr. Console: And went home the next day?

Patient: The next day, yes.

Dr. Console: And what happened then?

Patient: I was still having bleeding.

Dr. Console: Had the doctor said anything about coming back, do you think?

Patient: No. He said I should have a regular check-up with a gynecologist.

Dr. Console: Just like that? Have a regular check-up. When?

Patient: He said in another two weeks. I should see him or another gynecologist.

Dr. Console: And what did you do?

Patient: I didn't do anything about it.

Dr. Console: And he never asked you how you felt, or what had happened?

Patient: I never went back to him. For quite a while at least.

Dr. Console: But as you think about it now, as an adult, doesn't it strike you that he was taking quite a chance? He was running quite a risk.

Patient (smiling): Yes. For a person that age.

Dr. Console: For a person that age to have this procedure ...

Patient: Fourteen. Done without anybody knowing it.

Dr. Console: Done without anybody knowing it. And there are some dangerous complications of this procedure and you said he alerted you to the fact that you would bleed intermittently. How were you to determine whether the bleeding was a lot or a little, and would require going back to see him or not?

Patient: Well, I knew what a regular period was.

Dr. Console: Yes. ...

Patient: And I didn't feel anything that should send me back to the doctor.

Dr. Console: You didn't?

Patient: It was just regular periods after that.

Dr. Console: I see. And then at age sixteen you say you met a boy whom you liked and you had intercourse with him.

Patient: Yes.

Dr. Console: And then you said there were some other boys.

Patient: Yes.

Dr. Console: Were they always youngsters? Your own age?

Patient: No. Older.

Dr. Console: How much older?

Patient: Up to about twenty-two.

Dr. Console: And what thoughts did you have about the possibility of again becoming pregnant? You'd had the experience of being pregnant once, so you knew that you were a healthy girl.

Patient: Yes. I was sort of scared but they reassured me that they wouldn't get me pregnant.

Dr. Console: Yes. And since they were older their reassurances seemed to be enough for you.

Patient: Yes.

Dr. Console: Now this goes on, and then you went into nursing. How did that come about?

Patient: I don't know. I just chose something that I thought was easy. It didn't take such a long time to go through nursing. So I thought maybe I'd just do that.

Dr. Console: And ...

Patient: But it ended up that I didn't like it.

Dr. Console: What changed your mind?

Patient: I thought I wouldn't have to do things that I had to do. You know? What I thought was just an aide's job I had to do. I couldn't cope with it.

Dr. Console: You didn't like starting at the bottom (*smiles*).

Patient (*smiling*): No. Bedside nursing as a whole. That's what I didn't like.

Dr. Console: What kind of nursing were you thinking of?

Patient: I'd been in an operating theater several times and I liked that. I really wanted to be a surgical nurse. But you know, you have to do everything.

Dr. Console: To get there.

Patient: Yes. And ... I gave up so easily. I tried to stick it out for the whole year but I couldn't do it.

Dr. Console: Is that characteristic, do you think? That you ordinarily give up too easily on things?

Patient: Yes. If things aren't going the best, I give up.

Dr. Console: So you were in the nursing school actually for how long?

Patient: For a year.

Dr. Console: And it was during this period that you became depressed and took pills the first time.

Patient: While I was doing nursing. That wasn't the first time though.

Dr. Console: That was not the first time. When was the first time?

Patient: I was very depressed, for what I don't know. It was before I was eighteen. And—I took an overdose.

Dr. Console: Can you tell me what it means—"I got depressed"?

Patient: I just felt real bad. I didn't know what to do. I was restless. Everything was just upsetting me. I didn't want to see anybody. I didn't want to hear anybody. I was tense.

Dr. Console: But during this period you were with these older boys whom you say reassured you that they would take the proper precautions.

Patient: But still, deep down, I didn't really trust them.

Dr. Console: Deep down, do you find it hard to trust almost anyone?

Patient: Yes.

Dr. Console: Does this include your family?

Patient: Well (*pause*). Not really. I haven't told my family any of my personal business so I wouldn't really know if I could trust them or not.

Dr. Console: Well, without having told them your personal business, were there occasions, any events in which you came to the conclusion that either your father or your mother or both, couldn't be trusted? Couldn't be told things?

Patient: Yes. I thought they wouldn't really understand. So I'd rather not say anything.

Dr. Console: With your father as a dentist, before the family moved to the new borough—where was his office? Was it in the house?

Patient: No.

Dr. Console: Did you ever visit the office? During your first five years?

Patient: Yes.

Dr. Console: Under what circumstances?

Patient: About twice. I just went there. After school I went there one evening. For him to take me home. I was late going home from school and I didn't like going home alone. So I stayed there until he was finished.

Dr. Console: And while you were there what happened?

Patient: I sat in the waiting room.

Dr. Console: And people came in and out?

Patient: Yes.

Dr. Console: Do you remember anything about that?

Patient: I remember children crying. You know, in the waiting room. They were scared to go in. Just the normal things. You know, fear of going to the dentist.

Dr. Console: Do you have any memory of people coming out after your father had done whatever work he was supposed to do with them?

Patient: Well, they came out looking OK. Better than before. Maybe it wasn't that bad.

Dr. Console: So, as you remember it, there were maybe two occasions on which you made such a visit.

Patient: Yes, as far as I can remember.

Dr. Console: But you knew about your father's work and what a dentist does?

Patient: Yes.

Dr. Cosole: What do you remember? Your thoughts about it. Your father was a dentist and pulled teeth and drilled and so on. Do you remember anything? Having any feelings, any ideas about that?

Patient: No. That was just his job. I didn't think anything about that.

Dr. Console: You don't think a little kid would have all kinds of ideas about that?

Patient: Well, I guess he reassured them when they went in. He had toys in there. Different things to attract their attention.

Dr. Console: Did he work long hours?

Patient: Yes. 'Cause he also went to the hospital at times to work there.

Dr. Console: What about your mother? Was she pleased with the fact that he worked and went to the hospital and wasn't home?

Patient: Well, he got home quite early sometimes.

Dr. Console: He did.

Patient: Yes.

Dr. Console: So they got along all right.

Patient: Yes.

Dr. Console: No difficulty between them?

Patient: Only ... on Saturdays my father used to like horse-racing. And he used to bet on these horses. My mother didn't like that because she's religious and she doesn't believe in gambling. And, Saturday nights he would come home late and then they would have an argument. And I was scared that something might happen—because he had a gun. And you know, I knew he wouldn't really use it 'cause I knew my father well enough. But still I was scared to go to sleep from a very early age and I couldn't sleep well at nights. I would just lie there, looking and waiting. As if something was going to happen. But other than that, everything was OK. He's not a gambler anymore.

Dr. Console: But you say he was when you were a child.

Patient: Yes.

Dr. Console: And that your mother was distressed about this . . .?

Patient: Yes . . .

Dr. Console: And he had a gun, and you, while you knew he wouldn't, you had the thought that it could happen. . . .

Patient: Yes . . . it could happen.

Dr. Console: So you had some difficulty in sleeping.

Patient: Yes. Then sometimes, when I knew he was about to come home, I would pretend as if I was sick. Then my mother would stay with me. That would prevent an argument. You know what I mean? I would get more attention.

Dr. Console: Yes (*pause*). So that as a little kid you learned that being sick could take care of some other things?

Patient: Yes . . . it could be a camouflage.

Dr. Console: That's an interesting word . . . camouflage. What does camouflage mean?

Patient: You know, to cover up the real thing.

Dr. Console: To cover up the real thing and make it look like something else.

Patient: Yes (*long pause here*).

Dr. Console: Am I leading up to anything?

Patient (*after a slight pause*): I think that was the time when I had trouble sleeping and from then on I always had trouble sleeping.

Dr. Console: And 'till this day you have trouble sleeping? Hard to fall asleep?

Patient: Yes. And I wake up very often during the night.

Dr. Console: Do you have dreams?

Patient: Yes.

Dr. Console: What kind of dreams?

Patient: Oh—most of the times I have nightmares. Like I have these hallucinations. I told you about it last time. Should I repeat it?

Dr. Console: Well, a little more elaboration.

Patient: Like a creature standing over my bed, you know. It was there with outstretched arms, saying "Don't move. Don't you dare move." And I was stiff. I was stiff in the bed and I couldn't scream. I couldn't move. I think this is connected with what happened at fourteen.

Dr. Console: You *do* think it's connected?

Patient: Yes, I think so because it reminded me of the exact situation of the rape.

Dr. Console: Yes. You used almost the same words. He said to you, "Don't make any noise, don't scream" and you were frozen.

Patient: Frozen stiff.

Dr. Console: Yes. You say you didn't know this boy. You said he was looking at you and he wanted to dance with you. And for some reason you didn't like him and didn't want to dance with him. Would it be stretching things too much to say that at that time he was like a creature different from the other kids you liked and would dance with?

Patient: I wouldn't call him a creature. . . .

Dr. Console: But you would *dream* of a creature. And the creature had his arms outstretched.

Patient: Yes. And what he did . . . it reminds me of . . . it's similar to a creature. Right?

Dr. Console: Yes.

Patient: Because doing things like that . . .

Dr. Console: Yes. Against your will . . .

Patient: Yes. And even . . . two nights ago I had that terrible dream. The same thing happened. I was so frightened. I was so nervous. I just didn't know what to do. It was terrible.

Dr. Console: So here, eight years later you have the same dream. You tell me that the dream reminds you of and seems to be similar to the actual event at age fourteen.

Patient: Yes. That's what I think. I don't know . . . that's what I think.

Dr. Console: Now, the first time you were depressed and tried to hurt yourself, you swallowed pills.

Patient: Well, I took overdoses twice.

Dr. Console: Where did you get the pills?

Patient: When I couldn't sleep my doctor used to prescribe antidepressants and sleeping pills. But he wouldn't give me sleeping pills that often.

Dr. Console: How did you get enough if he didn't give them to you that often?

Patient: The first time I took all the sleeping pills I had. The next time, it was antidepressants.

Dr. Console: When was the wrist-cutting incident?

Patient: That happened last year. I was feeling very depressed and I went in the hospital. I spent two weeks there. The doctor said I could go home if I really wanted to go home. I was feeling very depressed. I was alone at home. My father was there too but he was asleep. I was in my room. I was crying. He didn't know anything about it. I was just there alone. And then I .. I didn't really know what I was doing at that time. I got a razor blade and I slashed my wrists.

Dr. Console: In the bedroom?

Patient: Yes. I was lying there on the bed and I saw all this blood going through the sheets and everything . . . and on the floor. And I was just looking at it as if it was nothing. Then my father came in the room and he saw me. He was shocked. And he took me to the hospital and they stitched it up. And I was admitted.

Dr. Console: Why do you think—you say you were in the house alone with your father. He was asleep. You were feeling badly. And you couldn't go to him? And say, "Father . . ."

Patient: I just couldn't. I was always close to my father. I thought I would burden him. I didn't know what was depressing me.

Dr. Console: You thought you would burden him . . .

Patient: Yes.

Dr. Console: And if you killed yourself, this wouldn't burden him?

Patient: It would, but that would be the end of it.

Dr. Console: Would it?

Patient: For a while it would bother him, but after a while . . .

Dr. Console: What's a while? What's a while, for a parent?

Patient: Well, at that time I wasn't thinking of anything.

Dr. Console: You say that you don't think of these things. And when we talked last time, I told you that you really don't have to think about them. That is, they don't have to be conscious. You tell me yourself that many of these things are subconscious, which means that they are there.

Patient: That means it's conscious, right?

Dr. Console: No. They are there, but the person is not aware of them. *Conscious* is aware. *Unconscious* is unaware. So you keep saying, "I didn't think of these things," as though, because, you didn't think of them, they couldn't possibly play any role in your behavior (*pause*). Do you spend all your time thinking about the rape at fourteen?

Patient: All my time? No!

Dr. Console: Do you spend *much* of your time thinking about the rape at fourteen?

Patient: No.

Dr. Console: And yet, it reappears time after time in your nightmare. Where is it coming from?

Patient: It's subconscious.

Dr. Console: Yes! And what are you saying when you say it's subconscious? You're saying, "I'm not thinking about it but I do ultimately fall asleep and I have the same dream on a good many occasions." So you say it's subconscious.

Patient: Yes. Dreams are usually from the subconscious. I know that dreams are supposed to be in your subconscious mind. That's how we dream.

Dr. Console: Yes. That's right.

Patient: It comes out.

Dr. Console: But for something to come out it has to be there in the first place, doesn't it?

Patient: Yes, but I'm not thinking about it at the time.

Dr. Console: Absolutely. I am agreeing with you one hundred percent. It can be there without your thinking about it.

Patient: Yes.

Dr. Console: And it can determine decisions you make, without your knowing why you're making the decision. You see, it's almost as if you're a little girl and there's a boy down the street whom you like. And you see him going to the store for candy and the idea suddenly comes to you that you want some candy. And you go to the store. You go into the store because you want candy, but behind it is what subconscious reason?

Patient: Because I want to see him.

Dr. Console: Yes. But you tell yourself, "I'm going because I want candy."

Patient: That wouldn't really be subconscious.

Dr. Console: What would it be?

Patient: That's sort of . . . (*laughs*) . . .

Dr. Console: We could make it a little more subconscious if your mother was aware of your interest in this boy and she strongly disapproved of him. And your mother said to you, "You will have absolutely nothing to do with him. If I see you having anything to do with him I will punish you severely." So when you tell her that you went to the store just to buy candy, it could be because you yourself were not at the moment fully aware of the desire to see him, because your mother had disapproved.

Patient: But still, I knew that he would be there, right?

Dr. Console: Yes, but you were just going for candy.

Patient: But still, I knew. It wouldn't be my subconscious because I knew he would be there. So I would be just fooling my mother.

Dr. Console: But you can see that the dream does come from your subconscious because you know that dreams come from there.

Patient: Yes (*pause*).

Dr. Console: Are your parents still alive?

Patient: Yes.

Dr. Console: And you write to them . . . talk to them.

Patient: My mother's here. She came just a few weeks ago to see me.

Dr. Console: Because you're in a hospital?

Patient: Yes.

Dr. Console: And what happened? What was the conversation?

Patient: She said I was looking OK. She thought I would be looking worse. You know. I told her I was OK, although I wasn't really. I told her I was fine. I try to put on my best to the outside, you know?

Dr. Console: Why?

Patient: You know, because I didn't want to hurt her. I didn't want her to feel sad.

Dr. Console: But she wasn't feeling sad. She came and said that you looked better than she thought you would. You looked OK.

Patient: Yes. But you asked me why I did that. If I had acted my real self, she would have said that I wasn't looking very good. You know? And she would have wanted to find out what's wrong. She asked me what's wrong. Asked if she could help me. I said, "No, you can't help me." I knew she didn't like that but I just had to tell her that.

Dr. Console: But let me ask you . . . who can help you?   .

Patient: Well, the doctors can help me.

Dr. Console: How can the doctors help you? Here you were in the general hospital for four months. You had all these tests ... all these examinations. You had an operation. And then they said that they couldn't find the reason for your difficulty and they wanted to discharge you. Yet you say, "The doctors can help me."

Patient: I mean here, in psychiatry.

Dr. Console: Why here?

Patient: Because, when I analyze everything, it could be psychological.

Dr. Console: When you analyze everything it could be psychological?

Patient: That's why I decided to go to psychiatry. And I'm trying along with the doctor to help myself. But it seems as if I'm getting nowhere because sometimes I'm OK and then all of a sudden I get very depressed. So I don't know. Maybe there's something else bothering me which I don't know about.

Dr. Console: Well, here I've seen you two times and while you're relatively quiet, I'm not aware that you're very depressed. Are you depressed?

Patient: I am depressed. But I try to hide it. Bottle up my feelings inside.

Dr. Console: But we've been having a nice little talk and you smile and so on. ...

Patient: Yes. People usually misinterpret me because of the way I look, you know? They think that nothing is wrong.

Dr. Console: Well, don't make the mistake of thinking that I will misinterpret you. I won't.

Patient: I hope not. Because most people do. I mean nurses and patients. And when they see me looking sad they say, "Oh she's pretending now." Like when I start crying and looking sad. One nurse said, "An hour ago you were fine, now look at the way you're acting."

Dr. Console: A lot can happen in an hour's time, in one's thinking.

Patient: Yes. I know *that*. I realize that. It upset me more because I was trying to act the way a normal person should act. Then I couldn't take it any more and I started to act the way I felt.

Dr. Console: Did you have the same kind of feelings when you were in the medical building?

Patient: No. I used to just act the way I felt.

Dr. Console: Well, in a way, in the medical building, you were kept pretty busy with all the things they were doing . . . the tests and procedures.

Patient: Yes. I was just myself. I didn't smile when I didn't want to. You know, I was just me. It was just me.

Dr. Console: But you suggest that you weren't as depressed as you have been on the psychiatry ward?

Patient: Yes. Maybe because at that time, on the medical ward, I hadn't told anybody about my problems. And then, sometimes in therapy, telling your problems affects you in different ways.

Dr. Console: Well, I don't know if it's entirely accurate to say that you were not telling them your problems. You were telling them of your physical problems and they were investigating your physical problems. And didn't they have a staff conference about you? Didn't you appear before a group of doctors?

Patient: On one occasion I did. But they only asked me what was wrong with me. Why I came in the hospital and so on.

Dr. Console: Was this immediately upon your coming in the hospital or after you'd been there a while?

Patient: About two months later.

Dr. Console: After about two months of being in the hospital you went before a group of doctors and they asked you questions.

Patient: Yes. "What do I think of my illness?" Things like that.

Dr. Console: I see. Do you remember what you told them?

Patient (smiles): I told them that I didn't know what to think because I'm no doctor and I can't tell what's wrong with me. I know that I have the symptoms. I had pain, which was real. And fever. And they said that it could be in my mind. I said that it's not in my mind. I remember telling them that. And they asked me something about living and I said that I couldn't care less. Maybe that's when they got the idea that I was depressed.

Dr. Console: Do you think it would have made any difference if, instead of their saying to you, "It's in your mind," they had said, "It's in your subconscious"? Do you think you'd have felt differently about it?

Patient: Yes. That means, it would appear to me, when you say it's in my mind . . . it's as if I'm pretending. But when you say it's in my subconscious, I don't feel that way.

Dr. Console: And you're not pretending. You have no control over it.

Patient: Yes. Thats right.

Dr. Console: Now what about that? You appreciate the fact that it could very well be in your subconscious, and that you are not pretending. All these things are happening as you say. When you have pain in your back, it *is real*. But, we can have real pain for deeper reasons.

Patient: Yes, I know that.

Dr. Console: Reasons that are not apparent to us.

Patient: I know. I know.

Dr. Console: Did you get any feeling of how the doctors felt about you and your case and your condition? In the general hospital?

Patient: Well, I thought most of them thought that I was just putting on an act, you know? I was very depressed. I started getting very depressed about that. They kept on taking my temperature every two hours . . . things like that. I thought, "Why should they be doing so much?" Every four hours would have been enough.

Dr. Console: Yes. Why *would* they do it every two hours?

Patient: Yes. So I was getting very depressed and I told a doctor there that I don't like the way they're acting because they think I'm not feeling any pain and they keep doing this to me and I don't like it. Well, he reassured me. He said I shouldn't worry and he said he believed me. He was the one who sort of perked me up a bit. I didn't feel that badly. But when they said they couldn't find any other thing to do but to operate, I said there must be something wrong because I'm still having the pain. So I agreed with the doctors to have the operation.

Dr. Console: Can you describe the pain to me a little more?

Patient: It's a pain. It's in the lower right side and it was always there and sometimes it got worse. I still have it occasionally.

Dr. Console: Am I correct . . . you've already had an appendectomy done?

Patient: Yes.

Dr. Console: And that was in the lower right side?

Patient: It was around the same region.

Dr. Console: So it can't be appendicitis again.

Patient: No.

Dr. Console: What else can it be?

Patient (laughs): I don't know.

Dr. Console (smiling): What else is *there*? (*pause*). Nursing student!

Patient (smiling): Well, when I had the fever I thought that maybe I had an abcess there.

Dr. Console: An abcess? Just *there*?

Patient: Somewhere along that area.

Dr. Console: But what is there along that area?

Patient: You mean here? (*points to her right lower abdomen.*)

Dr. Console: Yes. The lower right side.

Patient: You have your intestines and ...

Dr. Console: Yes ...

Patient: It could be a gynecological problem.

Dr. Console: It could be a gynecological problem. Because there are also the ...

Patient: The ovaries and tubes.

Dr. Console: But ovaries and tubes are paired. Right side and left side.

Patient: Yes, but one side could be inflamed.

Dr. Console: Yes (*pause*). You were in nursing school for approximately a full year?

Patient: A full nursing year.

Dr. Console: And did you have obstetrics and gynecology lectures? Did you have any classes in that?

Patient: Yes.

Dr. Console: What did you learn about the right side and the left side in obstetrics?

Patient: I don't remember. I just know where the different parts of the organs are.

Dr. Console: Where they are?

Patient: Yes.

Dr. Console: I'm more interested in your knowing what they do. What function they serve.

Patient: So, why do you ask me this question?

Dr. Console: Oh . . . I'm going to ask you a lot of questions (*smiling*). I'm going to talk with you again.

Patient (*laughs*): Oh boy.

Dr. Console: Because you and I are going to get to the bottom of this.

Patient: You know, I'm not able to think clearly, even when I try to read my books. My school books. I'm not able to concentrate. It's like reading something new. My mind is confused.

Dr. Console: You've had next to no difficulty in thinking and remembering and answering my questions here.

Patient: I mean when I start to read my books.

Dr. Console: Yes. . . .

Patient: It seems as if I don't know what I'm doing, you know?

Dr. Console: Now this is twice that I've been asking you questions. Any questions that you want to ask me?

Patient (*smiling*): Why are you so interested in asking me questions?

Dr. Console: Because I hope to help you to get at the bottom of this. To really understand.

Patient: And do you think that the questions that you ask me will help? The last questions . . . about where this part is and so on.

Dr. Console: Yes. Sure.

Patient: I don't see a connection.

Dr. Console: Rest assured that I'm not just making words. If I'm asking questions, I have a very definite reason.

Patient: I believe that.

Dr. Console: You see, the last time you said, "I knew you were going to ask that question." You said that it was the way I was questioning—I led up to it. And I'm still leading up to lots of things.

Patient: Yes, I know. Next time I guess you'll talk about something else. Sort of a different topic. You're sort of picking out each topic.

Dr. Console: Maybe . . . but we'll come back to some of the same ones too.

Patient (*smiles*): You'll put the same questions around in a different way, right?

Dr. Console: Maybe. But it won't be with any intention of fooling you. You will understand that I may be putting it in a different way

because I talk to a good many people and I don't precisely
remember how I put the question. So I put it slightly differently.
You'll know.

Patient: Do you think I should be in the hospital?

Dr. Console: For now? Yes.

Patient: Yes.

Dr. Console: Yes. What would you do if you weren't in the
hospital? Where would you go?

Patient: I'd go home. Maybe I'd find a job but still ...

Dr. Console: And get depressed?

Patient: I'm not sure of myself yet. Because I get so depressed. I
have to find out why.

Dr. Console: You do want to find out why?

Patient: Yes. I want to. I've been going on this way for so long.

Dr. Console: I will try to make these talks a little closer together so
we can get to the answers. All right?

Patient: OK.

Dr. Console: Thank you

Patient: Thank you too. *The Interview Ends*

The second session seemed to confirm many of the speculations
that had been made about the patient during the viewing of the
initial interview. After a two-week interval, she began the second
session with a spontaneous denial that there was any connection
between the rape and abortion at age fourteen and her present
symptom of hematuria.

It is apparent that Dr. Console wanted to obtain additional
history in the second session, to fill in the gaps that had been left at
the conclusion of the first interview. He learned more about the
death of the teacher when the patient was five years old. He then
proceeded to ask about the next major traumatic event and
inquired regarding the specific details of the party at which the
patient was raped. The patient described the incident as follows:

And, well, it so happened that I went upstairs to the
bedroom. I don't know what I went there for. I guess, maybe
... I don't know what I went for.

Her pause, followed by her obvious suppression of some additional thoughts, is most important and lends strength to the previous speculation that she may have unconsciously invited the rape.

Her assumption that she had become pregnant following the rape is also very interesting and may very well reflect her wish to become pregnant. She stated in this session that she was tested and found to be pregnant *a few days afterwards*, a determination that is virtually impossible at so early a time. Her description of the rape and the abortion again raises an issue that was mentioned in the previous chapter—one that may be vitally important in relation to the direction which this young woman's life subsequently took. To what extent was her behavior determined by an unconscious wish or fantasy to be repeatedly penetrated, probed and even impregnated by various distorted versions of her dentist-father? Such an unconscious wish may be the motivating force behind her need to present herself over and over again to physicians. Her offering herself for painful procedures both gratifies this wish and also serves as an expiation of her guilt for having such a wish, as well as her survivor guilt.

Despite the patient's bland and seemingly indifferent description of her father's dental office, there are good reasons to believe that his activities with his patients were of vital concern to her. Additional history obtained from the patient's first therapist revealed that the patient had indeed been her father's dental patient from the time of latency on, and that he had always administered anesthesia to her while working on her teeth. This makes even more understandable her seeking out surgical procedures that required anesthesia. The second interview also helps us understand better the patient's recurrent nightmares of a dark monster who approached her with arms and claws outstretched. We do not have her associations, but very likely contained in this dream is her wish for as well as her fear of penetration by a thinly disguised version of her dentist-father. The incident of the rape is remarkable not only because it seems to have been the result of an unconscious invitation by the patient but also because of her description of the young man's words at the time, "Don't move." These are words that might very appropriately be spoken by a dentist when a patient is seated in the dental chair, or by a physician about to perform an examination or operation.

The patient's compulsion to present herself repeatedly to a series of physicians and her demands that she be penetrated again and again now become more meaningful. Her demands in this regard were not limited to vaginal penetration, but also included the demand to be penetrated by almost any instrument in virtually every area of her anatomy. While on the medical and surgical wards she succeeded in having so many intramuscular injections of medication that her muscle tissue actually became fibrosed and by the time she came to the psychiatric ward, the nurses reported that it was difficult to find any area in her upper arms or buttocks that was not fibrosed.

During the course of the second session some of the patient's predominant defenses and resistances became more apparent, as well as her ability to use her body and illness as a "camouflage." It became increasingly evident as the session progressed that even an experienced therapist would encounter many difficulties in the treatment of this young woman.

The hospital in another state was contacted and more details about the patient's hospitalization there were obtained. She was extensively examined because of complaints of lower abdominal pain and it was not a cholecystectomy that was performed. *It was a culdoscopy.** The surgeon described the difficulties that she had presented to him. After many weeks of fruitless searching for the cause of her abdominal pain, he was about to discharge her but she insisted upon one last procedure—a culdoscopy. The surgeon was opposed to this idea, feeling that this procedure was not indicated at the time. The patient became insistent and in fact refused to leave the hospital until it was performed. The culdoscopy, therefore, was a demand that she made in return for her discharge. The surgeon reluctantly agreed and performed the culdoscopy, which revealed no abnormality. Only then did the patient agree to be discharged.

The surgeon remarked that he had never seen a patient who was as willing a recipient of pain as was this young woman, nor had he

* Culdoscopy—visual examination of the female pelvic organs by means of an instrument (endoscope) introduced into the pelvic cavity through the posterior vaginal recess or fornix.

ever met a patient who was as reluctant to be discharged from the hospital as she had been. He could not understand why so young and attractive a woman would want so fervently to remain in a hospital and submit to operative procedures, when there was presumably so much to look forward to in her life. He admitted that he was quite bewildered by her case.

CHAPTER NINE

Beyond The Initial Interview

Richard C. Simons, M.D.
Mark Rubinstein, M.D.

The basic format for this volume has been a series of initial interviews with five patients. Through the detailed discussion of these interviews, a great deal has been learned in depth about the lives of five individuals. And if we now reflect back over the five cases, perhaps we can also gain some perspective regarding the breadth of the issues that have emerged as well.

For example, a concern over *penetration* is one that, to varying degrees, is central in the lives of nearly all of our patients. The Roach Woman's fear of penetration is matched in intensity by the Suicidal Young Woman's compulsion to be penetrated. The Merchant Mariner experiences a need to penetrate virtually anyone that he can, of either sex, while the fear of penetrating someone else is quite overwhelming to the father of our Family In Distress.

The search for a parent is another fundamental concern that to varying degrees plays a crucial role in the lives of our patients. The Merchant Mariner searches for his dead mother in the ports and on the sea-going vessels of the world, while the Suicidal Young Woman seeks her father in her odyssey from hospital to hospital and in her repetitive relationships with physicians. And it may very well be that the man whose family is so troubled and whose sexual life is so barren is unconsciously struggling with a fear of finding the forbidden parent in his sexual activity, and therefore he must avoid such activity to the extreme. Even in his dreams, he is impelled toward a more passive form of contact in which he is nurtured.

Homosexual fears and wishes are concerns which many of these patients are dealing with on one level or another. The West Side Killer was in the throes of a savage homosexual panic, while one of the Roach Woman's major conflicts centered around unconscious homosexual strivings which are forbidden to her. The Merchant Mariner is constantly engaged in overt and compulsive bisexual activity, while our patient from A Family In Distress is enormously passive in his sexual life.

Survivor guilt is a constellation that is graphically portrayed by the Polysurgery Woman, by the Suicidal Young Woman, and the Merchant Mariner. In the first two patients, years of unremitting pain and countless operations characterize their lives and will probably continue to do so. The Merchant Mariner has spent an equal number of years wandering the world, drinking to the point of delirium tremens and avoiding any possibility of an enduring and close relationship in an effort to deal with his guilt. All of these people's lives have been dramatically affected by tragic events, the consequences of which they are largely unaware. The self-destructive direction of their lives has been and still is today determined by a pervasive and profound sense of guilt and by the never-ending question, "Why did I survive the other?"

We cite these parallels not merely to illustrate that many of the same fundamental dilemmas of human existence are found in people who have different presenting symptoms and who are of diverse backgrounds, but also to highlight the fact that these central motivating fears and fantasies emerged so strikingly in the course of an initial interview—in the course of a first encounter between a patient and a psychiatrist. That first encounter provides us with a rich source from which we may expand our knowledge and make sense out of what may at first seem incomprehensible. It enables us to increase our understanding of the person and his or her life's experiences. It is an encounter that has diagnostic implications and that hopefully has therapeutic value as well, because it is the very beginning of the patient's experience in psychotherapy.

Thus, beyond the specific details of the initial interview and all that it may tell us about a patient, issues emerge that are going to be crucial in the conduct of any psychotherapy. From the first moment of the first encounter between patient and therapist, a relationship is forming. In the course of that relationship all patients will bring their conflicts, hopes, fears and expectations to the treatment setting. They will eventually develop a transference to the therapist, and this transference will, at the same time, elicit in the therapist feelings from his or her own past. In every human relationship these phenomena will occur, but the nature of psychotherapy is such that the intensity and meaning of these transference and countertransference reactions will be greater than in other relationships of life. Whether providing a patient with the proper amount of support, understanding a patient's defenses and resistances, or introducing dynamic and genetic interpretations, the psychotherapist is dealing with a broad range of feelings in both his patient and himself.

This leads us to a fundamental problem for the future to which we hope this volume has implicitly addressed itself. As medicine in general has become increasingly specialized and technological, the patient as a unique human being has too often faded into the background. In the past it was often said that psychiatry was the one medical specialty where this was not the case, and where a unique dimension, rapidly disappearing in other specialties, still endured—that of the individual person and his or her inner world. But that may no longer be as true today as it once was. Today the psychiatric resident and the beginning psychotherapist are faced with a growing range of therapeutic modalities—such as psychopharmacology, behavior therapy, biofeedback, group and family therapy, crisis intervention, community consultation and many others—that place a premium on symptom relief and environmental manipulation, with a corresponding lesser emphasis on an understanding of the human being involved in these behavioral, interpersonal and community events. While there can be no doubt that many of these modalities are useful and indeed necessary in many situations and with many patients, it must be remembered that such therapeutic approaches are derived from models of mental functioning (neurobiological, behaviorial, sociocultural) that basically ignore dynamic considerations and bypass the intrapsychic dimension of human experience. These models are necessary and valuable, but if used exclusively they can lead to an overly mechanistic approach, with a consequent dehumanization of the inner world of the human being.

In this book we have attempted to address ourselves to the fundamental principles that a beginning psychotherapist must grasp in order to function effectively in whatever work he or she may ultimately undertake, or with whatever treatment modalities he or she may use in various situations. We have concerned ourselves in this book with the patient as a unique human being, raised in a specific family constellation, influenced by an equally specific sociocultural setting, with a rich and complex fantasy life that is the result of countless varied experiences from the time of birth on. We hope that we have demonstrated how much can be learned about a person in the course of a single interview and, through the use of videotape teaching, how much can be learned from a microscopic examination of a single interaction between a patient and a psychiatrist when they are both willing to expose themselves to such scrutiny. Hopefully the reader has had the opportunity to see a dynamic and empathic interaction unfold from the very first moment of contact, and has been able to critically view and appreciate that first encounter between two people that must form the foundation for the beginnings of any psychotherapy.

SUGGESTED READINGS

THE INITIAL INTERVIEW

1) Gill, Merton M., Newman, Richard, and Redlich, Fredrick C. (in collaboration with Sommers, M.) *The Initial Interview In Psychiatric Practice.* International Universities Press. New York. 1954. A very instructive and detailed dissection of the dynamics of initial psychiatric interviews. This book focuses primarily on the techniques of interviewing, and fosters an appreciation of the interaction between the participants in the interview.

2) MacKinnon, Roger A., and Michels, Robert. *The Psychiatric Interview In Clinical Practice*. W.B. Saunders. Philadelphia. 1971. This book describes the different types of psychiatric patients with whom an interview might be conducted, and elaborates on the techniques of interviewing as they may differ from patient to patient. It also deals with unusual situations such as the "telephone consultation." A fine book to help the beginner in approaching many different kinds of patients.

THE USE OF VIDEOTAPE
3) Berger, Milton M., Editor. *Videotape Techniques In Psychiatric Training And Treatment*. Brunner/Mazel. New York. 1970. A group of authors discusses many different aspects of videotape techniques in psychiatric training and treatment. Some of the papers are more technically oriented, while others are rich in clinical material and teaching approaches.

BEGINNING PSYCHOTHERAPY
4) Tarachow, Sidney. *An Introduction To Psychotherapy*. International Universities Press. New York. 1963. Dr. Tarachow's discussions with a group of residents cover a great many issues that are both theoretical and clinical. A very human and dynamic book that should be read by every beginning psychotherapist.

5) Colby, Kenneth Mark. *A Primer For Psychotherapists*. The Ronald Press Company. New York. 1951. A terse, well-written book that is indeed a primer filled with important basic information for the beginner.

6) Dewald, Paul A. *Psychotherapy, a Dynamic Approach*. 2nd Edition. Basic Books. New York. 1971. The book begins with a basic overview of psychodynamics and psychopathology and is followed by the major section dealing with psychotherapy. Well-formulated in helping the beginner structure and understand the essentials of psychotherapy.

ADVANCED PSYCHOTHERAPY

7) Langs, Robert. *The Technique of Psychoanalytic Psychotherapy*. Jason Aronson. New York. Volume I (1973). Volume II (1974). These two volumes are perhaps the most complete and detailed ever written on the principles and practice of psychoanalytic psychotherapy. They begin with the initial contact and interview, and proceed to cover virtually every situation in all phases of psychotherapy.

Name Index

Subject Index